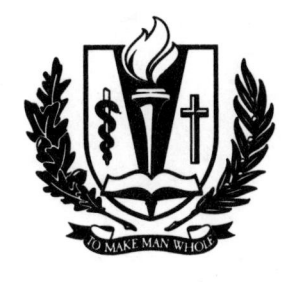

LOMA LINDA UNIVERSITY
School of Medicine

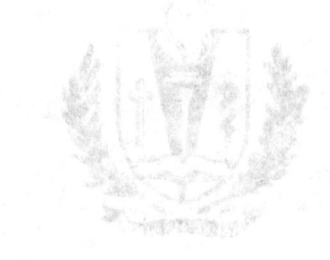

GRAND ROUNDS
DAILY DEVOTIONAL STORIES

A Collection of Stories, Poems, and Insights

by Students, Alumni, Faculty, and Friends

of

Loma Linda University School of Medicine

Commemorating the Grand Opening
of the new
Loma Linda University Medical Center
and
Loma Linda University Children's Hospital
2021

Edited by Donna R. Hadley

Copyright © 2021 by Loma Linda University Press. All rights reserved. No portion of this book may be reproduced, stored in a database or retrieval system, or distributed in any form or by any means—electronic, mechanical, photocopying, recording, or any other—except for brief quotations in printed reviews, without the prior written permission of the publisher.

Although every precaution has been taken to verify the accuracy of the information contained herein, the editor and publisher assume no responsibility for any errors or omissions. No liability is assumed for damages that may result from the use of information contained within.

Names have been changed or omitted as necessary to protect privacy.

Published by
Loma Linda University Press
Office of Academic Publications
Loma Linda University
Loma Linda, CA 92350
Printed in the United States of America

Copies may be ordered from
Amazon.com
Loma Linda University Campus Store
11161 Anderson Street, Suite 110
Loma Linda, CA 92354
Tel: (909) 558-4567
E-mail: campusstore@llu.edu
http://llu.bncollege.com.

Publisher:
Cover layout: Melinda Worden
Photographer: Jonathan Davidson
Compiler and production editor: Donna R. Hadley
Project manager: Alice Wongworawat
Project coordinator: Ezrica Bennett
Printer: Color Graphics, Anaheim, CA
Typeface: Adobe Jenson Pro

Library of Congress Control Number: 2021904914

ISBN 978-1-59410-002-4 (paperback)
ISBN 978-1-59410-001-7 (hardcover)
ISBN (e-book)

Cover Photo Credits

Front Cover:

This picture illustrates how the traditional style of conducting grand rounds changed during the pandemic from a large auditorium or amphitheater to small groups wearing masks. A team from LLUH's department of OB/GYN, takes a moment for prayer, and asks for guidance for the many patients they serve. Those pictured (clockwise, starting at top):

Parker Murray, University of North Texas HSC: Texas College of Osteopathic Medicine class of 2019
Resident, LLUH OB/GYN class of 2023
He is passionate about women's health, family time, avocados, beach volleyball, and traveling.

Jessica White, LLUSM class of 2017
Completed OB/GYN residency LLUH 2021
She enjoys photography, hiking, camping, indoor rock climbing, and beach walks.

Jeffrey Hardesty, LLUSM class of 1980-B
Completed OB/GYN residency LLUH 1985
Served at Penang Adventist Hospital in Malaysia from 1985 to 1993
LLUH OB/GYN faculty since 1993
Board-certified in female pelvic medicine and reconstructive surgery
He is grateful to LLUSM for the training received with an emphasis on whole person care, which has been an important feature of his medical practice; he continues to be committed to international medical mission service.

Joy Kim, LLUSM class of 2020
Resident, LLUH OB/GYN class of 2024
She delights in free time spent with family and friends, and hiking.

Heather Figueroa, LLUSM class of 2008
Completed OB/GYN residency at Grand Rapids Medical Education Partners in Michigan 2012
She is intentional about providing whole person care in a way that provides value and meaning to patients.

Priya Chakrabarti, UC Riverside class of 2018
Resident, LLUH OB/GYN class of 2022
She is "obsessed" with cats and has three of the cutest "monsters!"

Back Cover:

The landscape of the campus of LLUH is changed dramatically with the completion and opening of two new, state-of-the-art hospitals in 2021. They represent the culmination of Vision 2020, a capital campaign that raised more than $476 million.

Copyrights

Scripture quotations marked AMP are taken from the *Amplified Bible*, Copyright © 1954, 1958, 1962, 1964, 1965, 1987 by The Lockman Foundation. Used by permission.

Texts credited to ASV are from *The Holy Bible*, edited by the American Revision Committee, Standard Edition, Thomas Nelson & Sons, 1901.

Scripture quotations marked BSB are from the *Berean Study Bible*. © 2016, 2020 by Bible Hub and Berean Bible. Used by permission. All rights reserved.

Scripture quotations marked CEV are taken from the Contemporary English Version, Copyright © 1991, 1992, 1995 by American Bible Society. Used by permission.

Texts credited to Clear Word are from *The Clear Word*, copyright © 1994, 2000, 2003, 2004, 2006 by Review and Herald Publishing Association. All rights reserved.

Scripture quotations marked DRA are taken from the Douay-Rheims 1899 American Edition.

Scripture quotations marked ESV are taken from *The Holy Bible*, English Standard Version, copyright © 2001 by Crossway Bibles, a division of Good News Publishers. Used by permission. All rights reserved.

Scripture quotations marked GNT are taken from the *Holy Bible, Good News Translation*, Second Edition, copyright © 1992 by the American Bible Society. Used by permission. All rights reserved.

Scripture quotations marked GW are taken from *God's Word*. Copyright 1995 God's Word to the Nations. Used by permission of Baker Publishing Group. All rights reserved.

Scripture quotations marked HCSB are taken from the *Holman Christian Standard Bible*, copyright © 1999, 2000, 2002, 2003, 2009 by Holman Bible Publishers. Used by permission.

Scripture quotations marked KJV are taken from the King James Version.

Scripture quotations marked MSG are taken from *The Message*. Copyright © 1993, 1994, 1995, 1996, 2000, 2001, 2002. Used by permission of NavPress Publishing Group.

Scripture quotations marked NASB are taken from the *New American Standard Bible*, copyright © 1960, 1962, 1963, 1968, 1971, 1972, 1973, 1975, 1977, 1995 by The Lockman Foundation. Used by permission.

Scripture quotations marked NCV are taken from *The Holy Bible, New Century Version*, copyright © 2005 by Thomas Nelson, Inc. Used by permission. All rights reserved.

Scripture quotations marked NET are from the *NET Bible*, copyright © 1996-2006 by Biblical Studies Press, L.L.C. http://netbible.com. Used by permission. All rights reserved.

Scripture quotations marked NIV are taken from the *Holy Bible, New International Version*. Copyright © 1973, 1978, 1984, 2011 by Biblica, Inc. Used by permission. All rights reserved worldwide.

Scripture quotations marked NKJV are taken from the New King James Version. Copyright © 1982 by Thomas Nelson, Inc. Used by permission. All rights reserved.

Scripture quotations marked NLT are taken from the *Holy Bible*, New Living Translation, copyright © 1996, 2004, 2015 by Tyndale House Foundation. Used by permission of Tyndale House Publishers, Inc., Carol Stream, Illinois 60188. All rights reserved.

Scripture quotations marked NRSV are taken from the New Revised Standard Version Bible, copyright © 1989 the Division of Christian Education of the National Council of the Churches of Christ in the United States of America. Used by permission. All rights reserved.

Texts credited to Remedy are from *The Remedy Bible*. © 2020, Come and Reason Ministries. All rights reserved.

Scripture quotations marked RSV are taken from the Revised Standard Version of the Bible, copyright © 1946, 1952, 1971 National Council of the Churches of Christ in the United States of America. Used by permission. All rights reserved.

Bible texts credited to TEV are from the *Good News Bible*—Old Testament: Copyright © American Bible Society 1976, 1992; New Testament: Copyright © American Bible Society 1966, 1971, 1976, 1992.

Scripture quotations marked TNIV are taken from the *Holy Bible, Today's New International Version*. Copyright © 2001, 2005 by Biblica, Inc. Used by permission. All rights reserved worldwide.

Texts credited to WEB are from the *World English Bible*, published in 2000. The *World English Bible* is an update of the American Standard Version of 1901, and is in public domain.

All quotations from the writings of Ellen G. White are used by permission of the Ellen G. White Estate.

Abbreviations

The following abbreviations are used throughout this book:

Loma Linda University Health Entities

CME	College of Medical Evangelists (now LLUSM)
LLUBMC	Loma Linda University Behavioral Medicine Center
LLUCH	Loma Linda University Children's Hospital
LLUFMG	Loma Linda University Faculty Medical Group
LLUH	Loma Linda University Health
LLUMC	Loma Linda University Medical Center
LLUSAHP	Loma Linda University School of Allied Health Professions
LLUSBH	Loma Linda University School of Behavioral Health
LLUSD	Loma Linda University School of Dentistry
LLUSM	Loma Linda University School of Medicine
LLUSMAA	Loma Linda University School of Medicine Alumni Association
LLUSN	Loma Linda University School of Nursing
LLUSP	Loma Linda University School of Pharmacy
LLUSPH	Loma Linda University School of Public Health
LLUSR	Loma Linda University School of Religion
SACHS	Social Action Community Health System

Degrees

BA	Bachelor of Arts
BS	Bachelor of Science
BSc	Bachelor of Science
BSN	Bachelor of Science in Nursing
BSW	Bachelor of Social Work
CPA	Certified Public Accountant
DMin	Doctor of Ministry
DrPH	Doctor of Public Health
JD	Juris Doctor
LCSW	Licensed Clinical Social Worker
LMFT	Licensed Marriage and Family Therapist
MA	Master of Arts
MB	Bachelor of Medicine (British equivalency to MD)
MBA	Master of Business Administration
MD	Doctor of Medicine
MDiv	Master of Divinity
MHSA	Master of Health Services Administration
MN	Master of Nursing
MPH	Master of Public Health
MS	Master of Science
MSW	Master of Social Work
PhD	Doctor of Philosophy
PsyD	Doctor of Psychology
RN	Registered Nurse

With heartfelt gratitude

This book is dedicated to

*Our frontline and essential workers
during the
2020-2021 pandemic*

*Your commitment to excellence, values, and serving humanity
made you the tangible hands, feet, and face of Jesus to so many.*

From the Dean

Grand Rounds is the third and final book in the School of Medicine's *Rounds* series. The school's 112-year history is a remarkable journey of commitment to a mission—the same mission that exists today. The stories of that journey are invaluable to our heritage.

The first book, *Morning Rounds*, was written to commemorate the centennial of the founding of the School of Medicine. It looked at the past experiences of the school, as well as the mission integrated into alumni's and patients' lives.

Evening Rounds was compiled to celebrate the 100-year anniversary of the first graduates from the School of Medicine. The book came together in a way that showed the collective impact that numerous committed lives can achieve. The legacy of whole person care with generations of individuals practicing it changes both the practitioner and the patient.

Grand Rounds, the third book, coincides with the opening of the new LLU Medical Center and Children's Hospital in 2021. With the arrival of 2020, however, the world changed in impactful ways. New stories for this book came in that reflected the challenges and learning around these unprecedented times. *Grand Rounds* looks toward the future practice of our graduates. What does this future look like? What do we value that guides our lives and our practice of medicine? This book examines our stories within the context of our values—justice,* mercy, integrity,* excellence,* humility,* service, teamwork,* compassion,* wholeness,* gratitude, and humanity—through very real experiences. We equip our School of Medicine students and graduates to face a changing world through values integrated with excellence in medical education.

The stories woven together in these books illustrate how values turned into action can change lives and experiences of the people around us. While the impact of one person's experience is profound, all of these stories collectively is an inspiration.

— Tamara Thomas, MD
Dean, LLUSM

---

*Denotes a core value of Loma Linda University Health, presented and voted by the board, August 2020

Mission: To continue the teaching and healing ministry of Jesus Christ
Motto: To make man whole

Grand Rounds

Grand Rounds is a time-honored, regularly scheduled weekly meeting of health care professionals for the purposes of education, sharing ideas, seeking experts' opinions, and, most importantly, assuring excellence in quality of care. The patient's student or resident presents a particular patient's history, physical findings, imaging, and laboratory findings to the audience. The attending staff will ask further questions and opine on the diagnosis and next steps in management. Commonly a student/resident will have been asked to research the current medical literature and be prepared to give a presentation summarizing his/her findings. A jealously guarded tradition is that anyone can ask questions without being ridiculed. The defined roles of the learner and teacher become blurred, and even the most experienced professor acknowledges that everyone learns from each other.

Grand Rounds, the publication, embraces this learning process. In many of these stories, the authors will speak about what others have taught them. This is education at its best. The intention of this book is to capture and present these moments that have changed and will change lives forever.

Acknowledgments

LLUSM offers its deepest gratitude to the following individuals:

Hillary Angel—(communications specialist LLUSM) one of the behind-the-scenes people whose creativity has appeared in the beautiful graphic designs used for marketing this book. Her desire to assist in the perfecting of details throughout the text was crucial.

Author/Story Recruitment—The following individuals were essential in identifying which stories they heard that needed to be recorded in this book. In addition, they tracked down authors/stories, identified subjects that begged to be addressed and then helped write or rewrite submitted narratives as needed: *Ezrica Bennett, Morgan Green, Donna Hadley, Roger Hadley, Doug Hegstad,* and *Henry Lamberton.*

Ezrica Bennett—(administrative assistant LLUSM, *Grand Rounds* project coordinator) has been with this book since its inception. When 2020 brought new challenges for the book, her ability to switch gears and provide insights were most helpful.

Jonathan Davidson—(video and photography specialist LLUSM and LLUSMAA) through his lens he so brilliantly captured the vision and images for the front and back covers of this book.

Editorial Review Board—*Ezrica Bennett, Daniel Giang, Donna Hadley, Roger Hadley, Elaine Hart, Paul Herrmann, Henry Lamberton, Ricardo Peverini, Leo Ranzolin, Rhodes Rigsby, Tamara Thomas,* and *Alice Wongworawat.* Thank you for your advice in helping determine the tenor of the book while keeping it aligned with the mission of the school.

Donna Hadley—(volunteer editor) there are no words to express our profound thanks for the extensive labor of love in the journey of creating not only *Grand Rounds*, but *Morning Rounds* and *Evening Rounds* as well. To recognize the impact of a well-written short story is one of her many talents that has made all three books so compelling. Her vision to tell the story of Loma Linda University School of Medicine in this manner was fueled by her passion of personal narratives, her love of people, and her profound respect for LLUSM, the alma mater of so many whom she holds dear.

Roger Hadley—(dean emeritus LLUSM, senior advisor for *Grand Rounds*) spent countless hours obtaining and writing bios for the authors, contacting alumni and students to share their stories, copyediting, and along with *Rhodes Rigsby*, medical editing. His belief in and commitment to all three books were vital to each of them coming to fruition.

Acknowledgments

Barbara Couden Hernandez—(director of physician vitality LLUSM) was pivotal in providing publication support.

Lysenia Quijano—(senior executive assistant to LLUSM dean) with her vast knowledge of the campus and the individuals who are part of it, she was the go-to person for details and minutia needed for this book.

Elizabeth Venden Sutherland—with her expertise as a writer, she gave insights and direction when consulted by the editor.

Amanda Valencia—(project coordinator LLUSM) was always available to work wherever and however needed.

Carol Weismeyer—(former administrative assistant LLUSM and *Grand Rounds* volunteer) is a "veteran" of all three *Rounds* series books who has made countless behind-the-scenes contributions for each book. Her remarkable proofreading skills coupled with her half century of working at LLUH and knowing its history, made her an invaluable team member once again.

Marci Weismeyer—(*Grand Rounds* volunteer) has an incredible gift for paying attention to details, including fact checking and fact finding. Her writing skills, exceptional proofreading skills, knowledge of LLUH history and overall fund of knowledge helped assure the accuracy of this book.

Alice Wongworawat—(associate dean of finance and administration LLUSM, *Grand Rounds* project manager) has been involved in all three of the *Rounds* series books. Once again, she was key in keeping this project moving forward utilizing so many of her endless talents.

Melinda Worden—(VP for operations Review and Herald Publishing Association) and *Cavil Copy Editing* assisted with copy editing and created text layout. Always ready to lend a listening ear, they were a wonderful addition to the team.

Chip Wright—(digital education specialist LLUSM) from the day of his arrival was immediately all in, no matter the task at hand.

GRAND ROUNDS
DAILY DEVOTIONAL STORIES

The Loma Linda University Physician's Oath

Before God these things I do promise:

In the acceptance of my sacred calling,

> I will dedicate my life to the furtherance of Jesus Christ's healing and teaching ministry.

> I will give to my teachers the respect and gratitude which is their due. I will impart, to those who follow me, the knowledge and experience that I have gained.

> The wholeness of my patient will be my first consideration.

> Acting as a good steward of the resources of society and of the talents granted me, I will endeavor to reflect God's mercy and compassion by caring for the lonely, the poor, the suffering, and those who are dying.

> I will maintain the utmost respect for human life. I will not use my medical knowledge contrary to the laws of humanity. I will respect the rights and decisions of my patients.

> I will hold in confidence all secrets committed to my keeping in the practice of my calling.

> I will lead my life and practice my art with purity and honor; abstaining from immorality myself, I will not lead others into moral wrongdoing.

May God's kingdom, His healing power and glory, be experienced by those whom I serve, and may they be made known in my life, in proportion as I am faithful to this oath.

This oath is recited three times by LLUSM students in their academic journey: White Coat Ceremony, Freshman Dedication, and Commencement.

JANUARY

VALUES

"All of us celebrate our values
in our behavior."

JOHN W. GARDNER (1912–2002)
U.S. Secretary of Health, Education,
and Welfare, 1965–1968

January 1

New Year's Day

"Wherever the art of Medicine is loved, there is also a love of Humanity."
Hippocrates (460 B.C.–370 B.C.): Greek physician known as the Father of Medicine

Grand rounds. Just those two words conjure up images of pit amphitheaters with the semicircle of sage elders flanked by an ever-widening group of impressionable interns and fellows waiting for the next pearl to drop, or a herd of zebras* to thunder by, leaving a trail of new knowledge in their wake. But perhaps the concept of grand rounds is much more visceral, more personal, than we were taught to believe.

The elusive case perhaps is the case of diminishing hope. Those feelings of making a difference that blazed so brightly at the sight of those two significant modifiers at the end of our names, to the dampening of the flame as bureaucratic paperwork, insurance conditions, and malpractice defenses chip away at the fire and naiveté. Life not only changes us physically but also affects the perceptions of our craft. Yet in all this reality comes a chance experience, an interaction, an opportunity, no matter how seemingly small or inconsequential, to touch the lives of our patients and families. And there are even those opportunities to open up and be touched also—to have the light inside rekindled such that it is enough to rejuvenate and let us know.

Yes! This is why we serve; this is why we became physicians. We have so much more to offer: more compassion, more empathy, more knowledge, more of our God-given gifts, more love, more caring. Grand rounds is all of us, the entirety of our individual journeys as physicians and the volume of experiences we have gathered, created, and shared. The challenges, triumphs, frustrations, joys, and moments we felt failure or success—this is what we bring to the table. We are grand rounds.

*Zebra is the American medical slang for arriving at a surprising, often exotic, medical diagnosis when a more commonplace explanation is more likely.

Gayle Mitchell, LLUSM class of 1997, currently practices internal medicine in Los Angeles and Pasadena, California. She is involved in organizations that encourage leadership in future generations of physicians. This is dedicated to her late nephew Ashley (1986–2019).

January 2

> *"Jesus said, '"Love the Lord your God with all your passion and prayer and intelligence." This is the most important, the first on any list. But there is a second to set alongside it: "Love others as well as you love yourself."'"*
> Matthew 22:37-39, MSG

We were devastated. At age 3 our son, Chase, was diagnosed with Duchenne muscular dystrophy (DMD). With this news we truly felt as if we were mourning the death of a child, because our hopes and dreams for him were now shattered. Our new reality was that he would lose the ability to walk around 8 to 10 years of age, that everything that is a muscle would eventually give out, and that his life expectancy would be about age 15. For the next few years, although we were still reeling with the sadness of this diagnosis, we wanted to try to mirror the same joy and happiness that Chase had. Trying to answer his questions about his diagnosis as he grew was best met with saying that although his muscles were weaker than others, doctors were working to find a cure for DMD. Soon our little family of three became five with the addition of twin sisters, two more persons in his life that would love him.

We decided to mainstream Chase, so we sent him to a private Christian school. One day after school (he was in the third grade, a year before he began using a power wheelchair), as I was helping him into the car, he told me about a running race they had just had. He said he fell right at the start and could hardly get up. He then asked if he'd ever be able to win a race. Feeling a huge lump develop in my throat, I mustered up the courage to say that even if he'd never be able to be the fastest in a race, in the Bible Jesus says that when we get to heaven, the last shall be first, the weak shall be strong, so he would be able to win races in heaven! After a brief pause, Chase said with excitement, "Mom, I think maybe I don't want to be cured!" At that moment I realized how much he was looking forward to heaven.

During his freshman year at the University of Redlands, Chase was admitted to LLUCH Pediatric ICU. Even though he was struggling with labored breathing, we had no idea how much his body was failing. We were sad that Chase would be in the hospital over Christmas, but we made the very best of it. Unfortunately this was to be his last hospitalization; Chase's heart gave out, and he passed away on January 2, 2014.

I never really knew what kind of an impact this sweet young man had had until after he had passed away. His funeral was standing room only. After it was over I saw something that I will never forget as long as I live: his empty wheelchair in the foyer with a group of his close friends around it, just staring, faces somber. These were the boys that always pushed the limits in school, tested the teachers and their parents . . . need I say more? But the looks on those faces told me that Chase's impact will endure for years to come.

I believe Chase was an angel on this earth, sent to teach us humility and what is really important. He *lived* Matthew 22:37-39.

Caroline Boyd, LLUSD dental hygiene class of 1988, is married to Anthony "Andy" Boyd (LLUSD class of 1990). In addition to Chase, they are parents to twin girls, who are currently enrolled in college. In memory of Chase, Andy and friends Lance Weir and Bill Walton started Team Chase (a nonprofit) to raise money for disabled and challenged athletes to be able to participate in athletic events. To date they have sponsored seven athletes. #thechasechallenge #teamchase.net

January 3

> "All that the Father giveth me shall come to me; and him that cometh to me
> I will in no wise cast out."
> John 6:37, KJV

The giddiness I was experiencing could not be contained. I had taken three pregnancy tests that confirmed my pregnancy. It was surreal that after four years of trying to get pregnant, God had placed a new life in my body of 42 years. As the wife of a soldier, I saw the maternal fetal medicine (MFM) physician who did an ultrasound and confirmed that the "glob" inside the lining of my uterus was viable. Sadly, this would be my first and last visit with him. My husband was leaving active duty, and I would need to be seen by a civilian OB/GYN. The physician had a recommendation for someone who was qualified to continue my high-risk OB care.

The appointment was scheduled, and I sat in the lobby nervously waiting for the physician to see me. I found it strange that from the time I was called out of the waiting room to the obtaining of my history, urinalysis, hemoglobin draw, and vital signs, no one made eye contact nor introduced themselves. Hoping that things would be a little better with the physician, I read while I waited for him to come in. He kindly introduced himself and sat down on a stool in front of me. After waiting a few seconds, he proceeded with his soliloquy. He asked me if I had actually planned to get pregnant. He asked if I was aware of all the risks associated with a pregnancy at my age. The rhetorical questions continued, as he never allowed me to answer any of his questions. He took another breath and said that my pregnancy was too high-risk for him to care for as an MFM specialist. He walked out of the door without looking back.

My mind drifted to all the babies I had delivered during my family medicine residency at White Memorial Hospital in Los Angeles. I refused to have this happen repeatedly with other physicians. I would just deliver this little one on my own.

Later that day I met a labor and delivery nurse who raved about her favorite OB physician. I confided with her about my pregnancy and asked her to contact this physician to see if she would be willing to take my case. Within two hours the doctor who was recommended called me and put me at ease that my pregnancy at age 42 would be a breeze. Seven months later she delivered Orion Samuel. Eighteen months later she delivered Atlas Josiah—two healthy baby boys without complications or difficult pregnancies.

Jesus promised that anyone who "cometh to me I will in no wise cast out" (John 6:37, KJV). I am thankful for this promise. I am also thankful that there are physicians out there who are willing to see patients who others may discount. I challenge each of you not to give up or turn away that patient who may seem difficult or noncompliant. Be patient and Christlike—do not give up on them.

Sharon Michael Palmer, LLUSM class of 1999, is a family medicine physician, practicing primary care at Augusta University in Georgia. She is the hospice director and works with veterans. She is happily raising two spirited sons with her husband, Matthew. Her joy is teaching a kindergarten Sabbath School class.

January 4

"The practice of medicine is an art, not a trade; a calling, not a business; a calling in which your heart will be exercised equally with your head."
William Osler (1849–1919): Canadian physician and medical education pioneer

It's past 10:00 p.m., and my short legs are double stepping to catch up to the resident. I'm on acute-care surgery rotation of my third year of medical school, and it's our third trauma of the night. I am exhausted, and I don't know why I am there. In exasperation, I had prayed on my way to work earlier that evening, "Lord, please, no traumas. Please just two lap appies [laparoscopic appendectomies] and no traumas." And, of course, we had traumas back to back with no lap appies at all.

As we near the trauma bay, the nurses slide aside just enough for the resident and me to squeeze through. "Late 30s male, motor vehicle accident, ejected 10 feet from the car." I quickly scribble notes as we scan the patient for injuries. I notice dirt and blood all over the man's face. His eyes are bruised with a gash over his right eyebrow. His left forearm also has a deep abrasion. He loudly moans as we turn him to check his back, which gives me relief. He is in pain, but he is awake and able to talk.

The resident and I leave to work on our documentation. When we come back, the rush of people has already disappeared. We first work on stitching his arm. Afterward the resident hands me a pile of wet gauze and tells me to wipe the patient's face so that we can see what else we need to stitch. I nod and bend over to start with his forehead. He winces with my touch. "Sorry, sir," I whisper.

"It's OK," he replies slowly.

I notice how close this man and I am. Just a few short hours ago we were complete strangers, unlikely to cross paths. And now I am present in one of the most vulnerable moments of his life, when his clothes have been stripped, his neck is in a brace, and his torn face is in the hands of a medical student.

As I continue working in silence, he says, "Thank you for helping me." It makes me pause. Suddenly I realize why my prayer for lap appies was not granted. I realize why I am in the emergency department late at night. I am there for him. I am there for the patients that are under my care, for the next trauma patients who show up later. The health care workers in the hospital with me are there to help those that may otherwise die.

In small moments like these we can find meaning in our work. When I finally get into my car to drive home at 7:00 a.m, a huge smile spreads across my face. I let out a loud, happy squeal. I know that after a nice long nap, I will be ready to come back to the hospital, ready to meet and treat the next person. That is why I am there.

Eunice Marpaung, LLUSM class of 2019, is a resident at Tacoma Family Medicine in Washington. She is a Southern California native with Indonesian heritage. She still keeps in touch with friends from LLUH.

January 5

> *"For I, the LORD your God, hold your right hand; it is I who say to you, 'Fear not, I am the one who helps you.'"*
> Isaiah 41:13, ESV

As a physician, I am privileged to partake in unbelievable experiences and witness the raw emotions of patients and their families as they navigate some of the most vulnerable periods in their lives. In my attempt to understand their circumstances I find myself reflecting on my own experiences and God's Word. I too ask, "Why?" or "How?" or "What?"

Why did this happen?

How can they move on after this horrifying experience?

What can I say to help them in this trying time?

Three families come to mind right now.

The mother who finds out that her son is dying because the child's father with whom she left the child physically abused him. The grandfather who accidentally runs over his grandson with his car as he is backing out of the garage. The parents who lost their only two children in a blink of an eye after being hit by a drunk driver on their way to a family getaway.

Why did this happen? If only we could turn back time, we would do things differently—not work and take care of my son myself; check the driveway one more time before backing out; not go on that family getaway. But you can't always prevent accidents. That's why they are accidents, unfortunate incidents that happen unexpectedly and unintentionally, typically resulting in damage or injury.

How does one move on after this? I've heard "I can't do this." "I can't go back there." "I can't go on." "I can't hold on." Such agony and deep suffering.

What can I say to these people who are in tangible pain?

The lyrics of a song by Casting Crowns come alive and suddenly have deep meaning:

So when you're on your knees and answers seem so far away
You're not alone, stop holding on and just be held
Your world's not falling apart, it's falling into place
I'm on the throne, stop holding on and just be held
Just be held . . .

So in the quietness of the night when your soul is crying out, be still and know that He is God and that He will hold you. You don't even have to hold on, because He will hold you with His own righteous right hand.

Janeth Ejike is an associate professor in LLUSM's department of pediatrics, who practices pediatric critical care medicine. She has been married to her loving husband, Ugo Ejike, for 16 years, and they have two wonderful gifts from God in their sons, Gozie and Keneh.

January 6

"The best thing of all is God is with us."
John Wesley (1703–1791): English Anglican cleric, theologian, and one of the founders of Methodism

"Doctor, there is someone out in the lobby who says they really need to see you about something very important."

My heart sank. It was the very day before I was to start a six-week malpractice court trial, and I assumed this was another subpoena or legal discussion. I was a few years into my career in emergency medicine in a stressful work environment, and I had accumulated a couple of lawsuits. The legal world for physicians is dispiriting and demoralizing and moves far too slow. It feels unfair that the legal system is allowed years to retrospectively analyze and dissect split-second decisions made with incomplete data in chaotic situations. It felt like a nightmare to me. I began to second-guess my daily practice and career choice and fantasized about leaving medicine altogether. During periods of insomnia and worry, I prayed that God would help me through this trial, but any reassurance up until this time remained uncomfortably elusive.

Instead of another subpoena being delivered in the lobby, it was a former patient. She had been a previously healthy 38-year-old brought in by ambulance one month earlier. She had collapsed in her kitchen and hit her head. At the time of her arrival she was alert but amnestic and confused. She was also in cardiovascular shock. Quickly thin slicing the situation, I suspected she had suffered a pulmonary embolus and was concussed from hitting her head. I immediately sent her for a CT scan to confirm the diagnosis and to rule out any brain hemorrhage or aortic dissection before starting anticoagulation. Before we could get her onto the CT table she went into cardiac arrest. We performed CPR off and on for more than 30 minutes, intubated her, riskily administered a clot buster drug without a confirmed diagnosis, and threw every other Hail Mary resuscitation intervention at her. Long after the situation seemed futile, she regained a pulse and became stable enough for a CT scan, which confirmed a massive pulmonary embolus now showering everywhere throughout all lung fields without any hemorrhage in her brain.

She had walked out of the hospital a few days later in full recovery and was now, a month later, in the waiting room lobby with her 8-year-old daughter. She thanked me for a second chance to live with her family. I knew that this was God's answer to prayer and that He was going to see me through my malpractice trial, which He thankfully did. Medical practice can inflict some deep emotional wounds, but I am thankful for God's healing grace.

Fifteen years later I still keep that mom's note and her daughter's photo and drawing in my work briefcase for inspiration and confidence to keep fighting the good fight, to keep running the good race, and to keep the faith.

Matthew Underwood, LLUSM class of 1992, currently practices emergency medicine in Riverside, California. He is married to his wife of 31 years, Lynda Daniel-Underwood (LLUSM class of 1991), and they are parents to two grown children. He enjoys running, biking, hiking, and coaching high school basketball.

January 7

> *"God longs for your happiness and He has plans for your life."*
> Janet Fuller: contemporary Christian author

One Friday afternoon I decided to participate in the spiritual care practicum. In these practicums we are taught how to be a listening ear and offer spiritual care to patients. We pray before doing our rounds and ask the Lord to guide us to whom we need to see. I was with other students as we walked into a patient room and introduced ourselves. The patient was so touched by our presence alone that it brought tears to his eyes. As we were conversing with him, he told us that in the hospital he had been near death and had thought that his best friend would stick by him, but that the opposite had been true. He felt abandoned and alone. He said, "I just decided to let go of her and prayed for God to send me new friends, and here you girls came." He was so amazed by God's immediate answer to his prayer! He said that this was confirmation that God indeed loves him and cares for his every need. Tears fell down his face as he let the Spirit of God hug his heart.

We all felt the presence of God in the room. It was at that moment that I was able to experience what it is like to share hope. As I work toward becoming a physician, I want to be one who brings wholeness to my patients. Daily I desire to walk with God as He leads me to the brokenhearted so that I can share the joy of being His child.

On the wall above the patient's bed, I saw the verse "This is my command—be strong and courageous! Do not be afraid or discouraged. For the LORD your God is with you wherever you go" (Joshua 1:9, NLT).

I am ready to go wherever the Lord sends me, and I trust that He is preparing me for continued service in the ministry of healing.

Adwoa Wiafe, LLUSM class of 2021, is a family medicine resident at LLUH. She enjoys singing, listening to music, and being out in nature. She dreams of developing meaningful relationships with her patients and inspiring a positive change in the lives of those around her.

January 8

"May I remember that I am heir to the same diseases as my patients, must meet the same death, pass with them beyond the River, and may I go with a smile."
Stewart R. Roberts, MD: *"An Ideal of Modern Medicine"*

My medical career has spanned more than a half century, and I consider myself fortunate to be a product of the training program at LLU that holds forth the motto "To make man whole," as encapsulated in Jesus' teaching.

I marvel at the advances that I have witnessed during my journey. We can now diagnose and treat complicated diseases that not many years ago we lacked effective treatment options to offer our patients.

Since the advent of electronic medicine we now have extensive resources at hand to research, outline diagnostic plans, and provide up-to-date treatment protocol with strokes of computer keys. Rapid review of diagnostic data is readily available for fitting together the pieces of the diagnostic puzzle. No longer do we struggle with cumbersome paper charts.

These advances are not without drawbacks. There is the observation that more time is spent with the computer than face to face with the patient. With the computer interposed between the physician and the patient, subtle changes in patient facial expression, hand gestures, and other nonverbal elements of the patient history may be missed. These clues may be as vital as verbal replies in helping to form differential diagnoses. Further, the opportunity to demonstrate empathy with the patient may be missed, leading to failure to understand the patient's clinical picture.

As providers, we are at risk of becoming more mechanized; driven by protocols rather than paying attention to our patients as persons in need. As a result, whole person care is placed in jeopardy, and patients are more easily classified as "interesting cases" rather than God's children in need of more than a computer to address their total care.

In sympathy with my patients, I am not alone in appreciating my physician speaking directly with me rather than watching my words being entered into my computer file with little human connection.

I often read and ponder the "Physician's Prayer," by Sir Robert Hutchison:

"From inability to let well alone; from too much zeal for the new and contempt for what is old; from putting knowledge before wisdom, science before art, and cleverness before common sense; from treating patients as cases; and from making the cure of the disease more grievous than the endurance of the same, Good Lord, deliver us."

This message echoes the teaching from Jesus to treat our patients as we wish to be treated. He consistently met people in need with an attitude of loving-kindness and acceptance, and a demonstration of sympathy by His healing touch. His example should be the goal of every Christian physician.

Dale Isaeff, LLUSM class of 1965, is a professor in LLUSM's department of medicine. This story was based upon a patient care experience while he was a fellow in cardiology at Stanford University Medical Center.

January 9

> *"Behold, I am making all things new. . . . Write this down, for these words are trustworthy and true."*
> Revelation 21:5, ESV

Bella was a 42-year-old woman mandated to therapy for child neglect. She faithfully walked to her appointment with me each week, her hair tied in a large knot behind her head. Bella, for years, had been the victim of horrific domestic violence. It was the kind of violence Father Greg Boyle has said is perpetrated by people who are fighting the "lethal absence of hope." As with many clients, she didn't tell me her story for several weeks, nor did I ask to hear it. We both waited. During one session she told me she used to sing mariachi with her father. When I said I would love to hear her sing, without hesitating she stood, released her hair from its knot, and moved around the tiny room as she sang in full voice. She was full of light, power, and beauty, and I hoped she was remembering a part of herself she hadn't seen in a long time.

It was after that that she began to tell me her story of abuse, and later her story of getting away. She was rescued from imprisonment by a violent man when her mother sent a SWAT team and a news crew to where she was being held. Her mother hoped the news crew would keep the man from killing her daughter instead of releasing her to the police.

While she endured this abuse Bella did what many mothers in distress do: She sent her children to live with a family member with whom she believed they would be safer. Sadly, her children were abused in that home. Bella and I began the work of forming new chapters of her story, chapters that dared to include hope. She was not only coming to terms with her own trauma, but was also trying to accept that her children had been abused by people she had trusted. She now faced learning how to help her children heal as well. Child and Family Services had custody of her children, and Bella was fighting hard to find herself and to reunify with her children.

We worked together for months. She found a part-time job, took parenting classes, joined a gym, fixed a smile broken by repeated facial fractures, returned to church and Bible study, and attended support groups for survivors of domestic violence. She inspired me each time she came to see me. One day she came in, and I could tell something was different. Normally positive and hopeful, she was down and began to cry before she spoke. The social worker didn't want to return her children to her. After a long silence she started to sing a song by Mandisa, and I cautiously joined her: "You're an overcomer, stay in the fight 'til the final round, you're not going under, 'cause God is holding you right now." We finished that song and I started another, hoping she would keep singing with me. She did. It was Toby Mac: "I know your heart been broke again, I know your prayers ain't been answered yet, I know you're feeling like you've got nothing left, well, lift your head, it ain't over yet." The power of song to fill in spaces in ourselves when words alone cannot is a gift I am endlessly grateful for.

Bella did keep moving and was reunited with her children after a time. I'll never know what those moments meant to her. But I know they changed me and my capacity to keep moving through heavy darkness. Lift your head; keep moving; it's not over yet. "He who began a good work in you [or me, or Bella] will carry it on to completion until the day of Christ Jesus" (Philippians 1:6, NIV).

Tammy Hilliard graduated from LLUSBH in 2015 and works as a therapist in Redlands, California. When not at work, she enjoys running, yoga, golf, working in the garden, and spending time with her husband, Anthony (LLUSM class of 2002), and their two children.

January 10

*"Now in the morning, having risen a long while before daylight,
He went out and departed to a solitary place; and there He prayed."*
Mark 1:35, NKJV

Prior to entering medical school, I asked as many people as I could to describe the medical school experience. After my first week of classes I quickly learned that no description could prepare me for the challenges that would lie ahead. From the time I woke up at 4:00 a.m. to when I went to bed at 10:00 p.m., it seemed that every minute of my day was filled with studying. No amount of studying would help me remember the innervations, blood supply, and muscles of the superficial and deep back in anatomy. Moreover, I was the first person in my family to receive both graduate and undergraduate education. It was difficult to find people to identify with my experience. In spite of all of these challenges and shortcomings, I knew one thing: I would dedicate each moment in medical school to God.

During my first year I came across Mark 1:35, and it spoke much truth into my life. Notice that every word in that verse associated with Jesus is an active word, and that He did this of His own choosing. However, in order to truly appreciate this verse, we need to go back and read verses 21-34. Reading those verses, you can see that the previous morning Jesus had been teaching at Capernaum on Sabbath, and people were greatly attracted to the truths He was sharing, and He then proceeded to cast out a demon by His word alone! Talk about a powerful church program! Afterward Jesus goes to Peter and Andrew's house and heals Peter's mother-in-law. After Sabbath He spends the rest of the evening healing and casting out demons of all the people in the entire town! He spent every minute of His day ministering, serving, and healing those around Him. He must have been exhausted.

Going through these verses, I can see someone to whom I can relate. Furthermore, in spite of this, He took time to wake up early the next morning to pray. Why? The word "pray" used in Mark 1:35 in the Greek literally translates "to exchange wishes"—meaning during prayer Jesus surrendered His desires, burdens, and wishes in exchange for the Father's. He did this for us to show us how we can have access to the same power and will of God.

During my first year God continued to press upon my heart the need and desire to spend time with Him in the morning so that I too could surrender my burdens and desires in exchange for His. At first I surrendered only five minutes each day, but over time it grew. The most amazing part was that I covered just as much material each day, information became easier to absorb, and the long days did not seem so long anymore.

What about you? Do you feel as if you are at your end? Are you surrendering these things to God in exchange for what He has to give you? He promises that He has a similar experience in store for you.

Cristian Villegas, LLUSM class of 2021, is a resident in physical medicine and rehabilitation at LLUH. He enjoys spending time with family, reading, and hiking with his wife and dog. The Bible verse that gives him the most encouragement is Hebrews 2:17-18.

January 11

"But how can they call on him to save them unless they believe in him? And how can they believe in him if they have never heard about him? And how can they hear about him unless someone tells them?"

Romans 10:14, NLT

"Hi, Mrs. Smith, my name is Spencer Freed, and I'm a student physician here at Loma Linda University." I continued with my introduction and asked her if she was willing to share her story. With her rasp and quiet, yet soothing and gentle voice, she kindly agreed. This was not her first time here.

Five years prior, she had developed ascites from cirrhosis of the liver. She'd been waiting for a new liver until last week, when the doctors had told her that they'd secured one. However, soon after, they reluctantly informed her that the liver had been given to someone else. "I'm worried I'll just get sicker and sicker," she answered when I asked what concerned her the most, "and that I'll be in a wheelchair all my life with no new liver." The pain of coming so close to procuring a liver and then being denied was devastating.

In the middle of our conversation her husband came from the parking lot and proceeded to ramble on about the stressful parking situation he'd just been through.

"I can understand how that could be stressful for you," I said. He continued his tirade, but by allowing him to talk, I got insightful information about the family's predicament. According to him, his wife had not been acting like herself because of an increase in her blood ammonia levels. His mother-in-law had been helping by taking her daughter to the hospital, but that morning had slept in. Their 15-year-old son was having severe stomach problems, making it difficult for him to go to school. And to top it all off, the patient's husband had terrible back pain for which he felt he had no time to address. I could tell by this interaction that the stressed (the husband) was also a stressor (to the wife).

In an attempt to move back from this interruption to the purpose of my visit, I asked Mrs. Smith where she found strength in stressful times. "My caregivers and mother," she said. "They help me do errands and get groceries." She also found relief in making crafts for other people.

"That's great that you're able to focus on others in the midst of your pain," I said.

"Yep, it is," she responded. I offered to pray with her, for which she was quick to agree.

I was able to visit Mrs. Smith shortly before she was to have a procedure done. She glowed as she saw a familiar face and heard a familiar voice. "How are you feeling, Mrs. Smith?"

"Oh, a bit nervous, actually," she said. As the nurse and physician were prepping her for a procedure, she asked, "You're the one who prayed for me earlier, right?" I confirmed her guess. "Well, you're just standing there. Why don't you do something useful and pray with me?" I gladly took her hand and began to pray out loud. Mrs. Smith was so incredibly grateful for that prayer, as she squeezed my hand one last time.

I learned through this encounter that I naturally am nervous to offer spiritual care, but that patients who don't seem spiritual or religious may still be in need. I learned that the quickest way for a physician to reach the heart and soul for many of their patients is to help them look and reach outward from themselves to a supernatural reality. That is where peace and comfort in wearisome situations can always be found, whether they realize it or not.

Spencer Freed, LLUSM class of 2022, is from the Sierra Nevada foothills of Northern California, where he hopes to return one day to practice medicine.

January 12

> "The LORD turn his face toward you and give you peace."
> Numbers 6:26, NIV

Early in my intern year I began the overnight portion of my call shift with a flurry of calls regarding patient requests and complaints. As the night wore on I was told about multiple patients who needed to see me urgently, only to find that the true nature of their requests ranged from wanting to know what time they would be discharged in the morning, to a change in their diet, to checking their tuberculin skin test amid several other "false alarms." In my own weakness I became more annoyed with each new phone call. Around 3:00 a.m. I was called by the same nurse again requesting that I come see yet another patient. She said this patient was feeling short of breath. After having made multiple trips downstairs for requests that I felt had not been truly urgent, and having become more disbelieving with each, I had a hard time hiding the frustration in my face when I showed up to the patient's room. I was tired, I was perturbed, and worst of all, I was cynical. However, as I started examining the patient, I realized quickly that he was deteriorating. I immediately called for the proper support and began an ICU transfer. Despite our best efforts the patient passed away a few hours later from what we came to discover was a massive pulmonary embolus in the difficult-to-control state of liver failure.

Though I cannot point to a medical error that night, there is one thing I think about often: It could be that one of the last things that patient saw was my irritated, cynical face. A facial expression that said, "Why are you bothering me now?" An expression that questioned, "Is there really a problem?" I had transferred my building annoyance to a patient who did nothing to deserve it. I learned from that personal failure so many years ago the importance of encountering each patient with a clean slate and with a caring countenance. Since that experience, especially in my current procedural-based practice, my goal is that my face and words communicate care and comfort to each patient I treat, no matter my own feelings.

Recently my great-uncle was brought, as an emergency, to that same hospital where I had encountered that dying patient as an intern. He was in severe COPD, and his respirations were so rapid that he began losing consciousness. Time was short, and in those final moments I wanted to portray what I didn't those years ago. I held his hand, looked into his eyes with care and love, and spoke to him with the most reassuring tones I could muster. A few minutes later he was intubated, and soon after he passed away. There is a point where our earthly measures fail, and we can rely only on God to gift the "peace that passes understanding." I pray that in those final moments my countenance worked toward this divine goal and gave him peace.

Miriam Peckham, LLUSM class of 2011, currently practices diagnostic and interventional neuroradiology at the University of Utah Health in Salt Lake City, Utah. Her area of focus is the diagnosis and treatment of low back pain.

January 13

> *"Blessed are those who find wisdom, those who gain understanding, for she is more profitable than silver and yields better returns than gold."*
> Proverbs 3:13-14, NIV

In our role as physicians we often educate our patients as to the causes of certain disease processes and what can be done to remedy a situation, whether it be lifestyle changes, medications, or surgical procedures. We are supposed to be the experts and have spent years in learning, training, doing.

Then in walks a patient, and the roles reverse.

Kaylee developed viral cardiomyopathy as an infant and underwent a heart transplant at age 2. By the time she walked into my office with abnormal uterine bleeding, she was a sassy 14-year-old teen awaiting a second heart transplant. She had a phone in her hand and earbuds in her ears, and I'm not really sure she heard a word I said. But I heard almost everything she said in her conversations with her grandmother while I worked at the computer.

"I know what it's like to have a friend die! Johnny [another fellow transplant friend] might die!"

"Why me?" (She had the realization of the loss of her friend and her possible mortality.)

"Why do I have to have diabetes?" (a complication of immunosuppressants)

"Why do I have to bleed all of the time?" (another complication of immunosuppressants)

"Why did my mother let that man in the house?" (She was a victim of abuse.)

In her short lifetime she had experienced what most of us will never experience, never feel, never know. It was a window into the life of another human being, and she was teaching me. One who had experienced very unpredictable situations: illness, medical treatment, surgical treatment, friendship, camaraderie, all mixed with uncertainty.

Deal with it. Hang in there. Grow on.

Kaylee did receive a second heart transplant, and we were able to get the abnormal bleeding under control.

The last time I saw her she had just turned 18.

She announced to me that she was starting college the following week.

She wanted to become a nurse. She wanted to come to Loma Linda for training.

I was delighted, proud, and so happy for her. She had developed wisdom needed to deal with her situation—a God-given gift. She hadn't victimized herself, and had a vitality that was palpable.

Was I wise also? Or did I just know a lot?

Kathleen Lau, LLUSM class of 1982, is an assistant professor in LLUSM's department of gynecology and obstetrics. Her husband is Ricardo Peverini (LLUSM class of 1984). They have two sons, Daniel (LLUSM class of 2024) and Andrew (LLUSM class of 2023) Peverini.

January 14

"We are pressed on every side by troubles, but we are not crushed. We are perplexed, but not driven to despair. We are hunted down, but never abandoned by God. We get knocked down, but we are not destroyed."
2 Corinthians 4:8-9, NLT

I was walking through the pediatric emergency department's employee entrance, trying to reassure myself that I had only a few more shifts to go, and that "I could do this." I still carried a heaviness in my heart from the events the preceding night that I fear will always stay with me.

I remember that a trauma had come in from a motor vehicle accident. The ED fellow and one of the ED interns had rushed to the bedside, as the patient had had a cardiac arrest. Several patients were waiting to be seen, so I assigned myself to the next patient, but I couldn't help noticing all the commotion as I walked out of the physicians' workroom. The curtain was drawn around a patient's cubicle, but so many people were around the patient's bed that it could not be fully closed, and I glimpsed the body of a young boy lying in the bed as the team swarmed around him.

A short while later the ED fellow and intern returned to the workroom. I was typing my note from the last patient. I asked if the boy was all right. "No, he's dead," replied the intern matter-of-factly. I wasn't expecting to hear this, and the tragedy of this situation hit me like a punch in the abdomen. I muttered an "Oh" and returned to my computer. Inside, my heart sank. My thoughts became dark as I imagined this boy lying in the bed, eyes closed, his heart still inside his chest.

The ED fellow then walked in, looking defeated. She was discussing the case with the two attendings that night, and at one point she just broke down. She was fighting tears, brushing them away as if they were a nuisance. The attendings muttered words of condolences. She had just told the family that he didn't make it. She said she could stay strong for them delivering this devastating news, but was so overwhelmed by the emotions when she was out of their sight that she immediately lost that strength.

I mustered up the courage to give her a hug, and she hugged me back. I said, "I'm sorry," and I walked back to my computer. I buried my face in the screen, trying not to let my own emotions go unchecked, although I felt emotionally drained as the night went on, and I continued to overhear the bits of information that the fellow was providing to the attendings: he was 14 . . . his mother and twin brother were at a different hospital . . . it was a drunk driver . . . he was bradycardic at the crash site . . . the air paramedic's voice was shaking when he gave his report . . ."

I did not want to hear any more, and yet I felt that I had nowhere to go. I wanted to go home, to my safe haven, to wrap my arms around my own child and never let him out of my sight. The world suddenly felt like a dangerous place, and I vehemently wanted to protect him. As a mother I could not bear imagining the grief that this family would be going through now and for the rest of their lives and the number of people who would be adversely affected by this news. I just wanted to cry, to let my own sadness for the situation be released through my tears, but I couldn't. I felt an enormous pressure to be "professional." *What would my colleagues think of me if I shed tears for a patient I hadn't even been involved with?* I asked myself.

Somehow I made it through that night, but I couldn't get the image of the young boy's lifeless body out of my mind. It haunted me for endless nights afterward. I didn't want to be a part of a world where children died for no reason, where parents had to feel the anguish of losing a child, where brothers had to lose the bond of a beloved sibling, especially a twin.

I have found the only way to ease this pain is to lean on our loved ones for support. Sharing these feelings with others allows us to share this heavy burden and receive love, kindness, and understanding that eventually leads to healing.

Gina Henry completed her family medicine residency at LLUH in 2018 and is now a full-time family medicine physician serving her community of Thousand Oaks, California, in a dynamic outpatient practice. She is passionate about lifestyle medicine, physician wellness, and community service. She takes God to work with her every day for guidance and acknowledges that her patients are her greatest teachers.

January 15

> *"Know that you are never alone. God is with you, holding you, comforting you, and most of all loving you no matter what."*
> **Anonymous**

His yellowing eyes fixed fast upon me. "I'm afraid I'm not forgiven," Mr. Meyer finally stuttered, appearing simultaneously relieved and anxious at the admission. With a terminal diagnosis before him, his anxiety was growing. Together we sat—often in silence, sometimes with words—processing fears, accepting grace, and reaching for hope.

Together our journey continued as his health rapidly deteriorated. One morning I was called to his bedside for spiritual support following the decision to transfer Mr. Meyer to home hospice care. I slowly moved toward Mr. Meyer's bed as his wife fought back the tears beside him. Now weak and growing increasingly unresponsive, he opened his eyes in greeting and then fastened them intensely upon mine. After a few seconds my anxiety began to build as I felt the urge to look away, to share a scripture, or perhaps a nice thought to "fix" the sadness that had enveloped his hospital room. But resisting this strong impulse, I returned his gaze—staring softly into each other's eyes for the next 60 seconds or more as he searched my eyes for truth, for authenticity, and for strength. Sometimes gently nodding, sometimes simply staring back as my own eyes began to water, mirroring his. Then while peace and calm visibly washed over him, I offered a short word of prayer.

Upon request from the family (and within my practice as a chaplain), I left church and drove to his home that next Sabbath, being greeted by his family gathered there. For the past two or three days Mr. Meyer had been completely unresponsive. It was clear that soon he would pass. We gathered in the family room, around his hospice bed, and began to reminisce, sharing stories about "Pop" and all that he meant to us. Together, mixed with tears and laughter, we sang his favorite hymn once more. "Let's come close and surround him with our love," I invited the family, as together we placed our hands upon him and upon one another in prayer.

"Heavenly Father, today we come to You as a family," I began to pray. Suddenly Mr. Meyer's breathing drastically changed. Afraid he was choking, I opened my eyes, only to see his eyes also opened and fastened upon mine. "He's awake! He knows we are praying! He knows we are here!" his wife excitedly screamed. For the remainder of the prayer I kept my eyes open, returning his gaze, but this time seeing peace, forgiveness, and healing where fear had once dwelt. With the final amen, he closed his eyes, slipping back into unresponsiveness once more.

Many months have passed since this precious moment occurred, but as I reflect upon this experience today, the emotion I felt that day remains. Psalm 46:10 calls us to "be still, and know that I am God" (KJV). There are moments in life where words are not enough; where "perfect" answers fall flat. But in that moment—in the pain, in the turmoil, in the questions, and even in the joys—God in His compassion sits with us. He is not afraid of our questions; He is big enough for our doubts, for He has come as Emmanuel—"God with us" (Matthew 1:23, KJV).

Carissa McSherry, LLUSR class of 2020, graduated with her MS in chaplaincy and serves as the chaplain at SAC Health System, located in San Bernardino, California. She is deeply passionate about ministry, particularly overseas, and will almost never turn down a great adventure!

January 16

"Learn to do right; seek justice. Defend the oppressed."
Isaiah 1:17, NIV

I remember it as if it were yesterday. My life was new. I'd recently graduated from college, married, and started my first "real" job: organizing volunteers for the Loma Linda Ronald McDonald House. Little did I know, my life would soon change again.

At work I was honored to serve alongside people from all walks of life. People who volunteered countless hours to support families with critically ill children. Their commitment motivated me to use my free time to help other neighbors in crisis.

Accordingly, I trained to become a court-appointed special advocate, a volunteer who promotes the best interests of children in foster care. I was assigned to two young brothers, Jeremy and Luke. The boys, along with their seven siblings, were abandoned in an apartment with no running water, electricity, or food.

Jeremy and Luke were shy during our first visit. Bright eyes and curious smiles peeking from behind their foster parents, Lola and Joe. By the next meeting the boys greeted me with booming laughter and bear hugs. Full of life and promise.

Then something changed. Both boys struggled to maintain eye contact during one visit. They were unusually withdrawn, even lethargic. The behavior repeated during our next meeting, so I asked Lola and Joe about the difference. Having recently immigrated to the United States, the couple spoke in broken English. I gathered that they had recently gone to the pediatrician. Without a translator, the foster parents had tried to explain that the boys had some challenging behavior. Defiance. Hyperactivity. Inattention.

Without conducting any additional examinations or exploring alternate intervention, the pediatrician hastily ordered psychotropic medication for both boys. Taking pills to wake up in the morning and more pills to sleep at night, the children became shells of themselves. Lola and Joe weren't sure what to think. Surely the children needed medication if the doctor ordered it, right?

I wrote to the judge presiding over the children's case, opining that their behavior could be attributed to the traumatic circumstances that led to their placement in foster care, and not to some underlying behavioral disorder. And that even if a disorder existed, medicine may only mask symptoms—not cure the problem. I pleaded with the judge to suspend the medication until other treatment, including therapy, could be implemented.

Praise God, Jeremy and Luke were weaned from the drugs and received more appropriate support and intervention. They soon returned to themselves, even better versions of themselves. And best of all, their foster parents permanently welcomed them into their home. My life changed too. Inspired by Lola and Joe's selflessness and the realization that committing even a little time and attention can make a life-changing difference in another's life, I resolved to become an attorney and speak for the voiceless.

It's easy to become consumed with our own affairs and neglect the plight of our neighbors. Yet God requires that we do justice and defend the vulnerable (Proverbs 31:8-9; Jeremiah 22:3; Micah 6:8; Zechariah 7:9-10; 1 John 3:17-18). Indifference and inaction in the face of oppression or neglect offends God. He gave His all to us. We can give, even a little, to our neighbors. Our care can change lives and make them new.

Jennifer Williams is an attorney and writer, committed to lending her voice to the voiceless. She and her husband, Carlin Williams (LLUSM class of 2009), currently live in Charlottesville, Virginia, with their two delightful daughters, Olivia and Leilani.

January 17   Martin Luther King, Jr., Day, 2022

"It's not enough to have lived. We should be determined to live for something. May I suggest that it be creating joy for others, sharing what we have for the betterment of personkind, bringing hope to the lost and love to the lonely."

Leo Buscaglia (1924–1998): American author and professor in special education

In 2016, I was an intern at the Abundant Life Wellness Institute in Alabama. I often went with the doctor in the area, Dr. Marlo, to see patients at her clinic in Sumter County. One afternoon we received a call from the hospital next door as they needed a physician to help with an incoming patient. It was a small rural hospital, but I still found it odd that there were no other physicians readily available. Where were they?

Regardless, we went to see the patient they now suspected had suffered a heart attack. When we arrived, the patient was calm and alert. My eyes caught a glimpse of her hospital admission band. It was no more than a strip of paper with her handwritten information. *That's strange*, I thought, *I've never seen that before*. They moved her to another room to perform an EKG, and I watched as the nurses struggled to place the electrodes on the patient's skin because they kept falling off. In the end they settled for silver duct tape to hold them in place. Developing country? Not at all; it was right here in the U.S., and it was a clear glimpse for me of the condition of one of the poorest counties in Alabama.

Come with me to another moment in time.

It was the same year in a nearby county. We were driving for at least 45 minutes with nothing but trees in sight when we came upon a dirt road. There, tucked away, were two rows of trailer homes, and a small Black community. Our group had been there before, presenting children's programs with songs and Bible studies, but it was my first time. The kids, with smiling faces, bare feet, and the dirt of childhood, were so excited to see us. We sang with them, hugged them, played with them, and read the Bible together. I glanced around at the conditions of the homes they were living in. All were the same: broken, decaying, old, and seemingly unfit for people to inhabit.

Fast-forward to the year 2020. A pandemic has occurred, George Floyd has been killed, and I am painfully reminded of my own encounters with racism. What brought me through? What gives me hope? It is the dream I have of immersing myself in these same Black communities that I love, giving back with my acquired medical skills and knowledge, providing opportunities to learn life skills through programs, giving of my time and energy to communities rich in potential but lacking resources needed for them to flourish, and finally, offering them a friend and shelter in Jesus if He isn't one already. This is what motivates me when the world seems chaotic—the hope to one day impact and uplift the forgotten, just as Jesus did. Just as I would want someone to do for me.

"No, this is the kind of fasting I want: Free those who are wrongly imprisoned; lighten the burden of those who work for you. Let the oppressed go free, and remove the chains that bind people" (Isaiah 58:6, NLT).

Genise Browne, LLUSM class of 2023, loves teaching and inspiring children, swimming in the ocean, trying new vegan desserts, and enjoying a good laugh. It is her dream to one day become a rural physician in the South, providing hope and healing wherever it is needed the most.

January 18

"And pray in the Spirit on all occasions with all kinds of prayers and requests. With this in mind, be alert and always keep on praying for all the Lord's people."
Ephesians 6:18, NIV

Entering the medical field as an occupational therapist, I hoped that this career would be an opportunity for ministry. Attending Loma Linda University taught me the importance of caring for not only the physical needs of patients but also their emotional and spiritual needs. While working in a hospital setting, I began to really experience what it was like to connect with patients on a spiritual level.

One day is stamped in my memory because it had such a powerful impact on my life. I was working with a woman who had undergone orthopedic surgery for a joint replacement. As part of my evaluation I encourage patients to walk to the sink and do personal care or hygiene activities. While she was standing at the sink, I asked her what she was famous for, a question I learned to ask from Dr. Wil Alexander,* who pioneered whole person care at Loma Linda. My patient's answer was simple but beautiful: "God inside me." She told me that she had been involved in ministry for 40 years. We had a wonderful conversation during our time together, and I felt impressed to offer to pray with her, to which she enthusiastically agreed. We grasped each other's hands. Then something unexpected and surprising happened. Immediately after I finished praying for her, she spontaneously said a beautiful prayer for me that was so Spirit-led and heartfelt.

The patient's granddaughter was also present in the room. Both of them were such genuine people, and their words were very encouraging to me. They told me she has a prayer list with pictures that she lays her hands on as she prays for each person. She said she would put my name on her list, and had her granddaughter take my picture.

This experience was so rich, blessing me beyond words. I did not want to leave the room, because it was such a special moment. There is no question in my mind that this was a providential meeting ordained and planned by God for both of us. During my two years of hospital work I have had countless amazing experiences praying with patients, and on occasion they or a family member will pray for me. I am reminded time after time that it is always worth listening to that nudge of the Holy Spirit to offer to pray with patients. It is during these moments that I feel some of the most fulfillment in my daily work.

*Wil Alexander, founding director of the LLUH Center for Spiritual Life and Wholeness, was an exemplar and consummate teacher of bringing the grace, mercy, love, and hope of Jesus Christ's to the bedside of the patient.

Brianna Woodruff, LLUSAHP Master of Occupational Therapy class of 2015, currently lives in her hometown of Spokane, Washington, and works as an occupational therapist to help seniors in retirement communities stay as strong and independent as possible. Brianna enjoys bringing smiles to the faces of her elderly patients and making them laugh.

January 19

> *"A lit candle loses nothing when it lights another."*
> **Personal motto for Kim Carter**

When I entered this world, I was adorned with kisses and hugs and so much love. Everyone wanted to hold me, kiss my forehead, and squeeze my cheeks. I was wanted! Fast-forward 22 years: I was homeless, pregnant, and unwanted, living on the streets. I can remember how cold the nights were as I huddled in doorways, covered with newspapers, and hoped that I would not get an unwanted visitor in the night. It just isn't safe for a homeless woman to be on the streets. Then one day, like the good Samaritan, a woman approached me and told me that God had a plan for my life. She said He would never leave me nor forsake me. I remember thinking to myself, *I wonder if she's going to get me some breakfast. Can't she see that I am pregnant?* Well, what I got was a small devotional book instead.

I didn't even take the time to open it; instead, I put it in my purse. In less than a week I was in jail and on my way to prison for the first time. Things weren't looking too good for me—or so I thought. Once I made it to the main yard, I was given my few belongings, and there was the devotional book that I had been given! With so much time on my hands, I began to read it, and that is when I was able to open my eyes and my heart to see this was all a part of His plan for my life. Ephesians 6:17 says, to "take the helmet of salvation, and the sword of the Spirit, which is the word of God" (ESV).

Today I help other women recover from homelessness and incarceration. All that I have endured has strengthened my relationship with God and His purpose for my life. Isaiah 10:1-4: "Woe to those who decree iniquitous decrees, and the writers who keep writing oppression, to turn aside the needy from justice and to rob the poor ... of their right, that widows may be their spoil, and that they make the fatherless their prey! What will you do on the day of punishment, in the ruin that will come from afar? To whom will you flee for help, and where will you leave your wealth? Nothing remains but to crouch among the prisoners or fall among the slain. For all this his anger has not turned away, and his hand is stretched out still" (ESV).

Kim Carter is the founder and ambassador of Time for Change Foundation. Certified in accounting with an emphasis on not-for-profits, Kim was inspired to leave the corporate world in 2002 to start Time for Change Foundation in San Bernardino, California. Motivated by her own experiences as a formerly incarcerated woman, Kim made it her mission to help women and children make the transition from homelessness and recidivism to self-sufficiency. Today she is a powerful voice for women who bear the scars of poverty, homelessness, and incarceration. It is Kim's belief that by providing these women with training and the opportunity to develop life skills, in a nurturing and supportive environment, they will become independent, active participants in their communities. She aspires to the work of her idol, Harriet Tubman, by lighting a path and leading others to freedom from addiction and incarceration. Alongside her role as an executive director at Time for Change, she is also a motivational speaker, an advocate, an author, and more recently a developer of affordable housing. In 2015 she was named one of CNN's heroes.

January 20

> *"Even before they finish praying to me, I will answer their prayers."*
> Isaiah 65:24, GNT

During his senior year at LLUSM our son Stephen spent an elective month at Béré Adventist Hospital in Chad, Africa. Despite malaria and esophagitis Stephen thoroughly enjoyed the mission experience.

Stephen is a baroque music lover and had spent a month after his college graduation playing historic pipe organs in churches throughout Europe. He had planned his return trip to include a couple days playing organs again and wanted me to join him in Amsterdam for the adventure. With prior appointments in Korea, Taiwan, and Japan, I would be somewhere en route to Asia when Stephen would be returning through Europe. Sadly, I had completely ruled out joining him in Amsterdam.

God had other ideas. Several days before I was scheduled to leave, my travel agent called me and said, "Turkish Airlines has just canceled and refunded your flight from Istanbul to Seoul. We need to get you on another routing." As I hung up the phone, an idea popped into my head. Maybe I could take a flight to Amsterdam a day early and meet Stephen? I quickly found a one-way ticket to Amsterdam and arranged my flight to Asia from there. Everything fell into place—as if God had planned it. Stephen and I were both thrilled!

We met in the Amsterdam airport. Having already lost more than 20 pounds and now acutely ill on top of it, Stephen looked terrible and simply said, "I got sick on the plane, and I think the malaria has relapsed, but I've started treatment already. I'll be OK."

I suggested we get a hotel and he rest, but no—visiting cathedrals was much higher on his list of priorities that morning. We set out for a famous pipe organ in Haarlem, Holland. Somewhere in the city, as we were standing on a train platform, Stephen started vomiting over onto the rails and could barely stand.

We made it to the Grote Kerk in Haarlem, but by this point the fevers, chills, weakness, and overwhelming nausea made it impossible to continue. We found a hotel near the airport, but he kept on getting sicker, eventually becoming minimally responsive and confused.

Alarmed, I consulted with our oldest son, Jonathon, in his chief residency year at Johns Hopkins; he advised me to take Stephen to an ER. At the ER he was resuscitated with fluids, and a workup was started for his illness.

Eventually we left the hospital and went our separate ways, with Stephen returning to Loma Linda and me to Asia. Because he was still very sick, his flight was rather miserable but certainly memorable for him.

God knew Stephen would need help in Amsterdam, and He orchestrated events to allow me to be there for him. I stand in awe and love of such a great God who cares so much and divinely intervenes in the simple affairs of our everyday life!

Kandus Thorp is the grateful mother of two LLUSM alumni: Jonathon Thorp (LLUSM class of 2012) and Stephen Thorp (LLUSM class of 2016). She and her husband, Brad, are the cofounders of Hope Channel International, the official television network of the Seventh-day Adventist Church. They are retired in British Columbia, Canada.

January 21

"If we are afflicted, it is for your comfort and salvation; and if we are comforted, it is for your comfort, which you experience when you patiently endure the same sufferings that we suffer."
2 Corinthians 1:6, ESV

On January 21, 2014, our son, Matthew, was killed in a tragic motorcycle accident while on his way to a patient's home. Matthew had a passion for helping people. He didn't see his work as a physical therapy assistant (PTA) as a "job"—he really enjoyed the patients he worked with and took great joy in getting to know them personally. Working as a PTA was more than providing a service. For Matthew it was an opportunity to spend quality time with his patients. As long and hard as he worked, he always took the time to be with his family and stay connected.

Our hearts were filled when Matthew's bone marrow donation helped someone regain their quality of life. We are amazed how he helped people while he was alive and how he continues to do so today.

When you lose a child, there is no greater pain or grief. This was devastating, wrenching sorrow for my husband and me. Grief: shock, denial, depression, anger, confusion, lack of energy for living, and the feeling that you are drowning. You go through the motions of living but don't feel as though you are alive. Life is out of sync. For me, I also began stuttering.

After a few months I went to my doctor. I cried as I explained the loss of Matthew and the deep sorrow. I told him, and he could see and hear, that I was stuttering badly. I was totally surprised by his response. First of all, he said he had never heard stuttering after trauma. He wanted to put me on antidepressants and anxiety medication, which I refused. Then he looked at me and stated, "I am young; I have never experienced what you are going through, and I don't know how to help you." My brain could not process how my medical doctor could not have empathy. I asked myself, *Isn't that part of being a doctor?* I looked at him and said, "If you don't know about the loss of a child and the pain and sorrow that goes with it, you'd better learn."

More pain was endured by comments made to us. "He is in a better place." "God took him to build your faith." "God took him so someone else could be saved." "Just keep praying." "Don't be mad at God." "It is time to move on and get over it." "Start living; Matt would want that."

By the grace of God, we are who we are. We can't be the person others expect us to be. God did not take Matthew; it was an accident. God is love, God is compassion, and God is grace and mercy.

We are writing this so that others will read it, and even though they may never walk in our shoes, we want them to understand the power of words and the need to comfort those who have lost a child or someone they love. We need to teach others to understand pain and suffering, and how much unfailing love and compassion like our Lord's is comfort to those in great sorrow.

Jeanne Schrader is retired from California Polytechnic State University, San Luis Obsipo, where she was an administrative analyst. Jeanne and Michael's son, Matthew Lynn Schrader, graduated from LLUSAHP as a PTA in 2001. Jeanne and her husband volunteer at the LLUCH's NICU in memory of their son and continue to find purpose in helping others.

January 22

> *"Never be afraid to trust an unknown future to a known God."*
> **Corrie ten Boom (1892–1983)**: *Dutch author, involved in the Dutch resistance during World War II, and survivor of Nazi concentration camps*

In late January 2020 I began discussions with our hospital's leadership about the new viral pneumonia that was spreading in China. It seemed clear at that time that China would be unable to contain the virus despite unprecedented efforts to do so. I feared it was only a matter of time before this new virus would be in Malawi. These fears only grew in the weeks to follow, as we saw reports of overrun ICU's in Italy. My understanding at the time was that a substantial portion of even healthy people would become severely ill and require oxygen treatment to live. I struggled with the question of whether our staff and fellow missionaries would have access to even basic oxygen treatment if we were to experience this new illness. I have to admit that the thought crossed my mind to personally buy some oxygen machines while they were still available and save them for myself and those close to me who might need oxygen. However, to do so would have been playing into a poverty mindset and could have impaired our mission to treat the sick, teach by example, and show the love and provision we have that is in Christ.

In hindsight, it is now obvious how God answered our prayers and that our hospital's work is ultimately His mission. In fact, the local business community later came to us and offered to fund and procure whatever we needed to treat COVID-19. With their help we acquired numerous oxygen machines and other supplies to set up what Malawi's medical council later decided was the best-equipped COVID-19 treatment center in the country. By July COVID-19 patients had started arriving; many had severe respiratory failure and survived in large part because of the new equipment we were able to procure. As I am writing this in October and by the grace of God, none of our staff have become severely ill. Our experience is just one testament of many that reveal how God provides and that we should trust in Him as we aim to fulfill His mission.

Note: The following was posted on Tim's Facebook page on January 22, 2021:

Google "COVID cases Malawi." You'll see that cases disappeared in August. For months, we had no suspect cases, and speculated why we'd done so well despite minimal testing, mask use, or mandated distancing. In the last week of December, a visitor here tested positive before his flight home. It was the first sign of the latest explosion of cases that's quickly overwhelmed out fragile health care system.

Every day, Claire and I receive cold calls and requests from all over, wanting treatment in our rural hospital. Other hospitals still refuse to treat COVID or are full. We are told the central hospital can't manage to treat more than 70 COVID patients, and so it's turning them away. The best we can do for people whose lungs are failing is to stick two sets of nasal cannulas into their nose, each from a different close-by 10L concentrator, then stick a CPAP mask over the top. Our mini isolation ward worked well for the first wave that hit us in July. Now we're overwhelmed and need to make it bigger. However, we're facing the same limitations as other hospitals, with only a few oxygen concentrators and a sentiment among staff that COVID patients can't be treated in a hospital building for fear that the critical COVID patients are the main source of contagions, such as might be the case with Ebola. This is despite the fact that many people are already spreading COVID unknowingly, given we barely have enough tests for those being admitted. Our little COVID ward has six rooms with monitors, oxygen concentrators, and tiny home CPAP machines set up inside a hot, leaky tent set far away from any wards, surrounded by a swamp, storage unit, and a junkyard.

Claire and I were able to get away from the hospital for just two days in the last 36, a reality when we're the only medical doctors here . . .

Tim Gobble, LLUSM class of 2012, and his wife, Claire (LLUSM class of 2012), both work as deferred mission appointees at Malamulo Adventist Hospital, a rural teaching hospital situated among the tea plantations in the southern highlands of Malawi in Southern Africa. Tim is the only internal medicine physician at the hospital and just one of a handful in the country.

January 23

"And so, Lord, where do I put my hope? My only hope is in you."
Psalm 39:7, NLT

The sun streamed through the window as I entered room 7, belying the somber mood in the air. Jan lay quietly in the bed, nodding to acknowledge me. It was too painful to smile; her mouth was a mass of sores, a side effect of the chemotherapy she was taking for acute myelocytic leukemia.

When Jan had first been admitted several months earlier, she had quickly become a "favorite" patient, even though I knew I was supposed to treat everyone equally. From our initial meeting we had connected, sharing about our love of the Oregon coast and sand dollars. She laughed at my bad luck when I told her I had never been able to find one that wasn't broken. She told me that sand dollars were a symbol of hope to her. "The little pieces inside look like doves, a promise of better things to come."

On this particular day Jan's husband sat next to her bed, stroking her hand. Her teenage daughters hung back, watching from a distance. We had managed to get her a private room for this admission; it looked as though it might be her last.

I began my assessment and started to make small talk. Her husband asked me about my wedding plans—just one month away. Every admission, Jan had joyfully inquired about new developments. As we talked, I noted the multiple large bruises all over her body. As I listened to her heart and lungs, she winced at the slightest pressure on her skin.

"I'm so sorry you have to go through this," I offered. "It looks like you're pretty miserable."

She nodded her assent. Then she looked at her husband, nodding and raising her eyebrows. He smiled and reached down to a paper bag on the floor beside him. "She insisted on bringing this to you," he explained, handing me a small square box.

As I lifted the lid, my eyes filled with tears. There were two sand dollars. One was whole; the other was perfectly broken in half with three little "doves" sitting on a bed of cotton.

"It's a promise of hope for you," Jan whispered.

"And for you," I replied. "'Those who hope in the Lord will renew their strength. They will soar on wings like eagles; they will run and not grow weary; they will walk and not be faint.' That's your hope, Jan."

"I know," she smiled. "It won't be long now."

Kathy McMillan, MA, BSN, is the director of employee spiritual care at LLUMC. She and her husband, Jim (LLUSM class of 1986), live near Oak Glen, where they enjoy the bounty that grows in their garden and orchard.

January 24

"Let the words of my mouth, and the meditation of my heart,
be acceptable in thy sight, O LORD, my strength, and my redeemer."
Psalm 19:14, KJV

In my obstetrics and gynecology training I experienced a good share of difficult cases and even unexpected outcomes that to this day shape my approach to medicine and patient care. However, nothing has influenced me more than the overwhelming, never changing, endless love of God. In both my personal and professional life, I am a living testimony of His love's healing power.

Admittedly, the rigor of residency, fellowship, training in minimal invasive gynecological surgery, the devastating effects of a divorce, cases of advanced-stage cancers in some of my patients, and the general demand of instant-result/quick-fix healing in Western medicine have, at times, led me to a numbness, a desire to disconnect from reality, and a lack of compassion toward those around me. Time and time again I have to intentionally remind myself of Jesus' ministry of healing while He was on earth. He first attended to the physical needs of the people and then fed their souls. Always connected to His Father, with grace, compassion, and love. Always seeking His face.

I heard a sermon recently written by my childhood pastor, Doug Jacobs, called "The Colors of Love." Pastor Jacobs explained how each of us is a reflection of a color of God's love. A unique color that only I can give off to those around me. With this reflection comes great responsibility. Not just as a physician and surgeon attending to the physical ailments of my patients, but also as a possible influencing instrument for their eternity. I feel the same responsibility toward my 5-year-old daughter—the wonderful responsibility of sharing the colors of love.

I always remember Pastor Jacobs starting his sermons by praying Psalm 19:14 . . . and now, every time I scrub into surgery as I wash my hands, I pray the same prayer adding a personal twist:

"Let the words of my mouth, and the meditation of my heart [and the movements of my hands], be acceptable [to you,] O LORD, my strength, and my redeemer."

You see, in surgery I have to be perfect, as someone's life is in my hands. But I'm far from perfect. Only through His love in me can perfect love be manifested.

Astrid von Walter, LLUSM class of 2008, practices minimal invasive gynecologic surgery in Rockville, Maryland. She loves spending time with her 5-year-old daughter and has a passion for women's health. She strives to minister to her patients as Jesus did during His time on earth.

January 25

> *"You, therefore, have no excuse, you who pass judgment on someone else, for at whatever point you judge another, you are condemning yourself, because you who pass judgment do the same things."*
> Romans 2:1, NIV

Jim's life, at 26, was in tatters, with a recent loss of his only child from kidney cancer, a florid case of genital warts from a wandering spouse, and a realization that he had to come to terms with his sexual orientation. When he revealed his homosexuality to his parents, wife, and church, he was welcomed as poison ivy. Disowned by his parents, divorced from his wife, and disfellowshipped by his church, Jim had to face his reality that was so uncomfortable to so many. His Baptist upbringing and spiritual life was important enough to drive 60 miles to a church that would accept him and his love for Jesus.

I began seeing him several years later for his primary and HIV care because his "monogamous" partner of three years found other lovers.

For 12 years Jim came faithfully each month to tell his story to my junior medical school class. Besides discussing the care of the HIV patient, I would pose the questions: Is heterosexuality a choice? When do we choose our sexuality? Is this attraction to the same sex a choice?

It is easy to condemn a problem when it is not ours. As we read more carefully into Romans, especially the preceding verses, we discover the other sins that we might have, such as envy, strife, deceit, boastfulness, arrogance, and heartlessness.

As physicians, with many of us coming from conservative backgrounds, it can be hard to accept and be inclusive and treat all with competence and compassion regardless of religion, race, or sexuality. May we be quick to love and slow to reject. God's love gives us the capacity to embrace those we might quickly condemn.

Barbara Orr, LLUSM class of 1970, graduated at a time when there were only nine females in a class size of 87. Neither family medicine nor emergency medicine were specialties, both of which became fields of her expertise. She was one of the first members of LLUSM's family medicine department in 1980. She was the medical director of the family medicine clinic for 10 years. Her favorite job was director of student education, which she held for 14 years. In the early 1970s she worked with Wil Alexander in the emergency room and supported his ideals of whole person care, and continued to work with him throughout his tenure. She retired in 2010. Note: For Wil Alexander's bio, refer to the devotional on January 18.

January 26

*"Take my yoke upon you and learn from me, for I am gentle
and humble in heart, and you will find rest for your souls."*
Matthew 11:29, NIV

Mount Everest is the tallest mountain in the world—29,035 feet—and for many it has become a symbol or beacon for their greatest battles and goals in life. But in May 1996 eight mountain climbers died in one of the most disastrous attempts to climb Everest. The expedition guide was eager to get a client to the summit no matter what. In his desire to get his client to the top, earning a reputation for getting the most clients to their goals, he disregarded the proper time needed to get back to safety.

In our effort to help family members, friends, patients, students, employees, or employers achieve their goals or support them in times of need, we will make sacrifices. For some of us the sacrifice may be not making time to exercise, forgo going to church, having morning devotions, eating healthy meals, or getting enough sleep. The personal sacrifices seem endless when people are in need. In moments of crisis we will make great sacrifices for others, but what happens when we always live life in sacrifice mode? We eventually have our own crisis—or end up in the hospital—as a result of constantly sacrificing to keep things afloat. We may follow "love others as yourself" (see Luke 10:27), but neglect to love ourselves as we love others! It is like getting on a plane and hearing "Put your air mask on first before helping the person next to you." The problem with the analogy is that life has so many demands and unexpected challenges that it is hard to take care of ourselves as we should. Yet every time we push that hard, a price will be paid.

Before my wife, Elena, started LLUSM in 2012, we had the opportunity to be student missionaries in Nepal at Scheer Memorial Adventist hospital, church, and school in Banepa. It was so rewarding serving there. Elena helped in the hospital, I preached in surrounding churches, and we both taught English, Bible, and the crowd favorite, kickball. Before we left Nepal, we had a chance to climb to the base camp of Mount Everest. Along the way of that 12-day trek, I became totally exhausted—symptoms of mild altitude sickness—so I kept reminding Elena that we could just turn around, but she kept encouraging me to keep going. "We are closer than we will ever be," she would say. We made it to the base camp and saw the peak of Everest—it was spectacular!

The next day we started our descent. In her concern for me Elena pushed herself physically more than she should have. Without enough food or consideration for the cold weather, she was not able to pass up the allure to finally get to bathe after two weeks. That night she became hypothermic while waiting for the hot water, and collapsed in the teahouse shower. A little rest, a warm blanket, and good food helped. We thought of Mount Everest and the lessons we learned about taking care of ourselves, our marriage, and our spiritual walk all through her medical school journey and now during her residency.

What burdens are you carrying right now that are simply exhausting you? The Bible says that early in the morning Jesus started His day off right with prayer (Mark 1:35). What are some things you know you could do today to help yourself start off on the right foot while taking care of life's demands and supporting others along the way? Small changes can make a big impact on helping you summit your biggest goals.

Filip Milosavljevic, DMin, MDiv, is the young adult pastor at the Loma Linda University church. Elena (LLUSM class of 2017) is a radiology resident at LLUH. They have one daughter, Petra Rose Valentina, and one son, John Filip.

January 27

> *"Sometimes, all it takes is just one prayer to change everything."*
> **Anonymous**

I walked into my patient's room, smiled, and gave my usual introduction. "Hello, my name is Kristoff Foster; I'm a medical student working with the doctor. What brings you in today?"

"Well, I was told I may have a thyroid nodule, and wanted to get it evaluated." As she talked, I could see the expected furrowed brows indicating her frustrations. Upon talking to her, I discovered she had many more worries. From the children at home to her lack of proper sleep and constant fatigue, she wore years of stress on her expression. Her chief complaint? Chest pain, urination problems, shortness of breath, chest palpitations, abdominal pain, throat "weirdness." Each complaint was accompanied with a long-detailed history of what she felt, what she thought it was, and what she was worried it could be. Meanwhile her husband sat quietly beside her, reading a waiting room magazine.

I listened to her problems while fruitlessly trying to steer the conversation into a narrower frame. I had only perhaps 15 minutes to take her history, perform a physical exam, and come up with an assessment of her status, and potential plan that I could report to the attending physician—and she just kept on talking. I finished the interview and exam with a mixture of a bit of hidden personal anxiety from my own time restraints, and empathy for her issues.

With the physician in the room we discussed again her many concerns. A plan was made to find the causes of her symptoms, and the steps that were to be taken were carefully discussed. All the while the patient still wore her furrowed brows. Why? Perhaps healthy or pathological anxiety, perhaps fear or frustration, or maybe anger at her current situation could explain the expression of discomfort she bore as we discussed the options she faced moving forward.

Having compassionately addressed the patient's many concerns, the physician gave instructions to wait for the nurse, then exited the room, expecting me to follow. As my hand reached toward the door, I looked back. "Would you like to pray?"

Shocked by such a question, she was silent for a few moments, then replied, "Umm, yeah, sure, let's pray."

Holding hands, we prayed, "Lord, we know that ultimately healing comes from You, and we pray that as we try our best to maintain our health that You will bring that ultimate healing. More than that, God, we ask for peace. Peace that's beyond understanding. Peace through the storms that go on in our lives. Peace that only You can give, and that You have promised to give us. We pray this in the name of Jesus. Amen."

Our eyes opened, and for the first time in the encounter I didn't see furrowed brows on her face, but a hand wiping away tears. As I walked toward the door, her husband said, "Wow. I wish we could do that every time we came here." There are needs that only He can meet.

Kristoff Foster, LLUSM class of 2021, is a resident in internal medicine at Vanderbilt University in Nashville, Tennessee. He feels that he is still young on his journey in medicine and in life at the age of 25. However, he is beginning to learn of life's emotional, social, and physical difficulties through his own experience and that of his patients. He has personally discovered his walk through life to be a spiritual journey. He has found that in even the most difficult seasons of life, peace can be found in God.

January 28

"'What should we do then?' the crowd asked. John answered,
'Anyone who has two shirts should share with the one who has none,
and anyone who has food should do the same.'"
Luke 3:10-11, NIV

Years ago I had the opportunity to spend time with an advocate for the homeless. After seeing him give money to a homeless man begging, I recall asking him if he thought it wise to give money directly to such an individual. The skeptic in me argued that this man likely had a history of making bad choices and may just spend it on cigarettes or booze. The advocate acknowledged that this could be true and did not deny the toll that addiction plays in causing and keeping people homeless and impoverished. However, he finished by asking rhetorically, "What would I do with this money that would be so much more valuable than giving it to a homeless man?"

Working in the emergency department for 20 years, I have seen firsthand the results of poor choices. Such intoxicants as alcohol, opioids, and methamphetamines; poor diet; and lack of exercise make a large percentage of illness at least partially preventable. It is true that feeding an addiction is rarely helpful to an individual in the long term. However, Christ offered His grace and forgiveness unconditionally to all 10 lepers, despite knowing that only 1 would acknowledge His gift and be grateful (Luke 17:11-19).

I want for nothing materially. It is easy to rationalize my inaction in helping the poor around me every day, yet the Bible is clear on this point. We are to help those who are less fortunate. "If one of you says to them, 'Go in peace; keep warm and well fed,' but does nothing about their physical needs, what good is it?" (James 2:16, NIV). We can debate the best ways to do so, and we should be wise in how to share our limited time and money; however, we must share with those in need. In the case of helping the homeless, options exist, such as offering to buy food, handing out gift cards, and supporting local shelters. Those who are homeless feel continual rejection—they don't need more judging glances. They often lack the support and skills needed to succeed in modern society. What they could use is a demonstration of Christ's love. It costs nothing to show genuine concern with eye contact and a warm greeting.

Today, when you see someone unfortunate and struggling, ask yourself: What will I do with this money or my time that is better than helping a person in need? Let us pray that we find opportunities to share the wonderful blessings God has given us.

Torrey Laack, LLUSM class of 1999, currently practices emergency medicine at the Mayo Clinic in Minnesota. He is married to Nadia Laack (LLUSM class of 2001) and they have three sons. He especially enjoys caring for underserved patient populations and sharing his passion for medicine through teaching students and residents.

January 29

> *"Behold, now is the accepted time; behold, now is the day of salvation."*
> **2 Corinthians 6:2, KJV**

It was a typical busy Tuesday morning. Amid the chaos a call overhead announced "stroke alert" in the emergency room. The patient was whisked to the CT scanner and then to the angio suite. As I was helping the patient onto the table, this young woman, only 41 years old, stared at me with a look of fright and anxiety that I will never forget. She was hemiparetic and aphasic. I explained to her that she was having a stroke and that we would do everything possible to help her. Less than an hour earlier she was putting her little 3-year-old daughter down for a nap. Fortunately, a visiting friend who happened to be an emergency room nurse immediately recognized the signs of an acute stroke and called 9-1-1. By God's grace I was able to remove two clots from each of her M2 segments of her left middle cerebral artery. As I was helping her from the table, I asked her, "What's your name?" She was able to speak her name, and then a few minutes later with tears in her eyes she said, "Thank you."

This patient and her husband were not Christians, but the next day I was able to share Jesus with them. I told them about the health message and gave them some literature. It just so happened that I was assigned to present the children's story the following Sabbath at church. I asked them if I had their permission to share their story. They were more than happy to, and they even gave me a beautiful picture of their 3-year-old daughter. Then I turned to the patient and told her that God had given her a second chance at life and the most important thing that she could do was to raise her daughter well and acknowledge Him in all things. Then she reached over with her formerly paretic hand and shook my hand.

"Our time here is short. We can pass through this world but once; as we pass along, let us make the most of life. The work to which we are called does not require wealth or social position or great ability. It requires a kindly, self-sacrificing spirit and a steadfast purpose."*

Purpose in your heart to strengthen and bless others. Don't wait to do your great work for the Lord. Do it now, because tomorrow may never come.

*Ellen G. White, *The Adventist Home* (Nashville: Southern Pub. Assn., 1950), p. 32-33.

George Luh, LLUSM class of 1992, is an interventional neuroradiologist. He received a kidney transplant 28 years ago at LLUMC, and is thankful that God spared his life so that he can serve others. The Lord has blessed him with a lovely wife, two children, and the privilege of working with God to touch the lives of others.

January 30

*"Be strong and courageous. Do not be afraid or terrified because of them, for the
LORD your God goes with you; he will never leave you nor forsake you."*
Deuteronomy 31:6, NIV

A pounding echoed on the metal door of the boat and reverberated back to the room where my wife and I were sleeping with our family in our three bunk beds. We were on a medical launch on the Ucayali River in the jungles of eastern Peru, docked in a village named Charity. I looked at my watch: 1:37 a.m. on January 30, 2003. The pounding came again, and my wife saw, in the light of the full moon, a masked man outside with a gun in his hand gesture at a crew member whom he was holding. We sat huddled on our bunks, listening to the noises coming from outside the launch.

Remembering a previous incident in which people wishing to board and steal had seen angel "marines" on the launch and had aborted their thievery, we bowed in earnest prayer that God would send the heavenly marines to help us. Our whispered prayers reached a feverish intensity as we heard footsteps coming down the hall as the thieves gained entrance to the launch and neared our room. Flashlights pierced the darkness, temporarily blinding us as they entered.

"Who is here?" the masked men demanded. "All adults go to the main room, and leave the children here!" they directed, herding us to where the crew was being held by a man holding a rifle. We sat as instructed, swatting at the ever-voracious mosquitoes, and listening to the thieves going through the launch, stealing whatever suited their fancy.

"Where is the American doctor?" one of the thieves asked, emerging from our bedroom.

"I am the doctor," I replied.

"Come here!" he commanded. "Where is your money? We want money!" he demanded; the force of his question emphasized by the cold metal of his gun pushing into my temple.

With a quick prayer flashed to heaven I answered, "Here, I will show you where my money is," leading him to the boxes where we stored the medication to distribute to the long lines of patients who visited our daily clinics we held in the river villages. "That is where all of my money is. I bought these to give to your people. Do you need any medication?" He grunted in disappointment as he looked at the bottles and bottles of unfamiliar medicine and turned away, looking for more recognizable things to steal. For two hours we sat in the moonlight watching them steal our belongings. When they finally left, we said a tembling but heartfelt prayer to thank God for His protection over all of us.

Guillermo Gow-Lee, LLUSM class of 1988, currently practices internal medicine in Vancouver, Washington. He has a passion for missions, helping students, and hopes to continue spreading God's love in that capacity. He and his wife have three children: Vanessa J. (LLUSM class of 2019), Benjamin J. (LLUSM class of 2021), and Esther C. (LLUSM class of 2023).

January 31

> *"We have been made a spectacle in the whole universe,*
> *to angels as well as to human beings."*
> 1 Corinthians 4:9, NIV

Grand rounds means different things depending on where they are made. Where I was trained in medicine (South Africa), the weekly or twice-weekly professorial grand ward round carefully reviewed the diagnosis, progress, and charting of every patient. These or the impressive presentations on interesting cases and medical progress by the brightest and best were pivotal to learning, training, and ensuring best medical practice and saving lives.

Throughout my career there have been grand rounds of a life in medicine blended with ministry. It started with the decision either to study medicine or become a pastor. My mother prayed that I should become a missionary in the four corners of the earth—her prayer was answered, and I thank God for a faithful, praying mother.

In the early clinical years I struggled with my faith in the reliability of God's Word after being exposed to the arguments of brilliant scientists who found no place for God. But in a "grand round" experience at 4:00 a.m. one night, a young, vibrant Christian internist helped me to pray, "I do believe; help me overcome my unbelief!" (Mark 9:24, NIV). I turned around from the brink of becoming an agnostic and have never looked back. What a great learning experience that grand round was—the life saved was mine!

During national service as a physician (drafted and serving as a conscientious objector), while I was traveling to a remote village in northern Namibia, my vehicle detonated a nest of anti-tank mines. My driver was killed; I sustained relatively minor injuries and returned to work after three surgeries on my hand. On calling my mother a few hours after the incident to inform her that I was alive, before I could say anything she said, "You have been in an accident!" I was amazed at the efficiency of the army's messaging. I asked if they had called her. They had not. "At 12:45 p.m. I was compelled to my knees to pray for you," she said. The land mines were detonated at 12:45 p.m.—and the life saved again was mine! This unforgettable grand round taught me the evanescence of life and added two "better" practices to my life and ministry—urgency and gratitude!

In April 1993 my mentor, teacher, friend, and (eventually) patient, Professor John Barlow, a professed atheist, told me: "I have just been defending you on the university senate." He reported it had been mentioned that the perpetrators of Waco, Texas, were Seventh-day Adventists. He refuted this, stating, "I know Landless—he is a Seventh-day Adventist, and they would not do such a thing!" Another grand round experience—I am not sure of the life that was saved, if any, but I was reminded that as we are privileged to touch physical lives, we are at all times a "spectacle" to the onlookers.

These are a few vignettes from a life overflowing with gratitude and "grand round" experiences keenly looking forward to the heavenly homecoming of grand rounds, where we will hear, "Well done, good and faithful servant! . . . Come and share your master's happiness" (Matthew 25:21, NIV). Take time to review the "grand rounds" of your own life—they are compelling!

Peter Landless is an honorary alumnus of LLUSM who graduated from the University of the Witwatersrand, Johannesburg, South Africa, in 1974. He is a cardiologist, current director of Adventist Health Ministries at the General Conference of Seventh-day Adventists, and a LLUH board member. His passion is blended ministry. He is married to Ros, and they have two daughters, Bronwen and Jill.

FEBRUARY

↻ JUSTICE ↺

"Fairness is what justice really is."

POTTER STEWART (1915–1985)
U.S. Supreme Court Justice, 1958–1981

February 1

> *"I feel that there is nothing more truly artistic than to love people."*
> Vincent van Gogh (1853–1890): Dutch Post-Impressionist painter

Among the works of art on Loma Linda University Health's main campus, one piece that remains close to my heart is Hyatt Moore's painting *The Last Supper with Twelve Tribes*, located within the Del E. Webb Memorial Library. Depicting 12 followers of Jesus at His second coming, this image conveys a strong sense of unity: a dozen racially diverse individuals who likely would have never otherwise met one another find community through the central figure, Jesus Christ. Particularly during this cultural moment of extraordinarily high racial tension, it is refreshing to be confronted with an imaginative depiction of the reality of the unity that Jesus accomplished on our behalf. The cross makes every imaginable racial, sexual, gender, and worldview divide irrelevant. Paul said that "there is neither Jew nor Greek, there is neither slave nor free, there is neither male nor female; for you are all one in Christ Jesus" (Galatians 3:28, NASB). If Paul were writing today, I imagine he might say that "there is neither white nor Black, neither rich nor poor, neither young nor old. You are all one through the One who triumphed over the walls of hostility between you."

This unity doesn't imply a bland homogeneity or loss of individual identity; indeed, our uniqueness is redeemed through the cross. Jesus' call is both individual and terrifyingly absolute: He calls each one of us to complete surrender, to submit our whole selves to crucifixion with Him (Matthew 16:24). But through that very surrender we find resurrection, the complete and final redemption of who we were always intended to be. Furthermore, we find others who have done the same: "brothers and sisters and mothers and children . . . , along with persecutions; and in the age to come, eternal life" (Mark 10:30, NASB).

Jesus prayed that His followers would be one in the same way that He and the Father are one. Given the factionalism all around us, this is a cohesion that the world desperately needs to see. It would also be a powerful testimony to all those who do not yet consider themselves Jesus' followers: the reality that there is a path other than violence, demonization, and "us versus them." He has shown us a better way: unity through humility; unity through crucifixion; unity through self-giving love.

For this reason I see *The Last Supper* as a challenge, an invitation, and a promise. It is a challenge to see Christ all around us: in our neighbors, because they are His image-bearers (Genesis 1:27), and also in ourselves, because through the power of the Holy Spirit, we are called to embody Him (Galatians 2:20). It is an invitation because we have work to do, and indeed, God has prepared this work in advance for us (Ephesians 2:10). Finally, it is a promise: that the day will come when people from "every tribe and tongue and people and nation" will worship God (Revelation 5:9, NKJV). What He has commanded He has surely made possible, and we need only to abide in Him and run the race. May we at Loma Linda University Health run well.

Michael Z. Lee, LLUSM class of 2024, is a second-year medical student. He is trying his best to steward the talents and resources that God gave him. He intends to specialize in medical genetics.

February 2

"Verily, verily, I say unto you, He that heareth my word, and believeth on him that sent me, hath everlasting life, and shall not come into condemnation; but is passed from death unto life."
John 5:24, KJV

Thank you, Doctor!" The words took me by surprise. I was well aware that it was mere circumstances and two years of medical education that had placed me in the position of counseling this patient—a veteran with decades of life experience above me who could have easily claimed me as his granddaughter. What left an impression and gave me a deep sense of responsibility was the fact that the patient believed me—a young medical student with little clinical experience whom he had met just 10 minutes prior. Belief in whatever words I spoke that day would seem like a risk to take, if you were to ask me.

In stark contrast, our omniscient, all-powerful God invites us to believe His never-failing words. These are words that go out of His mouth and will not return to Him empty, but will accomplish what He desires and will achieve His purposes (Isaiah 55:11). Do we believe them? Ellen White once penned that Noah "gave the world an example of believing just what God says" (*Patriarchs and Prophets*, p. 95).

Believe just what God says.

His Word says that He cannot lie (Titus 1:2).

He says that He loves you with an everlasting love (Jeremiah 31:3).

He says that His thoughts toward you are innumerable (Psalm 40:5).

He says that He knows the number of hairs on your head (Matthew 10:30).

He says that He knows the plans He has for you (Jeremiah 29:11).

He says that He cares for you and to cast your burdens on Him (1 Peter 5:7).

He says that His strength is made perfect in weakness (2 Corinthians 12:9).

He says that nothing is impossible for Him (Luke 1:37).

He says, "Ask, and it will be given to you" (Matthew 7:7, NKJV).

He says, "Call to Me, and I will answer you, and show you great and mighty things, which you do not know" (Jeremiah 33:3, NKJV).

He says that He will complete the good work that He has started in you (see Philippians 1:6).

He says "All things work together for good to those who love God, to those who are the called according to His purpose" (Romans 8:28, NKJV).

He says "you are a chosen generation, a royal priesthood, a holy nation, His own special people, that you may proclaim the praises of Him who called you out of darkness into His marvelous light" (1 Peter 2:9, NKJV).

May our lives, too, give an example to the world of believing just what God says.

Shannon Fujimoto Calaguas, LLUSM class of 2019, is doing her residency in otolaryngology (ENT) at LLUH. She married her best friend, Daniel Calaguas (LLUSM class of 2013), on the palindromic date 02-02-2020 and enjoys being outdoors, cooking, and making music.

February 3

"You yourselves are our letter, written on our hearts, known and read by everyone. You show that you are a letter from Christ, the result of our ministry, written not with ink but with the Spirit of the living God, not on tablets of stone but on tablets of human hearts."
2 Corinthians 3:2-3, NIV

I walked into the Labor and Delivery room and introduced myself as I usually do: "Hi, I'm Dr. Alexander. I'm one of the OB doctors that will be taking care of you tonight." The patient was Black, and the room was filled with a number of her close friends and family whom she wanted to be a part of her labor experience.

As I said those words, the side conversations paused, and I felt everyone turn to look at me. I continued talking and letting the patient know our plan for the remainder of her labor course. It was hard to focus because I could hear her family whispering, "She's a doctor"; "She looks so young"; and (the most surprising observation of all) "She's Black." After moments of whispering, the patient's mother asked me, "Are you going to be the one delivering my daughter's baby?" "If she delivers before 7:00 a.m.," I responded. She then told her daughter she needs to get the show on the road. "My baby is going to be delivered by a Black doctor!" she said proudly with a huge grin on her face. "Go ahead, girl!"

At that moment it felt like I was a part of their family and they were cheering for me as my own family and friends have throughout my medical training. Throughout the night they would ask me questions about my age, how long I was in school, if I liked what I was doing, etc. Even in 2020 it is still not common for other Black patients to be treated by a physician that looks like them. They don't take it lightly when they encounter a Black physician, and I don't take it lightly that I am one.

I was able to deliver that patient's baby prior to my shift ending, and the energy in the room was unforgettable. Residency has been tough, and I am grateful for God providing me moments like these to keep me going and reminding me not to take my position for granted. Especially as an OB/GYN, I feel an even greater sense of responsibility when it comes to taking care of other Black patients, as the maternal mortality rate of Black women is three times as high as our white counterparts. I want my patients to feel reassured when they see me come into the room—that I am their advocate for whatever concerns they may have. I want my interactions with them to be reflective of the Spirit of Christ, who serves as an advocate for all of us, so that the impact from our interaction may not only encourage them through all of the turmoil of this world but also remind them of the world that is to come.

Kelcie Alexander, LLUSM class of 2018, is currently an OB/GYN resident at the University of Texas Health Science Center at Houston. She is so grateful for the strong support system she refers to as her "village" that continues to encourage and support her throughout her training.

February 4

"His angel guards those who honor the LORD and rescues them from danger."
Psalm 34:7, GNT

A bear standing and staring at me through the window of the car in which I was sleeping is my first memory of camping. My father reassured me with the above text, and I have kept this text in my mind throughout my life.

We have expectations of how our lives will go. Or at least I did. School, job, love, marriage, and babies. That's about how far I allowed my thoughts to go—because what comes after babies?

My boxes were all being checked off. Grandchild number 1 was coming; my life was on track. I was feeling great, participating in a "boot camp" exercise program, and getting my body ready for new expectations for this next phase of my life.

About three months before my first grandchild was to arrive, I started noticing a slight tremor in my left thumb. No big deal. But, when my youngest child noticed, I mentioned it to my neurologist husband, Gordon Peterson (LLUSM class of 1974), who said it was probably Parkinson's disease, which was later confirmed by a subspecialist.

Because I had not seen a doctor since I had had babies, I made an appointment for the next day with Adrian Cotton (LLUSM class of 1996), a general internist. Dr. Cotton listened to my lungs and heart while doing a general checkup. He said, "I hear a murmur." I assured him I'd had a murmur for as long as I could remember, and it had never been an issue. He went on to explain that when he was in medical school, they didn't have all the new technology they have today, and maybe we should get an echocardiogram "just to be sure." The next week during the echo, Dr. Bansal (LLUSM faculty) came in, and my "hearing" turned off. I was a cardiac nurse, and I knew what was being said; but my defenses would not allow me to "hear." Two days later my husband talked to Dr. Bansal. When I was told that I needed to have surgery because my mitral valve showed stage 4 regurgitation, I fell apart. This was not how my life was supposed to go!

I have learned through these events to accept the fact that I am not in control of how my life will go other than in the choices I make for myself and in my life with God. I know that we live in a "battle zone," and God "has to" allow the devil to show what his kingdom would be. God allows us all the freedom to choose for or against Him. If I allow God, He is guiding and protecting me. Psalms says that His angels watch over me during all the phases of my life, not changing things to give me all the "goodies" while keeping all "the bears" away, but helping me deal with life on this earth.

Myra Peterson is a retired registered nurse and is married to Gordon Peterson (LLUSM class of 1974). February 4, 2014, was the date of her heart surgery.

February 5

> *"On that day, when evening came, He said to them,*
> *'Let us go over to the other side.'"*
> Mark 4:35, NASB

It was a week before I was scheduled to take USMLE Step 1, and I couldn't shake the idea of failure from my mind. Anxiety and fear plagued me daily. This insecurity came not only from the exam that would determine the rest of my life, but also from the scholastic year prior. To say that my second year of medical school was challenging is an understatement. Every test cycle I wondered if this time God would work a miracle. But each cycle ended in tears, as I saw exams I barely passed and those I failed. I felt incompetent, unworthy, and undeserving of my spot in medical school. In those dark moments I could not imagine Match Day, graduation, or even residency. I felt as if I were alone, drowning in waters of uncertainty.

In Luke 8:22-25, NKJV, Luke described a similar situation of doubt and despair among the disciples of Jesus. One day Jesus told His disciples, "Let us cross over to the other side of the lake." And as they started their journey, a violent storm developed that threatened their lives. These fishermen who have sailed through many a tempestuous water before were now afraid! In desperation they cried out to Jesus saying, "Master, Master, we are perishing!" Jesus in response stood before the storm and rebuked the raging waters, and they were stilled. The disciples were in awe, but Jesus simply asked them, "Where is your faith?"

Like the disciples, I felt overwhelmed by my circumstances. Though I have navigated through many academic storms in the past, nothing compared with what I was faced with at that moment. However the God who called me to start this journey to medicine never left my side. Although I felt as if I were drowning, He was still in the boat with me. Since then, as in times past, God has brought me through each and every situation, reminding me that any difficulties in my life were no match for His power. Today I can testify that by the grace of God I made it through second year, passed Step 1, passed Step 2, matched to a residency, and finally graduated! Even though each milestone came with its own raging waters, God continued to remind me that He is in control. He has taught me not to lose faith during adversity. "For God has not given us a spirit of fear, but of power and of love and of a sound mind" (2 Timothy 1:7, NKJV). Before the storm began, Jesus said, "Let us cross over to the other side." Therefore, He will see it through.

Sharmila Price, LLUSM class of 2017, currently practices as an internal medicine hospitalist in Kettering, Ohio. She enjoys traveling and spending time with family and friends. February 5 is her birthday.

February 6

> *"The LORD is good, a stronghold in the day of trouble;*
> *he knows those who take refuge in him."*
> **Nahum 1:7, ESV**

During the years I practiced OB/GYN, I learned many things from my patients. Something that took me quite a few years to realize was that my goals and the patient's goals were not necessarily the same. This was realized when I took care of a patient named Saramma in our Ottapalam Hospital in South India. She presented as 39 years old, married 13 years, never having been pregnant. With the help of some medication I had brought in my suitcase (medicine not yet available in India) we were able to help her conceive after five months of treatment. She was ecstatic, that is, until 33 weeks when she came with ruptured membranes and premature labor and delivered a 3 pound 7 ounce female. The baby died with abdominal distention after four days. Since we had no pediatrician, or the ability to do cultures for infection, we were pretty much in the dark about the exact reason for the baby's death.

Saramma and her husband took their baby home to their village for burial, and though they conceived once more, she had a miscarriage and at age 43 she finally gave up on ever having a child. Nevertheless, I continued to see more and more infertility patients from Saramma's village, 30 miles away.

When I would ask them who recommended our hospital, the answer was almost invariably, "Saramma sent me." Sometime later Saramma came again, and we asked her, "Why, when you lost your only baby, do you continue to send patients to us?"

Her answer startled me: "You don't understand, Doctor. For most of my married life I had been the butt of jokes, with neighbors accusing me of not being a good wife for my husband, because I had not had a baby. When I would walk down the street, they would point at me and gossip to each other about my childless status. But after we had our baby, even though we had to bring her home and bury her, whenever someone would remind me that I had no child, I would correct them: 'Yes, I *do* have a child! She is lying in her grave in the churchyard over there!' Now I can hold my head high, and am given respect from my former critics, all because you helped me have my baby."

Until then I had thought of Saramma's experience as a medical failure. She opened my eyes to the fact that in her opinion, it was a social success!

Mary Small, LLUSM class of 1966, practiced OB/GYN in southern India for 14 years following residency. She was an associate professor in LLUSM's department of gynecology and obstetrics until her retirement in 2004. She retired to the Olympic Peninsula, Washington. Her father, Carrol Small, and brother, David Small, are also graduates of CME class of 1934 and LLUSM class of 1962, respectively.

February 7

> *"Call to me and I will answer you, and will tell you great and hidden things that you have not known."*
> Jeremiah 33:3, ESV

Do you know what I can do with a bridal gown?" My daughter was changing her mind after alterations; this dress did not work for her, and she was deciding a week before the wedding to find a different one. "It has never been worn, and I would like to donate it."

A close friend and I were having lunch, and while I contemplated my daughter's question, the fleeting thought from high school days of *Wouldn't it be exciting to work in the wedding business with joyous brides and assist in making dreams a reality?* flashed through my mind. And then: *Why not?* This first bridal gown donation could be the catalyst for a new offering for the students who come to the Little White House (LWH).* We could have a bridal boutique on campus! So I said, "Yes to the dress!"

The ads went out to the LLU Medical Auxiliary members and the vintage dresses started arriving. One member's sister closed a bridal shop, and we received 20 gowns from her. Another local salon receives sample gowns from surrounding areas and gives their proceeds to cancer research. They heard about the Little White House project and called us when they had too many dresses hanging on the rack to see if we could use them. We then received 25 more wedding gowns!

In February of 2015 we held the first bridal boutique event. Little White House sparkled with flowers and candles and a miniature wedding cake; the volunteers could not wait to welcome our campus brides. These young women went into the dressing rooms with armloads of gowns and friends; they emerged as gorgeous, glowing beautiful brides. Many found their special dress.

Now picture a freshman medical student engaged to be married in May rushing in just before closing time. Her story: health challenges, little money, found a dress before school started; waited for sale after Christmas; dress gone. She remembered that in Matthew Jesus tells everyone not to worry about what to wear because the flowers are clothed more beautifully than even Solomon, and aren't we worth more than the flowers? She realized that God really did want to give good gifts, and she wanted to do His will; He would find a way for a beautiful dress to happen. The first dress she tries on is a perfect fit and is BEAUTIFUL. As the LWH mothers ooh, ahhh, dote, shed a few tears, and toast her with a "Yes to the dress," she says, "I know that God answers prayers, but I never expected Him to answer it this way."

*The Little White House, part of the LLU Medical Auxiliary, provides students on the LLUH campus with needed items for setting up a home as well as clothing. Students "shop" for free from the community's generous donations. To date, the Little White House has given away 40 wedding gowns. If you are inspired by stories like the one above and have a gown in a closet or box that you are ready to share, consider donating it to the Little White House: www.llumedaux.com or 909-558-4639.

Jolene Hilliard (née Lang) graduated from Union College with a BA degree in English. She taught at Loma Linda Academy while her husband, Dennis (LLUSM class of 1975), attended medical school. Mother of three and grandmother of four, she has worked at the Little White House as co-chair for six years. Growing up with a bargain-hunter mother, she and her mother found her wedding gown c. 1972 on sale for $135!

February 8

*"The steps of a good man are ordered by the LORD: and he delighteth in his way.
Though he fall, he shall not be utterly cast down:
for the LORD upholdeth him with his hand."*
Psalm 37:23-24, KJV

I chose to become a general surgeon because I felt the Lord's call to do overseas missionary work. During my fourth year of residency I decided to do a fellowship in surgical oncology. After I completed my five-year general surgery residency, I then did a two-year research fellowship at Johns Hopkins in Baltimore, Maryland. One of the reasons I believe God was leading me into surgical oncology is that I would be able to maintain my general surgical skills to be useful in the mission field. After completing the research fellowship at Johns Hopkins, I applied for a surgical oncology fellowship. However, I did not match! I was devastated. I knew the Lord was leading me into surgical oncology, but why didn't I match? I was discouraged and confused. Out of nowhere I received a call from a surgical oncologist at Wake Forest University in North Carolina. He tells me they are starting a surgical oncology fellowship, and they would like to interview me for the fellowship. I interviewed and was given the fellowship position in surgical oncology. God was ordering my steps, and my dream was alive again!

During my final year of fellowship I begin applying for jobs in the Maryland area. I accepted a job at a hospital in Washington, D.C., and signed a contract. In March of that year the hospital said they had to rescind the contract because they had to put a freeze on hiring because of financial constraints. I was again devastated. I had a wife, three children, and no job. I was reminded of an Ellen White quote: "We have nothing to fear for the future, except as we shall forget the way the Lord has led us, and His teaching in our past history" (*Last Day Events*, p. 72). I was not as discouraged this time, because I remembered what God had recently done for me in obtaining the fellowship.

The next month I was reading a surgical journal, and there was an article written by the chief of surgery at the Anne Arundel Medical Center in Annapolis, Maryland. His email address was at the end of the article. I emailed him to ask if he had any job openings for a surgical oncologist. He asked me, "How did you know we were interviewing?" I didn't; I just felt compelled to reach out to him. He interviewed me and offered me the job. I have now been working there for six years. This chief of surgery is a surgical missionary and is part of an organization called PAACS (Pan-African Academy of Christian Surgeons). I recently did a two-week mission trip in Malawi with PAACS training surgical residents in Africa. This group of Christian surgeons does not believe in just doing mission trips, but has started eight residency programs in Africa to train surgeons. Loma Linda University is the accrediting body for these residency programs. Talk about a full-circle moment! God truly ordered my steps.

Naeem Newman, LLUSM class of 2004, currently practices surgical oncology in Annapolis, Maryland. He has a passion for spreading the everlasting gospel through healing the sick and preventing illness with diet. He was the speaker at the 2019 LLUSM Annual Black History Vespers and Dinner.

February 9

February 9, 2011... The day I found myself in a family support group at the Behavioral Medicine Center. I had driven past that facility for more than 20 years, always thinking about "those poor people" that had loved ones there. I now had someone there, and I was now one of "those poor people."

It took me almost three months from that day to set foot in my church. I had been a part of that faith community for over 25 years; not only a part of it, but active and involved. I raised my children in that community, and over the years, it became our home church. So one would think that going back during one of the darkest points in my life would have been, if not easy, at least a welcoming and safe place. I was somewhat nervous and apprehensive; but in all honesty, I wanted to go. So I did. Before the song service was over, I ran out of church.

When I got home, I sat down and what I couldn't articulate verbally, poured out from my heart onto the piece of paper in front of me. Here are those words.... Here is my experience....

> I am one that just lost my job; I am one that seeks comfort in food;
> I am one whose marriage is no more; I am one that cuts herself in the darkness;
> I am one whose child is not here in church; I am one living with addiction;
> I am one with an eating disorder; I am one whose child was expelled from school;
> I am one struggling to make ends meet; I am one suffering from depression;
> I am one that just walked through these doors; I am one living beyond my means;
> I am one whose health is fragile; I am one whose life is crumbling;
> I am one whose only companion is loneliness; I am one who has been here since cradle roll;
> I am one at church with jeans, t-shirt and tattoos; I am one attending public school;
> I am one in leadership and always upfront; I am one in designer clothes;
> I am one attending a Christian private school; I am one in the back pew;
>
> I am here... but I might as well not be. I am invisible. I sit next to you, but I am not seen; I am afraid to share my truth, so you don't know my story. And if I do, you don't know what to say. I sit next to you, but do you see me? All I need is a smile, a hug, a caring word, encouragement, and for you to look me in the eyes; not whisper behind my back. All I need is grace and compassion; I don't need to be judged, all I need is acceptance and love, because of the journey that I walk today. I am here next to you. Where are you?

Tears were running down my cheeks as I finished writing. My pain and loneliness were excruciatingly real to me; and they were ripping my soul apart. But I sat there basking in my pain, reliving that morning's church experience, and resenting what should have been, my thoughts gave way to reflections. How many times had I sat next to someone, saw their tears rolling down their face, and looked the other way? How many times did I join in conversation about someone else's misfortune, and never asked if I could help? How many times did I see that hesitant visitor, and walked past them with barely a shadow of a smile? How many times did I judge someone because of their clothes (nice or not), cars, lifestyle, or demeanor, and never took the time to know them? How many times did I feel sorry for a parent whose child was hurting, but froze in place not knowing what to say? Many times; perhaps too many times. I found myself wishing for

Continued on lower half of February 10...

February 10

"A joyful heart is good medicine."
Proverbs 17:22, ESV

I was rescued tonight. Junk mail to go through. Photos to edit. Bills to pay. Dishes to wash. Photos to edit. Thank-you notes to write. Laundry to wash. Did I mention photos to edit?

Clicking on the phone's "answer button" connected me to a very recognizable voice from more than 45 years ago. The conversation started, and 114 minutes later it ended because the worker bee in me said I had to. I really didn't want to.

The topics went from high school reunions to new and old friends, from aging parents to precious grandchildren, from old vacations to future escapades. I could have gone to bed earlier. Had more chores done. Been better prepared for tomorrow. But I didn't. Sometimes it's healthier and more fruitful to listen to a friend. Sometimes your life is more fulfilled when you are rescued from the day-to-day grind and share your heart with a good friend that you rarely talk to but you know is one of those lifetime friends.

So I will wake up tomorrow grasping for energy and wondering why I didn't hit the sack earlier. My stomach will hurt from all the underexercised laughter muscles that were used, but my heart will be full. My apologies for all the deadlines I missed. Sometimes it's best if we just stop our lives and pick up the phone.

Cyndee Pelton, LLUSN class of 1985, affirms that pediatric hematology/oncology nursing stole her heart after graduation. She currently is LLUCH's pediatric oncology clinical trials coordinator and volunteers as a photographer at a rescue dog and cat facility. She is thankful for the night she picked up the phone and spoke with her high school friend Patricia Roberts Aldrich.

Continued from February 9 . . .

something that I, perhaps, had been unable to extend to others. I had needed something that morning that I did not receive; but I was not the first one, and as I write this, I am sure that I will not be the last one.

I learned that day that in giving is when I receive. In extending grace, compassion, friendship, and love to others, is when I am blessed with grace, compassion, friendship, and love. While you may not walk in my shoes, and I may never walk in yours, we can walk next to each other and lean, if we need.

Life has a way of teaching us and inviting us to grow. We must be open to the lessons and learn, because as we emerge from them, we are one step closer to what we are meant to be. It is my hope, today, that I am more aware, sensitive, and compassionate; and less paralyzed when it comes to extending grace, compassion, acceptance, and love to the person next to me, for they might need it today as much as I did that day.

(Written on April 28, 2011)

Ester Boloix-Chapman came to LLUH more than 35 years ago and currently works in central administration. She thinks of herself as a "repurposed" employee. That ordinary day in February 2011 turned into an extraordinary one—an unforeseen gift of a never imagined journey. She lives "one day at a time," walking in hope, and living in gratitude.

February 11

> *"Earth has no sorrow that Heaven cannot heal."*
> Thomas Moore (1779–1852): Irish lyricist

A life-threatening infection was rapidly spreading through her body from a gaping wound on her foot. Several of her organs were already shutting down, and her speech was incoherent. I was four hours into my second 24-hour shift as a third-year medical student when I found myself in the emergency department with my senior resident assessing a woman I will call Joan. After only a few minutes my resident declared that she would need an emergency leg amputation. I was shocked as I looked at the woman before me, who seemed merely confused. How could someone with so little outward evidence of injury be so close to death? As my resident went to prep the OR I stayed with Joan to try to explain to her that she was going to lose her limb. I felt it was the least and perhaps only thing I could do as a student in that situation. I couldn't tell if she understood me, and I couldn't help feeling as though she was trying to tell me something important, but the sounds coming out of her mouth were not making any sense.

After several failed attempts at finding any of Joan's family or friends, we took her into the OR for an emergency amputation. That afternoon I watched with dismay as Joan's organs slowly declined in the ICU. I watched as doctor after doctor tried to come up with a life-saving solution. When the night team took over, I realized that my fears were becoming true. No one expected her to make it through the night. All I really remember is sitting in front of Joan's large glass door, wishing that I could do something, so I prayed. Not with words, because I had none, but I cried out to God with an ache I had not experienced before. An ache that I had for someone I had had one unintelligible conversation with, yet in that moment my life seemed so wrapped up with.

Deep in the night the code was called. The quiet room turned into a bustle of activity. I found myself in the group of people taking turns doing chest compressions—the whole time wondering how I could show Joan how much I wished I could have talked to her and learned more about her. The time of death was called, and the room went back to the quiet stillness that it was before. There were no family members or friends to tell, just several residents upset about the unfortunate situation, and one questioning medical student. I found myself wondering how I could show this woman, who had in one day found a significant place in my heart, that she had made a difference in my life—especially when I didn't even know what that difference was. This is a question that I am still asking myself today. But one thing that I know is that the lessons that I learned from Joan in regard to the pathology, physiology, and pharmacology will stay with me forever. Not only will the scientific lessons stay with me, but so will the lessons I learned from how I react to human suffering, life-threatening situations, and death. I hope to incorporate these lessons that I learned from Joan into the care of my future patients—showing them that they have made a difference in my life and that they have helped me to take one step further in my education as a lifelong student, physician, and friend.

Whenever I would walk past Joan's room in the days that followed, I'd often remember that night. Death became very real for me that night. But with death there is hope. A hope that there is something beyond the grave. A hope that the questions of suffering and pain will all be answered, and we will live forever with the ultimate Physician.

Heidi Spady, LLUSM class of 2020, is an emergency medicine resident at LLUH. She has a passion for global health and enjoys skiing, rock climbing, and playing Spikeball in her free time.

February 12

*"Be the one who nurtures and builds. Be the one who has an understanding
and a forgiving heart, one who looks for the best in people.
Leave people better than you found them."*
Marvin J. Ashton (1915–1994): businessman and Utah state senator (1957–1961)

At the end of my first year of medical school I was following the neurology team around the hospital during rounds. One day I followed the team into the room of a patient who had been showing some strangely inconsistent neurologic symptoms for the past few days. The patient, a young man in his late teens, was lying in the bed with a deadpan look in his eyes while his concerned family sat around the bed.

The attending doctor on the team introduced himself to the patient and offered a hand to shake that the patient weakly took without changing his facial expression. The doctor proceeded with the relevant tests from a standard neurological exam. He checked the patient's pupils and eye movements, his sensation, and reflexes throughout his body, and he even held out a finger and asked the patient to touch it with his toes. Then he checked the patient's coordination by holding up a finger and asked the patient to move his own finger back and forth between his nose and the finger. The patient jabbed a finger out, but missed the doctor's finger by a wide margin. Without changing his expression at all, the patient then attempted to move his finger back to his nose but ended up just poking himself in the ear. Back and forth the patient's finger went, missing both the finger and his nose and just kept poking himself in the eye, neck, or ear, demonstrating a finding called ataxia. Next, the attending asked the patient to stand up to check his balance. The patient lurched and swayed back and forth as the attending stood by to catch him should he fall, but the patient never did, a finding called astasia-abasia.

At this point the attending had the team follow him into the hall, where he gave us the diagnosis: The patient was faking! While it was disconcerting that the patient presented with finger-to-nose ataxia, he was able to shake the doctor's hand and touch his finger with his toes, and he had astasia-abasia, all findings that require the same neural circuity involved in the coordination test. I'll never forget my excitement at catching the patient red-handed! Nor will I ever forget what I learned that moment when I condemned the patient: The concerned doctor instead looked beyond the how to ask why. He had the family leave the room too, so that he could talk to the patient in private to ask him what he was going through and if he needed help.

The attending recognized that it wasn't his job as a doctor to judge the patient for his mistakes or just to cure his body, but to work together with the patient to help him in mind, body, and soul. Jesus is like that too! Just as He cured and ministered to the demon-possessed, the sick, and the sinners, Jesus cared for the minds, bodies, and souls of all those in need and calls us to do the same.

Michael Moores, LLUSM class of 2021, is a former electrical engineer who enjoys reading, microelectronics, and weightlifting. His father, Donald (LLUSM class of 1987), and grandfather Arthur (CME class of 1953-B) contributed to the two previous Rounds Series devotional books.

February 13

"Again he entered the synagogue, and a man was there with a withered hand. And they watched Jesus, to see whether he would heal him on the Sabbath, so that they might accuse him. And he said to the man with the withered hand, 'Come here.' And he said to them, 'Is it lawful on the Sabbath to do good or to do harm, to save life or to kill?' But they were silent. And he looked around at them with anger, grieved at their hardness of heart, and said to the man, 'Stretch out your hand.' He stretched it out, and his hand was restored."

Mark 3:1-5, ESV

The poor man remembered the terrible day when his fingers became stiff, and then he could not bend his wrist. Gradually his arm shriveled until it hung limp and useless at his side. He could no longer work. Jesus responded to this man's hope and faith in His healing power with love and compassion rather than conforming to the Pharisee's letter of the Sabbath-keeping laws.

As a hand surgeon I have seen many withered hands. The causes may be on account of nerve paralysis, muscle atrophy, or both. To repair a withered hand, one must repair the nerve or do a nerve graft and often a tendon transfer from another muscle must be done. To properly treat a withered hand may take several surgeries, but even with all these surgeries it is rare to recreate a perfectly functional hand.

During a lifetime, fingers flex and extend millions of times. One-fourth of all bones in our bodies are in our hands—actually 29 in total. Picking up a piece of bread, for instance, involves moving more than 50 muscles and 30 joints. A piece of finger skin, the size of a postage stamp, contains several million nerve cells that detect the temperature and texture of anything we touch. This is why lovers like to hold hands.

When we approach Jesus and offer ourselves to Him and His purposes, He stimulates atrophied nerves and restores action. He holds life in the hollow of His hands, which are the safest and strongest hands in the world. Those hands were cruelly nailed to a cross with spikes driven through His nerves and tendons for you and me. Do we appreciate the scarred hands of Jesus and what they have done for us?

My favorite picture of Jesus shows Him with outstretched hands welcoming those who come to find peace and joy. "Come unto me, all ye that labour and are heavy laden, and I will give you rest" (Matthew 11:28, KJV). His hand knocks at the door of our hearts. He will heal not only our withered hands, but our entire body and soul.

Virchel Wood, CME class of 1960, was a professor in LLUSM's department of orthopedic surgery. For his pioneering and international work as a hand surgeon, he was awarded LLUSMAA Honored Alumnus in 1999, received the LLUH Distinguished Service Award in 2004, and was named LLUSMAA Alumnus of the Year in 2007. Note: Dr. Wood hand-delivered this story for Grand Rounds, when stories were first being collected. He passed away peacefully on April 16, 2020. February 13 is his birthday.

Valentine's Day
February 14

> *"For I am confident of this very thing, that He who began a good work in you will perfect it until the day of Christ Jesus."*
> Philippians 1:6, NASB1995

Life doesn't always go the way you think it will.

When I first moved to Loma Linda and started medical school, I had my life planned. I would pass all of my classes my first year, and for second year I would get married to my long-distance fiancé. After school we would work in the same residency program and start our family. Then all of a sudden my fiancé broke off our engagement with a phone call, and I failed my first set of exams. I couldn't catch up fast enough, and by Christmastime I realized that I would need to repeat the year. All of a sudden my plans were falling apart. I wasn't going to be a wife, and I might not even get to be a physician. I knew God had put those callings on my heart, but I was watching them slip away.

Months later I realized that God was asking me to hold His promises with open hands. I needed to believe that whatever happened, He would fulfill His calling for my life. But it wasn't going to be the way I wanted Him to. It would be in His timing and through His guidance, and I was going to learn how to trust Him more because of it.

That year was the hardest year of my life. I learned to rely on my family and friends to give me the love and support I needed to make it. I learned how to seek community and invest in a church. I learned to ask for help and accept my personal limitations. And most important, I learned that God wanted me to find my worth in Him alone. It didn't matter if I became a physician or a mom. I was His, and my purpose in life was to bring Him glory in whatever situation He put me in.

Two years after my plans fell apart, they started to come back together. I finally passed first year with the help and encouragement of so many people. Last summer a diesel mechanic who serves on the worship team with me asked me out for coffee, and just a few weeks ago he asked me to be his wife. My life looks so different today than I thought it would two years ago, but it is so much better. I now have a solid community of friends and mentors, a faithful and God-fearing future husband, and a deeper trust in the Lord. I know I have many more ups and downs in my future, but now I'm ready to trust God and follow wherever He leads me.

Maddison Pearl Ulrich Hussey, LLUSM class of 2021, is currently a resident in psychiatry at Prisma Health Greer Memorial Hospital in South Carolina. She loves coffee shops and going on walks with her new husband and her old pug.

February 15

> *"'Meaningless! Meaningless!' says the Teacher. 'Utterly meaningless! Everything is meaningless.'"*
> Ecclesiastes 1:2, NIV

When I was a child, I would often grumble about being forced to make my bed. To my 7-year-old mind, my parents were coercing me into doing something completely meaningless. The careful work I spent in the morning folding my blankets and tucking in the sheets would rapidly be undone that same night as I tucked myself into bed to sleep. What is the point of making the bed if it is necessarily going to be messed up?

This question of meaning has stuck with me through the years, although it no longer concerns my bed. I have often grappled with what gives meaning to my life and human life in general. We are born, we live, and we die. Some lives are longer; some are shorter. Some are filled with joy; others with sadness. But no matter what type of life, they all end the same way. We can try to live a life filled with service to others, a life that really makes a difference, but nearly everyone is forgotten within a few generations. What then is the point of life? Sad people may be cheered up, but sadness will afflict them again. Sick people may be healed, but their health will not last forever. Hungry people may be fed, but hunger will always return. What then is the point of even trying?

I ultimately found my search for meaning in Jesus. He is fully God, yet fully human. As a human, He felt the meaningless of life just as deeply as we do now. He rejoiced with life and cried with death. He provided comfort to the suffering. He, more than anyone, knew the futility of life, and yet He chose to have compassion on the sick, knowing full well that His physical healing was only a temporary respite from the suffering of this world. Jesus' earthly ministry was meaningful, not because He provided temporary rest from physical suffering, but because He is the permanent rest from all suffering.

It is with this on my mind that I strive to become a physician. Yet despite how hard I work or how skilled I am, I will be unable to help everyone. However, like Jesus, I can rejoice with life and cry with death. I can provide comfort to the suffering. As the Teacher states in Ecclesiastes, there is no meaning in this earth alone, but my meaning comes from Him who created this earth. I can find meaning in continuing Jesus' healing ministry while pointing toward Him who is the source of meaning and the end of death and suffering. My meaning is not through the actions that I do, but through the actions of Christ.

Ethan Miles, LLUSM class of 2022, enjoys dabbling in athletic things even though he finds little success in them.

February 16

> *"'My grace is sufficient for you, for my power is made perfect in weakness.'*
> *Therefore I will boast all the more gladly of my weaknesses,*
> *so that the power of Christ may rest upon me."*
> 2 Corinthians 12:9, ESV

You are in acute liver failure, and you have a brain tumor." Waking up groggy from the toxicity in my body and hearing these words was a shock, to say the least. How could I, a seemingly very healthy 44-year-old woman, be so suddenly diagnosed with such life-threatening illnesses? As I sit here writing, I admit that the question has seared my mind on way too many occasions. On a deeper level, how could God allow this to happen to me? I was happily married with an 11-year-old son. I had a life to live. This is not what I signed up for, God! And knowing and believing that my God's intentions for me are only good, how could these diagnoses possibly be the best story of my life? It's just so much easier to scream and yell and wallow in the sadness. However, this was not the story I wanted for myself. To accept the story and to receive it and to walk it—well, now, that's something I could never do on my own. This is where God enters. One moment at a time, even when the road ahead may be dark.

I have to trust that the best story is being written by the Author, not by me or by any fancy ideas and plans that I may have for my own life. Some days I struggle with wondering what the future holds, and some days I live in each and every moment with immense perspective. It's a step-by-step journey. I have learned more about God during this time than I could have ever learned otherwise. He is faithful to all He has promised. He is good, not because He gave me a miracle, but simply because He is God. That's enough. And even if I would not have survived my liver failure or my multiple brain tumor surgeries and treatments, He would still be good because He is God. This is His story being written through my life, and all I want is for Him to be glorified.

In the words of Nancy Guthrie, from her book *Holding On to Hope*:

"But because I believe that God's plans for me are better than what I could plan for myself, rather than run away from the path He has set before me, I want to run toward it. I don't want to change God's mind—His thoughts are perfect. I want to think His thoughts. I don't want to change God's timing—His timing is perfect. I want the grace to accept His timing. I don't want to change God's plan—His plan is perfect. I want to embrace His plan and see how He is glorified through it. I want to submit."

Shani Judd Diehl, LLUSAHP BS occupational therapy class of 1997, and her husband, Byron (LLUSD class of 2002), are local business owners of Diehl Orthodontics in Redlands, California. Since 1995 Shani has been a vocalist with the Heritage Singers, an American gospel group. Shani currently homeschools their 15-year-old son, Matthew Judd, while enjoying music, travel, golf, and skiing together with her family. February 16 is the day she had neurosurgery to remove her brain tumor.

February 17

"Now faith is confidence in what we hope for and assurance about what we do not see."
Hebrews 11:1, NIV

My origins are not exotic or sensational as many expect when I say I am Haitian, born and raised. There is no special childhood story of deprivation or victory against great odds. My parents are professionals, working in academia and health care. I did not move to the United States in search of a better life from an impoverished environment. That is not my story. We moved in mid-2001, and eight years later I graduated college with job offer in hand, while my dad labored over his studies. The future was bright, and so was the hope of creating my own home in this country.

Both in high school and as an undergraduate, I was surrounded by international and American students, each with a unique story, though often peppered with financial woes. Many prayers centered on tuition and the stories of miraculous ways God intervened in a particular situation. Those stories felt foreign to me at the time, as I was cocooned away from the family's finances, as most Haitian kids are. Nevertheless, those stories echoed a much urgent reality in our family, something that soon evolved into a yearly scourge: an unstable immigrant status with no end point in sight. For 16 years while in the United States, I moved from visa to visa, each with its detailed forms, inconvenient deadlines, increasing fees, but never promising stability. Creating a home seemed impossible, especially after my parents returned to Haiti at the end of their studies.

The absence of an end to these visas and a drawn-out promise of an immigration law overhaul created doubt bordering on pessimism about the possibility of ever creating a home. I did not reach the point of hopelessness until the 2016 unwelcoming political climate, which had been simmering in the background of American sentiment, became apparent. It worsened because the stakes had become higher: I had been accepted into medical school two years prior.

At the start of my fourth year, the visa that had once protected me from deportation was suspended, leaving me four months short until graduation. My student loans were denied, and I soon found myself understanding far too well the tuition-centered prayers of my classmates back from my undergraduate days. God's grace, displayed through local food pantries and family help, enabled me to begin my last year in medical school. It also began with the most supportive individuals who brought their best tools to my aid. Friends shared their personal stories of resilience, family prayed and fasted, classmates advocated, faculty advised, and even strangers formed a network to raise awareness for the plight of immigrant students.

My visa was extended, granting me enough time to graduate. It was the answer to many prayers, though the specific path ahead is uncertain.

Christelle Miot, LLUSM class of 2018, is an internal medicine resident at LLUH. She is the middle child of two teachers and is also passionate about education. She would like to encourage all immigrant students to pursue their dreams and become a channel through which God's blessings can flow to others.

February 18

LLUSM Family Day—Dedication, 2022

> *"As a prisoner for the Lord, then, I urge you to live a life worthy of the calling you have received."*
> **Ephesians 4:1, NIV**

I found myself in an unfortunately familiar situation. Tiptoeing down the stairs in the middle of the night, I was bone-tired. In my first months out of training I was trying to adapt to attending practice. I had been consulted as the "expert" on things I'd never heard of, asked to perform procedures I'd only read about in books, and worked night and day. But when the hospital called, there was nothing to do but put on my scrubs and leave my husband and daughter yet again.

This particular patient was a 5-year-old girl whose leg was starved of blood flow because of compartment syndrome, which occurs when the muscles in the leg swell significantly, compressing the nerves, veins, and arteries inside the fascial envelopes. The treatment is to cut the fascia open, relieve the pressure, and let circulation return. This little girl's toes were deep purple, and her foot felt like ice. I had the team prep the OR while I drove to the hospital.

I felt sick. A case like this would be relatively simple in an adult, but felt momentous in a child. But this was also a culmination of the past months of feeling insufficient. I felt like a bad mom, a lousy wife, an imposter trying to fit in where maybe I didn't belong; attempting to do everything but doing it all poorly. There's no way I was the best person to be treating this patient. Who did I think I was even to attempt it?

I scrubbed at the sink, said a prayer, and walked to the OR table. I held my patient's foot while I marked out the incisions. Her foot wasn't much bigger than my daughter's. The same chubby ankle; the same flip-flop tan. I can say only that I was granted a divine perspective in that moment: I was up for yet another night in order to save this perfect foot. That is why I endured the long years of medical school and surgical training and why I had to trust that God had brought me here—all because of that 5-year-old's foot.

Being a doctor is a vocation, a deep calling. Paul tells the Ephesians to "live a life worthy of the calling you have received." What does that mean for a career in a technical profession such as medicine? Developing professional competency is the primary focus in training. But competence without character is arrogance. What will undergird and anchor a physician is character. Empathy developed, kindness cultivated, thoughtfulness intentionally nurtured: These are the deep roots of identity you put down in the soil of God's calling. To be clear: Excellence is still critical. Character without competence is irrelevant. Being worthy of your calling means you go through the technical training to become excellent at what you do. But when I wake up in the middle of the night, questioning the purpose of it all, I must remember it is the calling that gives meaning and motivation to everything else. It is the calling that gives peace when fear of technical insufficiency creeps into my heart. It is the calling that makes me the hands and feet of Jesus to people who are frightened and hurting. While my own family slept peacefully at home, it was a 5-year-old's foot that God used to remind me of the calling I have received.

Kristyn Mannoia, LLUSM class of 2011, is a vascular surgeon at LLUH. She graduated along with her fantastic husband, Daniel Ng, an emergency medicine physician. They have two delightful daughters, Maia Anne and Naomi Rose, and enjoy barbecuing and gardening together. She spoke at the 2019 LLUSM white coat ceremony.

February 19

"Jesus answered her, 'If you knew the gift of God and who it is that asks you for a drink, you would have asked him and he would have given you living water.'"
John 4:10, NIV

Traditional interpretations of Jesus' noontime encounter with the Samaritan woman at the well in Sychar usually suggest that she was a "shady lady" who came to draw water despite the midday heat, solely to avoid the disapproving looks of neighbors. There is an old legal maxim that "silence means assent" and it is true that her failure to deny Jesus' assertion that she'd had five husbands and now was living, unmarried, with a lover affirmed his summary of that part of her life. But many aspects of their interaction point to another possible explanation for the unusual behavior of a complicated woman.

Where was she and what was she doing, we may wonder, on the cool evenings when most townswomen were at the well drawing water? Up to no good? Or was she listening somewhere quietly in the shadows outside the place where the men of the community met for intellectual discussions in which she, as a woman, could not participate—but to which she could listen. Evidence for this possibility can be found throughout the story.

First, perhaps because of the life experience Jesus referenced, she was not afraid to talk to strange men. She may have been poor and seen an opportunity to profit: He was thirsty; the well was deep; she had a waterpot; He did not. But as their conversation [of which we have only a fragment] progressed, it became clear there was more to it, and to her, than that. She acknowledged Jesus' authority ("Sir, I perceive that thou art a prophet" [John 4:19, KJV]), but it did not impede her inquiry. Instead, it intrigued her. Here at last was an intelligent man with whom an intelligent, though [probably] illiterate, woman could speak of weighty matters.

Second, she was informed, and she spoke with confidence. She knew her history ("Our father Jacob...gave us the well, and drank thereof himself, and his children, and his cattle" [verse 12, KJV]). She was aware of theological conflict ("Our fathers worshipped in this mountain; and ye say, that in Jerusalem is the place where men ought to worship" [verse 20, KJV]). She understood the uncertainty and significance of events to come ("I know that Messias cometh, which is called Christ: when he is come, he will tell us all things" [verse 25, KJV]).

Third, she had credibility. When she went into the town and told the men of her conversation with Jesus, they did not dismiss her report as the ravings of an ignorant, immoral woman. They listened to her; they believed her; and they followed her to Jesus ("Then they went out of the city, and came unto him.... And many of the Samaritans of the city believed on him for the saying of the woman" [verses 30, 39, KJV]).

Jesus understood and appreciated the woman's hunger for answers to spiritual questions, and He took her seriously. She listened, and He was able to tell her things He had not yet shared with his own disciples: that true worship is a matter of spirit, not geography or group identity; that He alone is the source of "a well of water springing up into everlasting life" (verse 14, KJV).

Donna Carlson, LLUSM class of 1969, is a retired pediatrician and attorney living in Redlands, California. She loves teaching and for many years participated in the Orientation to Religion in Medicine class for first-year LLUSM students. Currently she directs a Law and Medicine seminar course for senior LLUSM students.

February 20

"For this reason he had to be made like them, fully human in every way, in order that he might become a merciful and faithful high priest in service to God, and that he might make atonement for the sins of the people."
Hebrews 2:17, NIV

As a gastroenterologist I'm constantly amazed by the variety of diseases I've encountered in my practice, but none more amazing than the patients who have a liver transplant.

Because of a shortage of donated livers in California, where I practice, patients usually have to have liver cancer or be near death to receive a donated liver.

The liver transplant teams are the ones that make the miracles happen. But as the patient's primary gastroenterologist, I have a different type of role consisting of diagnosing, treating, and keeping their liver disease under control, hoping to hold off cirrhosis and subsequent failure. If cirrhosis does develop, then I take on the role of patient advocate where I present my patient's case to the liver transplant committee and try to convince them of "my" patient's qualification for a life-saving transplantation. If approved and my patient receives a successful transplant, my "near death" patient will usually have a miraculous turnaround and often will experience a fairly healthy life.

One of my young patients had severe primary sclerosing cholangitis (narrowing of ducts that drain the liver). Her pain was so severe that it required large doses of narcotics. In the early days of transplantation, patients needed to accumulate enough points to qualify for a transplant. Hospitalizing a patient for an extended period of time was an effective but expensive way to accumulate points, but in those days doctors had more latitude, and I kept my patient hospitalized for more than six months until she finally received her transplant. She did well and a few years later gave birth to a healthy baby boy.

Another case involved a young African female refugee in her 20s with hepatitis B and D who then developed liver cancer. She refused even to discuss the possibility of liver transplant despite the need to have it done before her liver cancer grew too large. After exhaustive efforts she acquiesced and agreed to the transplant. Since her window of opportunity was closing, I sent her to Louisiana to obtain a fairly speedy and successful transplant. She later apologized for giving me such a hard time and was grateful that I didn't give up on her.

Being an advocate for my patients has helped me better understand Christ's role as our advocate before God. Christ willingly took on our human nature to undergo trials, temptations, and even death so that He could take on the role as advocate for us. Even though we are sinners deserving of death, He is able to plead our case so that we can spend eternity with Him. That's even more amazing than a liver transplant!

Nathan Kam, LLUSM class of 1983, is a retired Northern California Kaiser gastroenterologist who is now scoping at Kaiser in Hawaii. His wife, Serena, graduated from LLUSN class of 1982; their son, Chris, is a hospital chaplain; and their daughter, Kelli Kam (LLUSM class of 2017), completed her internal medicine residency at LLUH in June 2021. Her career plans include working as a hospitalist at MC Wisconsin.

February 21

> *"Whatever you do, work at it with all your heart, as working for the Lord, not for human masters."*
> **Colossians 3:23, NIV**

A few weeks after finishing my internal medicine residency, I am finally taking some time to reflect on the journey. I still have days that I cannot fully fathom that I am done with that stage of my life. As many say, the days are long, but the years fly by. There were moments when it seemed it would never end, but when I look back at it all, it seems to have gone by incredibly fast. I have had the privilege to interact with many patients and families, many of whom will remain in my memory for the rest of my career. I saw sadness and death; joy and life renewed. I cannot erase from my mind the vivid memory of the patient that coded right in front of my eyes as we were preparing to place a central line in him. I can still hear the screams of his daughter as she yelled, "That's my dad! Do something!" and we did everything in our power to resuscitate him but were unable to. It was in moments like this that I would feel utterly helpless—when I would have to turn to the family, having nothing more to offer than my sincerest condolences.

Then there were days when patients would be blessed with new life. I remember the young man that we diagnosed with severe pneumonia whom we did not think we would be able to extubate. He had no family or friends that would come to visit him, and we became his family throughout those weeks in the ICU. I hoped and prayed for a miracle, and a few months later he walked out of the hospital.

I saw how easy it was to start feeling calloused and jaded. After a while you start protecting yourself from the emotional pain that watching patients and their families suffer takes on you. It is even more difficult when they look to you for an answer and you have nothing to give them.

I have gained an incredible amount of medical knowledge during my training. But the greatest lessons I leave with is not the medicine. I realize that it can be challenging dealing with all the uncertainties that face a physician. However, sometimes patients don't need you to have all the answers—they just need to know you care. It is an honor to be able to serve as God's hands and feet in this incredible ministry, and my prayer is that as partners with Christ, all those around us may see and feel His love and compassion for them.

Adegbemisola Daniyan, LLUSM class of 2015, is currently working as an assistant professor of medical education at California University of Science and Medicine in Colton, California. She completed an internal medicine residency at Kaiser Permanente Los Angeles Medical Center, which was followed by a fellowship in community medicine at Kaiser Permanente Fontana. She is grateful for the opportunity to continue to grow in her walk with God and for the many lessons learned on the journey of becoming a physician. Her interests include wellness for all levels of medical education training and beyond, as well as attempting to address the many health disparities in the community.

February 22

> *"And what does the LORD require of you? To act justly and to love mercy and to walk humbly with your God."*
> Micah 6:8, NIV

Believe it or not, this is the Bible verse that brought my husband and me together. It was listed on his online dating profile, and it had become a sort of life motto for me. He was a public urban educator in Koreatown Los Angeles for more than a decade, and I was a therapist and an aspiring academic researching the effects of power on gender, race, ethnicity, and spirituality. Together we have spent time personally and professionally wrestling with what justice, mercy, and humility look like in relationship, ministry/work, and in our cultural context.

From my lens as a relational therapist, I can't help seeing justice, mercy, and humility as relational realities. My guess is that the Lord requires this of us because we are inclined to engage in ways, consciously or unconsciously, that are unjust, unmerciful, and lacking in humility. As a Taiwanese American woman, it is not hard to recall the countless experiences I've had with racism and other types of microaggressions ("Where are you from? Your English is so good!"; "You're Taiwanese? I love Thai food!"). It is easy to feel mistreated, minimized, invisible—that these experiences are unjust. It is much harder to come to grips with the ways that I might do the same to others—unknowingly, unintentionally. With my privilege (having a high level of education, U.S. citizenship, being cisgender, heterosexual, able-bodied, and Christian) there have been countless times that I have unknowingly spoken or acted in ways that have harmed others.

A previous institution at which I worked had a large population of deaf students. Each semester I had at least one deaf student in my class. As a hearing person, I had never considered my hearing privilege and the ways that I engaged in audism (believing that hearing people are superior to deaf people) and the ways I could perpetuate this as a professor with students. I learned how to work with interpreters, captioned the videos shown in class, tried my best to make sure other classmates included their deaf peers in group work, and took a beginning level American Sign Language class. Without this sort of effort, the learning experience would not be as equitable for all students, deaf and hearing alike. There were many instances in which I made mistakes and offended students along the way, but was blessed with deeper connection with and understanding of my deaf students and colleagues. It required much mercy (compassion and forgiveness) and humility extended to others and to myself.

When we talk about -isms/phobias (racism, sexism, homophobia, xenophobia, etc.), there is often much emotional energy, discomfort, guilt, or shame. It is hard to move toward addressing these sociocultural issues of justice when it's uncomfortable. It takes the hard work of humbling ourselves, extending mercy to engage in justice work. It is so much more difficult to do than say, but I can understand why God requires all three of these together.

Jessica ChenFeng, PhD, LMFT, is an associate director of physician vitality at LLUH. Growing up in Los Angeles in a Taiwanese immigrant family and in the Asian American Christian church has shaped her research and clinical work around sociocontextual issues, such as gender, race, generation, and spirituality. She loves New York in the fall, Seattle in the summer, baking sourdough bread, sewing clothes, and lightly sweetened jasmine milk tea.

February 23

"Yet those who wait for the Lord *will gain new strength; they will mount up with wings like eagles, they will run and not get tired, they will walk and not become weary."* Isaiah 40:31, NASB

The first of two bells to roll call had just sounded. Fourteen-year-old Gordon Riffel moved toward the lineup place where the Japanese guards had piled up their weapons and were doing their morning calisthenics. He heard the roar of an airplane and looked up. The word "rescue" was clearly written on the fuselage. Suddenly, as he scanned the sky, he could make out the shapes of opening parachutes. As gunshots rang out, Gordon raced back to hide in the barracks that had been the Riffel "home" for the past 14 months. Unbeknown to him, the previous night Filipino guerrillas and American soldiers had infiltrated the camp parameter, and, upon the signal of the paratroopers jumping, they began shooting the guards.

Gordon, his parents, and two sisters had been American prisoners of the Japanese for the past 33 months, being moved from camp to camp and finally taken to Los Banos, where more than 2,100 prisoners of war were interred. Word of an imminent massacre of these POWs reached the Allied forces, and a daring rescue was quickly planned and accelerated when it became known that the Japanese had already dug an enormous ditch and set up a machine gun at one end. Another camp had just been liberated, and the Japanese were determined that they would wipe out Los Banos before the Americans could arrive. As the first liberating GI strode into Gordon's barracks, yelling for everyone to get out and get down to the beach, my dad's first thought was *big, fat, and juicy*, because the young soldier looked so healthy, and Gordon was so hungry. The Japanese had been systematically starving and killing their captives, with victims dying daily. Miraculously, God had provided a chicken that laid a daily egg for Gordon's family for several months without ever cackling. This additional protein was the difference between life and death, and was just one of many miracles they experienced.

This dramatic and daring rescue was successful beyond even the most optimistic scenarios. Providentially, not one of the POWs was killed in the rescue, which necessitated a double trip across the Bay of Manilla by huge amphibian tanks. The rescue took six hours and has been heralded by General Colin Powell as "the textbook airborne operation for all ages and all armies."

A major source of encouragement was Psalm 91, which Gordon and his family memorized and repeated often, living for rescue. Once back in the States, Dad and his sisters caught up quickly with their schoolwork, and eventually all three graduated from LLUH, with the girls becoming nurses (Retta Snider, LLUSN class of 1953, and Dorothy Huff, LLUSN class of 1954) and my dad becoming a physician. After a two-year stint in the U.S. Army, Dad accepted a call to the "mission field" of Missouri and spent the next 39 years in solo general practice. He delivered more than 3,000 babies, reattached digits, casted countless broken bones, taught physicians how to do surgery, and made numerous house calls. His patients could always count on him to pray with them and point them to Jesus, who is his refuge, strength, and ultimate rescuer.

Krista Woodruff, LLUSN MS class of 1977, RN, is the daughter of Gordon W. Riffel (CME class of 1955). February 23, 1945, was the rescue date from the Los Banos Japanese prison camp in the Philippines. Krista is the wife of Roger D. Woodruff (LLUSM class of 1981) and the mother of three: Michael K. D. Woodruff (LLUSM class of 2018), Brianna L. Woodruff (LLUSAHP Masters of Occupational Therapy class of 2015), and Jonathan.

February 24

*"For the word of God is alive and active. Sharper than any double-edged sword,
it penetrates even to dividing soul and spirit, joints and marrow;
it judges the thoughts and attitudes of the heart."*

Hebrews 4:12, NIV

I walked into Bob's room on my post-op morning rounds with my resident. Bob was a 30-year-old who had severe juvenile diabetes that had never been well-controlled. He had recently had a leg amputated at the Jerry L. Pettis Memorial Veterans Medical Center and had been admitted to LLUMC in need of a second amputation, which we had done a couple days earlier. On this day his father was in the room, and I immediately realized he had been reading aloud to his son, who was already nearly blind from diabetic retinopathy. I was pleased to see that his post-op recovery was progressing well.

After completing the medical part of the encounter, I asked what they were reading. Bob's father told me that while his son was hospitalized at the VA, his regular nurse had begun discussions about his illness, how he was dealing with it, and whether or not he had any religious beliefs. She got them started listening to a popular radio preacher who offered a copy of the Bible with a commentary in exchange for a contribution to his ministry. They had done this. Not knowing any other place to begin, he had started at Genesis 1, reading aloud to his son for several hours each day. They were already up to Joshua—in the King James Version.

I immediately asked if they would like to have a more modern translation, one easier to read and understand. I gave them a copy of the New International Version the next day, along with a suggested reading plan starting with the Gospels of Mark and John, and then reading about the early church in the book of Acts and then on through the rest of the New Testament.

Bob was transferred to the medical service soon thereafter, and I didn't see him again for several months. During that subsequent encounter, Bob's father told me that they had continued regular Scripture reading and that as a result, both had made a personal commitment of faith in Jesus Christ. Bob's parents had been divorced for years. His mother suffered from severe rheumatoid arthritis and had been living in Florida. Bob and his father both had recognized Christ's call to love and serve and had invited her to come back to California to live with them. She had done so and had also been led by their example into a life of faith in Christ.

I haven't seen or heard from them since. I'm very much looking forward to my next encounter with Bob and his father, as well as meeting his mother for the first time.

The Word of God is sharper than a surgeon's scalpel (Hebrews 4:12)!

William P. Bunnell is a professor and former chair of LLUSM's department of orthopedic surgery.

February 25

*"When pain is to be born, a little courage helps more than much knowledge,
a little human sympathy more than much courage,
and the least tincture of the love of God more than all."*
C. S. Lewis (1898–1963): British writer and lay theologian

One major lesson I learned from being a medical student is never to underestimate our influence. In the first week of my third-year rotation, one patient I met gave me the privilege to see her vulnerability. She was being treated for a diabetic foot ulcer that slowly festered into life-threatening osteomyelitis. After multiple trips to the operating room for debridement of the infection, the team of physicians I worked with said that an amputation was necessary. Unfortunately, no matter what the treatment team said, she adamantly refused an amputation. As trust began to break down between her and the team, I witnessed her initial friendly attitude sour into anger. Days turned to weeks as her physical and emotional condition worsened.

One day after work I decided to take extra time to visit her, and simply listen to whatever she had to say. When I arrived, she solemnly shared that she had agreed to an amputation a few minutes before I had entered. During the conversation I realized the cross that she had been carrying on her heart. One month prior, her husband had passed away. She had been so preoccupied with her hospital stay that she hadn't been able to process or talk about her loss. Not only was she suffering physically, she was also grieving the fresh loss of her husband. No matter how much pain relief medication was given to her, nothing could alleviate her emotional suffering. She burst into tears, grieving the loss of her limb and husband. At that moment I felt moved to offer a prayer. She accepted. I praised God for providing me the opportunity to meet and listen to her inspirational story, and asked Him to empower her with even more courage to face her trials. Then before leaving, I extended a hug. Later I realized that in an environment in which the majority of physical touch is for an objective physical examination, a hug transforms a sick patient back into a person.

When I saw her the day after her amputation, her transformation was like night and day. She thanked me and introduced me to her family, explaining what I had done and prayed for a few days ago. "This is going to be my testimony to God," she exclaimed.

Throughout life countless people have questioned, "Why?" Why did they get sick? Why do they suffer? No matter how much medical knowledge and experience I gain in this lifetime, I will never be able to provide an absolute, satisfying answer. However, I think I have discovered why it hurts so much.

Suffering and death were never intended by this world's Creator. When God made humans, we were meant to experience peace, love, and growth—not loss or death. This world has been distorted so much that unnatural suffering is now seen as natural. However, we are not helpless. We have a God who can turn our darkest moments into strength and use His children in unsuspecting, powerful ways.

Respectfully submitted anonymously by a LLUSM student.

February 26

> *"I was taught that the way of progress is neither swift nor easy."*
> Marie Curie (1867–1934): Polish-French physicist and chemist and
> only Nobel Prize Laureate to win in two scientific fields

Donald B. McCormick, PhD, was a fear-inducing figure. Chair of Emory University's biochemistry department, he held in his hands the fate of the future careers of all of us first-year graduate students. His qualifications were monumental. With more than 300 peer-reviewed publications, and the winner of the National Westinghouse Science Talent Search in 1950, he was one of the world's experts on vitamin B_6 metabolism.

I was one of those graduate students, and vividly remember being in awe of Prof. McCormick as my cohort. We began working our way through the classes and laboratory experiences that would eventually lead to our PhD degrees. One memory is of myself and my friend Wendy, both graduates of Southern Missionary College (now Southern Adventist University) in Tennessee, standing in Prof. McCormick's office while he stated, "I believe training women is a waste of time, because they will decide to get married and have children and leave science. However, because I am required to, I will train you, and I will train you well." Indeed, about 50 percent of PhD students in the biomedical sciences nationwide do leave before completion of their degrees, either by their own choice or that of their programs, and Emory was pretty close to the national norm. Furthermore, national data proves that many of those who do complete the degree drop out of the pipeline before establishing their own laboratories. Was McCormick correct? Was training us a waste of time?

Fast-forward about 15 years. I have my PhD, discovering and publishing on the first enzyme that "proofreads" the process by which ubiquitination tags proteins for degradation, and am now an assistant professor at Georgia State University. I am about halfway through the seven years that are so critical for promotion and tenure, after which I will either become an associate professor or lose my job. And I have a secret: I'm pregnant.

I am shopping for just the right dress in which to give my progress report seminar. At this seminar all those involved in the decision as to whether or not I am good enough to make associate professor will be attending, critically listening to what I present, and deciding if I have been sufficiently productive. I am concerned because I know that my paper production has been less than desired. I didn't work on Friday nights or Sabbaths, and I had to leave before 6:00 p.m. each day to pick up my 4-year-old.

The dress had to be just right. A good color for my skin tone, probably a V-neck, and—this was most critical—a loose fit overall, with an undefined waistline and a pattern that would distract from my overall profile. I carried at the forefront of my mind the stories I had been told by other women, including the woman whose dean (also a woman) had removed her from tenure track the moment she revealed that she was pregnant. Certainly, any woman who would choose to have a child (let alone two!) was insufficiently dedicated to science and should be removed from the competition sooner rather than later.

I found a dress I liked, and the seminar went well. As it turned out, most of my female colleagues had already guessed my secret (you know, that glow) but none of the men had. I did end up earning the promotion, though it was a close call, and the process was full of anguish. I am now the proud mother of two awesome adult children, Joe and Lorelei, and am blessed to serve as a professor and associate dean in the Loma Linda University School of Medicine, where I search for better ways to treat cancer, and try to figure out why some people can live such long and healthy lives.

Thank you, Prof. McCormick, for training me well, and no, it was not a waste of your time.

Penelope Duerksen-Hughes, PhD, is a professor and chair in LLUSM's department of basic sciences and translational research. She enjoys learning about the world, figuring things out, and finding ways to make things work better. She and her husband, James, have two adult children.

February 27

"Unless I see the nail marks in his hands and put my finger where the nails were, and put my hand into his side, I will not believe."
John 20:25, NIV

The MRI was black and white, a grayscale. White matter, gray matter, globular structures scrolled on my computer screen. Diffusion-restriction, laminar necrosis, basal ganglia-thalamic injury . . . and bilateral subdural hemorrhage, acute on chronic—pathognomonic: nonaccidental trauma. This is a brain beaten, asphyxiated.

On rounds, when I look through the sliding-glass doors into her room in the pediatric intensive care unit, I see a light on her head: unwashed hair, sheen of sweat on her forehead, metallic staples transecting what was once her hairline.

Her hands are dystonic and tremulous, clenching bedsheets as if grasping for something she lost—or someone who can help her reach and find what she cannot see. Up close, I see her lips quiver undecipherable vibrations, as if reverberating something now distant and past.

Purple, blue scalp; yellow, brown scabs; red, abrased skin—her flesh and blood surprise me. She is not a brain but a child. Three years old. Not pathology but life that's changed. A story snuffed out, a bruised reed drying. Cracked lips trapped in infancy. And skin that feels like my daughter's skin, soft cheeks, a nose, a mouth, a chin.

There is disease, and then there is child abuse. Heads broken in by human hands, childhood aborted by ruthless power wielded against innocent persons. Breaking faces, bodies tumbling down the stairs, skin scalded by boiling water, belt marks on their backs, contusions impregnated deep inside their bones until they lose the will to cry.

Terror and tenderness face me facing her. Should I hold her hand for just a second longer? Will she find me with her fading eyes? Can I ever look away? Or can I stay—here where it all intersects, desperately caring, helplessly present, daring and defeated, praying in a quiet whisper, "My Lord and my God!"

Young-Min Kim is an assistant professor in LLUSM's department of pediatrics who joined the faculty in 2016. An alumnus of Washington University, he completed his residency in pediatrics and neurology at St. Louis Children's Hospital, Barnes Jewish Hospital, and Washington University in St. Louis. He is the father of three children.

February 28

> *"Love . . . your neighbor as yourself."*
> Luke 10:27, NKJV

"Love your neighbor as yourself."

It is hard to argue with that advice. It is also hard to argue that the world would not be a markedly better place if our neighbors all followed that advice.

Of course, there are a lot of ways to be loving. Such words as kindness, generosity, patience, empathy, and compassion come to mind. Given a chance, we probably treat our neighbors that way most days.

It might have been an easier admonition to accomplish had the story, recorded by Dr. Luke nearly 2,000 years ago (Luke 10:28-37), ended there. But a lawyer asked a clarifying question: "Who is my neighbor?" (Luke 10:29, NKJV). Jesus' response in the parable of the good Samaritan is certainly familiar to us all.

The dramatic story includes a crime, an assault, life-threatening injuries, and acts of indifference and disdain. It concludes with brave and generous acts of neighborly love.

And that neighborly love is described in terms that are not only very specific, but also very relevant to us today. Your neighbor is anyone who needs your help. Recognize your biases, both conscious and unconscious. Love responds, even if the time or place may not be convenient. Love reacts to injustice. Love reaches across racial and ethnic divides. Love takes risks. Love requires no reward. Love leverages your resources. And love restores health and saves lives.

We might reasonably imagine that we could be nearly as loving as the hero in that story. In the same circumstances, we too might be willing to act and to sacrifice. But are we willing to apply those lessons to our everyday personal and professional lives? Can we love in that way most days, or even every day?

For those of us in the medical professions, the story sets a particularly high standard. Not only did the Samaritan provide the emergency care and the emergency transportation; he paid the retail rate for the acute and post-acute care that the traumatized traveler required.

And even if we are consistently willing to come to the aid of the obviously traumatized, are we committed to look for and help those whose trauma is much less obvious? Are we committed to do our very best to understand and prevent the trauma in the first place?

Stated another way, do our neighbors include those who don't enjoy the advantages of a good education or a good job? Do our neighbors include those who suffer the mental and physical health impact of adverse childhood experiences? Do our neighbors include those who are trafficked? Do our neighbors include those who experience health inequities? Do our neighbors include those who are victims of injustice? Do our neighbors include those who suffer from systemic racism?

The parable suggests that the answer should be an unequivocal yes.

Together let's commit to make our homes, our workplaces, our schools, our places of worship, and our communities places that love like that. Places where love shows. Places where neighbors that need the most love get the most love.

Let's be committed to love our neighbors—all of our neighbors—as ourselves.

Loren Hamel, LLUSM class of 1980-A, MHSA, is president of Spectrum Health Lakeland in Michigan. He has served as a family physician, university professor, and vice president of medical affairs. He is most proud of his role in instilling a culture of love and respect at Lakeland Health and in setting aside a multimillion-dollar endowment fund to address health equity. Loren is married to Ann Hamel, PhD, DMin. They share seven children and nine grandchildren.

MARCH

⌘ MERCY ☙

"I would like to share with you two simple truths: there is nothing that cannot be forgiven and there is no one undeserving of forgiveness. When you can see and understand that we are all bound to one another—whether by birth, by circumstance, or simply by our shared humanity—then you will know this to be true."

DESMOND TUTU (1931–)
South African Anglican cleric, Nobel Peace Prize Laureate, theologian, and anti-apartheid and human rights activist

March 1

"But Jesus bent down and started to write on the ground with his finger. When they kept on questioning him, he straightened up and said to them, 'Let any one of you who is without sin be the first to throw a stone at her.' Again he stooped down and wrote on the ground. At this, those who heard began to go away one at a time, the older ones first, until only Jesus was left, with the woman still standing there."
John 8:6-9, NIV

I often wonder what Jesus wrote on the ground that so deeply affected each of the accusers of the woman taken in adultery. How did He target so many people with so little writing? Did He just write the sins down and let the accusers pick out their own guilt? Did He write each accuser's name and then his sin for all to behold? I wonder....

Or did He write down names—names of people who were hurt by the action or inaction of an accuser, beginning with the highest-ranking priest and then down the line? He would not even have to write the name of the accuser, just the name of the injured soul and, perhaps, the accuser's offense. Adultery? False accusations that led to condemnation? Robbery of a poor widow in the name of religion?

Someday Jesus will have a list of names for each of us. Each of our lists may show the names of those who suffered our actions or inactions, be it to an individual, a class, or a race. Perhaps you would recognize many of the names and your offenses against them. But the verb "would" allows a conditional alternative: We would not find the names of the maimed, because the nearer we let Jesus draw us to Him, the fewer names, if any, remain to be written. He forgives our sins and tells us, "Go and sin no more" (John 8:11, NKJV).

However, Jesus will still have names on our list, the names of those that we helped bring closer to Him by feeding the hungry, by relieving the thirsty (particularly with the bread and living water of life), by clothing the naked, and by visiting the sick. Our educational system, our churches, and our view of Jesus need to grow sheep rather than goats, sheep with blessings rather than sins next to the names on their lists.

Jeff Cao, LLUSM class of 1971, is a professor in LLUSM's department of pathology and human anatomy. He was LLUSM teacher of the year in 1991, 1999, and 2007. He received the Distinguished Academic Award from the LLUH President's office in May 2020 (publicly awarded in May 2021 due to the COVID pandemic). He has had the honor of serving as a pathologist and as the director of the human systemic pathology course at LLUH since 1977. He now works half-time as medical director of four of the outlying clinical laboratories of LLUH and assists the new pathology course director, Cody Carter (LLUSM class of 2013), who "is doing a great job running the course and participating in the development of the new, integrated curriculum."

March 2

> *"Brothers and sisters, we do not want you to be uninformed about those who sleep in death, so that you do not grieve like the rest of mankind, who have no hope."*
> 1 Thessalonians 4:13, NIV

They're going to text a picture from the top to me!" I excitedly told my friend at work on Tuesday as we talked about my husband, Jim, and daughter, Whitney, as they were hiking up Mount Whitney that day. I had left them at Lone Pine Sunday evening, and Monday morning they called as they were driving to the base, telling me it was a beautiful sunny day.

On Tuesday evening I began to receive horrifying texts from Jim, which had been sent earlier in the day but were unable to be transmitted until he had returned to town. Whitney had died peacefully in her sleep during the night at Outpost Camp. Jim was incapacitated by grief, sorrow, and guilt, and as I made my sad journey to meet him, our dear friends Jan and John (LLUSM class of 1986) Sturges flew down from Coeur d'Alene, Idaho, to support us. Our lives were devastated, never to be the same.

During my long and painful journey of grief I have learned a few things about life, death, and the events in between. First, life is fragile and precious. It is a gift from God of an unknown number of years. It may be 18, like Whitney's, or 105, like my grandmother's. During those years, we the living need to make the most of this gift, to live in honor and memory of those who did not have the gift of a long life.

Second, after a tragedy, life goes on whether you want it to or not, but God will sustain you through your grief and pain. He and His envoys, who may include people you don't even know, will overwhelm you with love and support. As I was waiting at the Lone Pine Airport for the helicopter to bring Whitney's body down, I began to receive texts and emails from people who had heard the terrible news, and I remember being strangely comforted by these electronic expressions of support. As time went on, letters, flowers, and cards poured in, some from perfect strangers. These heartfelt messages came from people who understood and sympathized with our pain. I have kept and treasured them to this day.

Third, there is more to life than the days we have on this planet. Thankfully, we can look forward to an infinitely better world than we can ever imagine (Revelation 21:1-4). Jim and I have purchased cemetery plots adjacent to Whitney's, and there are some days when I want to go there and take my rest alongside her, to escape the pain of her loss. But there are more days I am reminded of God's many gifts and guidance in our lives. His blessings are abundant, although we cannot always choose the details or timing. We are not privy to the plans He has for us (Jeremiah 29:11), nor do we always understand His ways or thoughts (Isaiah 55:8-9), but we can be confident in the promise of His coming, when we will be reunited with our loved ones for eternity (1 Thessalonians 4:13-18).

Marilene Wang, LLUSM class of 1986, is a professor of head and neck surgery at UCLA. She and her husband, James Watson (LLUSM class of 1986), have been blessed to have two daughters, WayAnne Watson (LLUSM class of 2020) and Whitney (March 2, 1997–December 15, 2015).

March 3

> *"Dear Friend, I pray that you may enjoy good health and that all may go well with you, even as your soul is getting along well."*
> 3 John 2, NIV

I want you to remember the tagline: Thrive 3J2. Why? Because it pleads for you to have good health, as well as an encouragement to experience a peaceful "whole person" life.

The dictionary defines "thrive" as "to prosper" (to grow vigorously) or how to live (to progress toward or realize a goal despite or because of circumstances).

As health care providers we want our patients to, well . . . "thrive" in the sense of enjoying good health with a prosperous life. But as LLUH's motto asserts that we are here "To make man whole," the second part of 3J2 includes the fact that an authentic "whole person care" provider is interested in her/his patient's soul. Thus, just as the definition of health includes more than absence of disease, the definition of "thrive" [3J2] includes more than good health.

To many the word "shalom" means peace. However, just as the broader definition of "thrive" means more than good health, shalom means more than "peace." Shalom embodies having complete peace—a feeling of contentment, completeness, wholeness, well-being, and harmony (the absence of agitation or discord).

Proverbs 18:21, NIV, tells us that "the tongue has the power of life and death." So if we tell one of our patients at the end of a clinic visit that we want them to "thrive," or if we tell them "shalom," we are imparting a blessing: for him/her to have prosperous health as well as your desire for their soul to experience complete peace ("contentment").

But health care workers personally need to "thrive" and to personally experience "shalom." Too many health care staff today are frazzled and feel their life is similar to a hamster on a never-ending cycle of work that never gets them anywhere. More than 50 percent of health care workers are experiencing burnout. Too often we fail to take time for self-care to help us "thrive" in the face of poorly designed work systems that overburden us working in often fragmented, inefficient settings. The answer may lie in the expression "Physician, care for yourself." A functional corollary to "thrive" for health care professionals is "joy." Joy is more than the absence of burnout. It is the result of an intellectual, behavioral, and emotional commitment to a meaningful and satisfying life of service to others.

So, remember Thrive 3J2, as well as "shalom." Why? Because in order for us to accomplish our task as health care professionals to help our patients "thrive," as well as for us to live a life of complete peace.

Dwight C. Evans, LLUSM class of 1973-B, is an associate professor of medicine/endocrinology in LLUSM. He recently completed 16 years as the CMO at Veterans Affairs Loma Linda Healthcare System. He is an "honorary" associate director of the General Conference of Seventh-day Adventists Health Ministries Department, participating in consulting (during the past 27 years) on quality improvement implementation in 10 divisions. His wife, Helen Staples Evans, is the senior vice president for patient care at LLUMC. Their son, Jonathan, is a 2019 LLUSM graduate and an internal medicine resident at the University of California, Irvine.

March 4

> *"Whatever work you do, do it with all your heart.*
> *Do it for the Lord and not for men."*
> Colossians 3:23, NLV

Today's political and social climates have brought racial tensions to an all-time high. While racism has never truly gone away, for some, it has been easier to ignore, as they were not being confronted with it on a daily basis. People often point to America's progress and use the election of a Black president as evidence that "we" as a whole were doing better, for how could racism exist when the face of our country proved otherwise. What seems to be almost every day now, the news reports that yet another Black life has been cut short prematurely, only adding to the ever growing list of people who have become household names. As these stories come more into the spotlight, it becomes increasingly clear that Black people are often undervalued simply because of the color of their skin.

Racial injustices and microaggressions seep into every aspect of society, including medicine. Unconscious biases are stereotypes or judgments formed about groups of people, usually negative, that influence an individual's behavior and may be opposite to consciously stated values. There are countless examples that Black physicians face on a daily basis both from patients and co-workers. It can seem as minute as being called by another Black colleague's name when you two look nothing alike. It can manifest as being called by your first name even after introducing yourself as the doctor because you are young and female, while, in the same breath, the white male in the room is addressed as doctor. Black female physicians are often called everything from nurse to care partner to respiratory therapist, because it has not even crossed the individual's mind that a young Black female could possibly be the doctor, capable of providing care to the patient in front of her. There needs to be intentional, recurring dialogues about unconscious biases and microaggressions within medicine in order to eradicate these injustices and create a culture where everyone is valued.

Nevertheless, pursuing medicine has been one of the greatest blessings of my life. The privilege of taking care of a person and his/her family during one of the worst moments of their lives is unmatched. Throughout the journey, I felt as if I were one of the few Black faces stepping into unfamiliar waters, and if I just slipped up or failed once, I would ruin the chances of others behind me with the same dream. I had imposter syndrome, comparing myself to classmates and coresidents, sometimes feeling as though I did not measure up, despite doing well. I kept waiting for someone to see right through me and announce that I did not belong.

Throughout all of this, God always provides a light in the darkness. During moments that I may be frustrated, He sends me encounters that rejuvenate me and remind me of His calling in my life. I have had numerous experiences in which I am greeted with smiles and excitement for a doctor that "looks like us." It is an honor, but it should not be a surprise or shock to see a minority provider; it should be commonplace.

Despite whatever difficult encounters I may face, I strive to do everything to the best of my ability, as though it were unto God, for that is what I am called to do.

Victoria Magloire, LLUSM class of 2018, completed her pediatrics residency at Monroe Carell Jr. Children's Hospital at Vanderbilt in Nashville. She is in a pediatric emergency medicine fellowship at Norton Children's Hospital in Louisville, Kentucky. She has a passion for global health and increasing minority representation in medicine.

March 5

"Nothing but grace makes a man so humble and, at the same time, so glad."
Charles Spurgeon (1834–1892): *English Baptist preacher, author, and philanthropist*

It was an evening in the emergency department sometime in the early 1990s, a time when I still developed some anxiety when seeing a patient whose sexual identity was "different." This was especially so, as in this case, when the patient's anatomy belied the stated sexual identity. Even though the designation LGBTQ+ did not exist then, at least to my awareness, it was my practiced habit to take extra time and effort when encountering patients who so identified themselves.

Before leaving the workstation to see this particular patient, the nurse shared the patient's female sexual identity with me. The name was feminine, and I took a moment to fix my mind toward the use of feminine pronouns such as "she" and "her" to help the anticipated interaction be respectfully appropriate. The chief complaint was testicular pain.

In the exam room all seemed to go well. Through the history and physical there was not a glitch. Correct introductions were used, and a friendly acceptance seemed present from both of us. When the exam ended, and I pulled up the sheet and blanket before sitting down to speak, physician/patient rapport seemed good enough to anticipate a high patient satisfaction score. Most important, I hoped to provide competent care with empathy.

Whether it was the usual pressing backlog of patients to see or just my unfortunate relaxation into habitual routine will never be fully clear to me, but as I took off my exam gloves and reached for the stool on which to sit, and then explain the diagnosis and recommendations, the words "well, guy" slipped from my lips. What an error! The room seemed still, and time moved slowly, as our eyes locked in a gaze of surprise and pregnant emotion. My thoughts reeled with questions and frustration regarding my error and what I feared would be a patient encounter that would rapidly deteriorate. A quick apology did not seem adequate. I felt that patient respect and empathy seemed to have vanished. What happened next shocked me, and to this day still causes me to smile.

Without seeming to miss a beat, my patient's eyes left mine, and looking down toward her just-examined and painful scrotum, she said, "That's an honest mistake," and smiled! I took my first breath since finishing the exam. Time began moving again. My apology could now be spoken. And I realized I had experienced grace from the most unlikely source.

When my best intentions had run amuck, my patient reminded me of my Savior. Christ did not ever categorize people or decide to be respectful to some but not others. Many years later I am still grateful because one patient reminded me of God's wonderful grace.

William R. Shawler, LLUSM class of 1973-B, is mostly retired after 44 years in emergency medicine. He has enough time to hike, bicycle, and wade waters for fly fishing, but is not fully retired, because it is so wonderful to be a physician and try to help people. He is married with three children, seven grandchildren, and one nearly perfect Labrador retriever.

March 6

"Be anxious for nothing, but in everything by prayer and supplication, with thanksgiving, let your requests be made known to God; and the peace of God, which surpasses all understanding, will guard your hearts and minds through Christ Jesus."
Philippians 4:6-7, NKJV

My husband, Reggie, is an avid golfer. He plays, reads, watches and talks golf. January 24, 2017, found Reggie at Torrey Pines, San Diego, watching a golf tournament. He had a successful and enjoyable day, but having walked excessively, he returned to his motel exhausted. The next morning, feeling no better, he proceeded home. He realized he was thirsty, and pulled off the freeway at an *ampm* store. With his drink in hand, he pulled up at the stop sign before entering the freeway on-ramp. The next thing he remembers is waking up in an ambulance heading for Palomar Hospital.

When our son, Brandon, and I arrived, we pieced the story together. Reggie had had a cardiac arrest at the stop sign. Some wonderful "good Samaritans" noticed him. Unable to open the car door, one broke the right back door window, climbed in, turned off the ignition, and unbuckled the seat belt. Reggie was pulled out of the car and laid on the ground, where a nurse did chest compressions. Miraculously, the fire station was across the street, so paramedics arrived soon after.

We tried to contact the two "good Samaritans" through the CHP, but were unsuccessful. We returned and had a moving experience thanking the paramedics, and found out that they don't usually have people return and thank them. At the *ampm* store we asked if they remembered the event. Yes, they did, and the person who broke the window was working over the freeway. We were surprised to find, not an ex-EMT, as we had been told, but a homeless, Black man who lived in his truck.

In December of 2017 Reggie again had a cardiac arrest while greeting at church.

In February 2018 Reggie had his third cardiac arrest at home. Statistically surviving three cardiac arrests outside a hospital setting is one in a thousand. The decision was made to have a LVAD, or left ventricular assist device, placed. Once the decision was made, we were at peace. Staff and friends shared prayers, comfort, and best wishes. Reggie voiced, "Whatever happens, it will be OK." On the morning of the surgery Brandon and I went to the hospital to accompany Reggie to the OR. His surgeon personally came and prayed with us; preoperative staff prayed. We were bathed in prayer and felt that "peace which surpasses all understanding."

The nine-hour operation went well, and his recovery was uneventful. Now six months later, if you ask Reggie how he is, he will say, "Better than wonderful." We are so grateful for the wonderful LLUMC staff, whose exceptional care has made this journey successful. Psalm 9:1, NIV, means so much more to us now. It says, "I will give thanks to you, Lord, with all my heart; I will tell of all your wonderful deeds." And so we do. Every. Single. Day.

Janette Whittaker-Allen was born in New Zealand. She received her nursing education at Sydney Adventist Hospital, and later completed a cardiothoracic course at the Royal North Shore Hospital in Sydney. After working with LLUH's overseas heart surgery team in Saigon, Vietnam, in 1974, she immigrated to the U.S., where she worked for more than 40 years in LLUMC's cardiac services, including serving as a heart transplant coordinator. She is now retired. March 6, 2018, was the date Reggie received his lifesaving LVAD implant at LLUMC. He carries a battery pack 24/7.

March 7

> *"I will give them a heart to know that I am the LORD, and they shall be my people and I will be their God, for they shall return to me with their whole heart."*
> Jeremiah 24:7, ESV

Tapita woke up from her sleep in the mud hut in the remote village in Malawi, Africa. Everything was so quiet. The grown-ups had gone to prepare the maizefields and her mother had left to get water at the river and firewood. Oh! She was so hungry. Her stomach was rumbling. There had been so little mielie meal (maize porridge) for the family last evening—so many mouths to feed, so many family members.

The last maize crop had been poor because of lack of rain. Her parents had not had the strength to extend their garden either, and the soil was not yielding as before. She moved around. On a rock next to the neighbor's hut she saw a few bread leftovers. Wow! She was so lucky. That would ease some of her hunger pains until her mother came back and was able to cook. Suddenly her father appeared. He had been visiting some men in one of the huts farther away. They would drink and play games while the women did the hard work.

"Where did you find the bread?" he angrily asked. Tapita was 6 years old. She had to learn the difference between right and wrong. Her father had never heard of Jesus or God. He knew only the gods that appeared in the trees, the rocks, the sun, and in the thunder and lightning.

When Tapita arrived at the hospital and I met her, her father had carried her through the jungle in rough terrain for four hours. Both of her hands were severely swollen; burned, double the size of the hands of a 6-year-old. She was supposed to learn not to steal from others—her dad had wrapped rags on both hands, dipped them in paraffin, and used his matches.

We worked for weeks treating her burns and moved every little finger to prevent contractures. We were hoping to be able to send her home with hands that could work in spite of scars. Her father stayed by her side during the day and slept under her bed at night. During hospital worship times and Sabbath School, both father and Tapita learned to love Jesus. He experienced forgiveness and gained understanding, through love from God, how to bring up his precious little girl. He thanked Malamulo Hospital staff for showing Jesus to his little girl and to him. They returned home healed, filled with God's love in their hearts.

Bjørg Irene Harvey Hellsten is a retired nurse anesthetist and former hospital director of nurses. She was born in Norway and currently resides there. She has served in Nigeria, Malawi, Botswana, and Lesotho between 1969 and 1990. She has one son and three lovely grandchildren living in the USA.

March 8

"My chains are gone; I've been set free. My God, my Savior has ransomed me."
"Amazing Grace (My Chains are Gone)," Chris Tomlin (1972–):
American Christian singer and songwriter

I was working the night shift at the county hospital. It is there we take care of prisoners as well as individuals from the community. In one specific section in the hospital prisoners come in and out from the emergency department. I picked up the chart and walked to one of those rooms, where the guard let me in.

There lying in the hospital bed was a man in an orange jumpsuit. His hands and feet were chained together, and he looked extremely nervous. I introduced myself and began asking him about the issues he was facing that day. He started to tell me about his back pain. His anxiety was palpable, and I could clearly discern his discomfort from the way his voice quivered and his eyes darted back and forth.

I decided to pause my medical evaluation for a moment, and instead asked him why he seemed so worried. He began to share his story. He told me that two weeks earlier he had been arrested for a DUI. Not only was he drunk, but he hit someone while he was drunk. My patient began to shake as he spoke. I put my hand on his shoulder and began to ask him more about how he felt. He expressed his deep fear to me. Most notably, he kept on repeating, "I just want to be forgiven! I just want to be forgiven! I really messed up! I just want to be forgiven!"

As our conversation continued, I asked whom he wanted to be forgiven by. I asked if he desired forgiveness from the person he hurt. He was clear: He desired not only their forgiveness but forgiveness from God!

There was a heavy burden on his heart. I asked him about his faith background, and he told me that he was a Catholic. I began to talk to him about Jesus. I shared with him that Christ promises us complete forgiveness from all of our faults and mistakes if we only ask. "You can be forgiven today," I said, but when I asked him if he believed me, I could tell he was on the fence.

He was still engaged, so I offered to share an analogy with him. "Just as your hands and feet are chained," I said, "your heart is chained and burdened by the weight of your mistake. But God promises that He can break those chains and set your heart free. Do you want God to break the chains that are on your heart? He may not break the physical chains you have on you, but he can set your heart free. Today. Right now." He began to weep and said yes. So I prayed with him, and he accepted the forgiveness of Christ into his heart.

Many of us are like this prisoner: Our hearts are burdened and chained. Maybe it's because of the mistakes we've made toward others or maybe because of the mistakes others have made toward us. But just as God broke the chains on his heart and set him free, God can break the chains on your heart too!

Matt Dalley, LLUSM class of 2019, is currently an emergency medicine resident at LLUH. Matt has a passion for spreading the love of Christ both in the hospital and in his everyday life. He can often be found preaching for local churches and having Bible studies with his friends. In his spare time he enjoys soccer and surfing.

March 9

"Therefore be imitators of God, as beloved children."
Ephesians 5:1, ESV

I never realized how sweet the innocent inclination of a child to imitate was until I had one of my own. Less than four weeks after giving birth to our miracle baby girl on March 9, I developed a facial paralysis that left me with a half smile. Workup of the paralysis revealed that some time before becoming pregnant, I'd suffered a potentially life-threatening brain bleed. Miraculously, my body had formed a protective AV fistula. During and after delivery, blood flow to my facial nerve was compromised, leading to paralysis. In the midst of having a newborn and during the COVID-19 pandemic I had to be hospitalized and undergo urgent cerebral vascular coiling. Throughout this experience I was filled with a multitude of emotions. My eating, drinking, and speaking was impaired. I felt that any picture of me with my newborn would be "flawed" because of this half smile. Yet I also felt an overwhelming sense of peace seeing God's protection throughout it all.

Only 12 days later, on April 12, 2020, shortly after my husband, our 4-week-old daughter, and I had fallen asleep, our house in Chattanooga, Tennessee, was hit by a tornado. We quickly took shelter as our bedroom windows shattered. While we hid in the closet and the storm was passing, I held my daughter close. I watched her peacefully sleep and again felt a similar peace I'd felt just a few weeks prior. A feeling that everything would be OK—that God's hand was protecting us.

The next few months were full of chaos. But more important, they were humbling. They were filled with an outpouring of love and generosity from those around us. We were constantly reminded of how blessed and fortunate we truly were, despite the recent events. We had each other, we had our safety, and we had our miracle baby. A child we had longed for, prayed for, and were finally blessed with after a long journey of infertility. She is truly a miracle, and her imitating skills remind us even more so of our many blessings.

This sweet daughter of ours has learned to imitate my half smile. She has learned a smile that is a mirror image of my paralyzed smile. And while I was initially devastated about having this half smile, seeing my daughter's imitation of it is a constant reminder of our many blessings and how the Lord has protected us over the past few months. It's a reminder of the peace He provided us when we needed it most. A peace that only He could give.

Ashley Evans Fedusenko, LLUSM class of 2016, is currently a hospice and palliative medicine fellow at Wellstar Kennestone Regional Medical Center in Marietta, Georgia. She recently completed a family medicine residency at Erlanger Hospital in Chattanooga, Tennessee, her childhood home. Her husband, James, graduated in LLUSD's class of 2016. Prior to medical and dental school, she and James were both registered nurses.

March 10

"I can do all things through him who strengthens me."
Philippians 4:13, ESV

In the spring of 2012 my family and I were enjoying a ski vacation. My twin daughters, Francine and Melanie, who were 7 at the time, and my son, Joshua, who was 5, were all enrolled in ski lessons one day. My wife and I were skiing together. Francine, our best skier out of the three, had been up and down the slopes throughout the day with her group.

In the late afternoon the weather had turned cold, and it had started snowing. A few minutes before it was time to pick up the kids from ski school, my wife received a call on her phone. She went pale, stood up, and quickly walked toward the ski patrol. "Francine fell off the chair lift; she's in the first aid station downstairs!" As we entered first aid, I asked the ski patrol clerk where our daughter was. He pointed to the ambulance outside. I asked him if he knew how far she had fallen. He said, "Thirty feet." Fear immediately set in.

Francine was in the ambulance with a c-collar on, her right wrist in a cardboard splint. I kept on asking her: "Are you all right? Are you in pain?" She would respond by saying, "I'm fine, Dad." But she seemed to be so quiet and was wanting to sleep as we rode to the local hospital.

As we entered the ER, I felt sick. The fear of the future set in as the ER doctor evaluated my daughter. He said that she appeared to have no neurological deficits, but had a closed, deformed right wrist fracture that would need to be reduced. He was ordering a pan-CT scan.

As we transported my daughter to CT, I began to panic. Francine was somnolent and seemed in shock. As the CT tech helped me put on a heavy apron, I prayed to God to give me the strength to look as if I were not afraid and to have dry, calm eyes. As they positioned her, I held her hand and told Francine that I loved her. She managed to smile as I began to feel an assurance. I then prayed with Francine, "God, we know in the Bible that it says that even when a sparrow falls, you know. God, we know You are here with both of us. Please watch over Francine; heal her, and help her not to be in pain. Amen." As I ended the prayer, I sent a silent prayer: *Please let Francine live.*

"The radiologist is at the control panel looking at your daughter's scan," said the technician as we transferred her onto the gurney. I introduced myself as he started reading her scan out loud: "No C-SPINE injury, small pneumothorax, small pulmonary contusion, grade 1 splenic rupture. Left kidney laceration. No free abdominal fluid. Nondisplaced left pelvic fracture. No thoracic or lumbar spine injury." I looked at the radiologist and said, "Thank God!" How could anyone fall from that height and still be alive or have no neurological injuries? My anxiety and fear turned to thankfulness.

Francine spent five days in the hospital. She had no hematuria, and was able to walk after two days of bed rest. Two liters of O_2 was reduced to room air; IV morphine was stopped and PO ibuprofen started. With a new toy panda in her arms and a promise of a puppy when we got home, we made the drive back home. She stayed home from school for one week, but was eager to get back to school. She was right-hand dominant prior to the fall. However, with a cast on, she started writing with her left hand. To this day she writes with her left hand—the only thing that changed with Francine!

When the stresses of work and life—sick patients, difficult schedules, and family challenges—become overwhelming, I always stop and think about that day. My outlook on life changed completely the day she fell. I had experienced intense fear and panic, which was replaced by a calm that God gave me. "I can do all things through him who strengthens me." All we need to do is pray. Oh, by the way, we named the puppy Bo!

Matthew Ho, LLUSM class of 1996, is a Kaiser Permanente emergency room physician. His wife, Candice Ho (LLUSM class of 1999), is a pediatrician at UCLA. They live in Los Angeles with their three children.

March 11

> *"Home is not where we live; home is where we belong."*
> African proverb

There's something special about home, or at least a healthy home. Home gives us a place where we feel accepted, where we are allowed to be who we are. A place where we feel a sense of belonging. But sometimes the place we call home can be devoid of that feeling of belonging. Especially when the focus is on differences rather than similarities. Let's discuss one of the things that differentiates us.

The way we speak is shaped by so many different factors . . . how and whom we learn the language from. Some of us learn from our parents, others from teachers, or friends, and some even learn from watching TV. The environment in which we practice using the language also shapes how we ultimately speak a language.

I have experienced and observed an unconscious bias against people who speak with an accent, at least what we deem to be an unacceptable accent. In reality, every single person speaks with an accent. And I mean everyone. But society has chosen to classify some accents as "acceptable" while others are "unacceptable." I call this accent bias.

The body language, the reactions, and the treatment of someone who speaks with a different intonation than ours, as they speak and share, sends a certain message. It comes across that just because a person says certain words or phrases differently from the "acceptable" intonation, they don't know what they are talking about. Therefore, they must not be as intelligent. Or the surprised "You're so articulate!"

Trust me, I understand the need to communicate and to understand what is being said. Remember though, that communication is a two-way process. There's the listening end, too. Listening without judgment. Listening to understand, not to find fault. Remember that when you speak, the other person is also having to adjust their listening process to hear you, because you too have an accent to them. Communication is easier when we all speak the same language, in exactly the same way. But it's not by accident that we all speak differently! That's not the way God designed it, and I believe it was on purpose! God created us all in unique ways, with different tongues to add color and flavor to this world. One way to overcome this bias, which may be counter to how some approach this, is to spend more time speaking to or listening to persons who speak differently from you. Let us become aware of our unconscious reactions to others who speak differently than we do. Let us embrace our differences and appreciate our differences and uniqueness. Life would be colorless without them.

Emily Ndlela, MBA, CPA, currently serves as assistant vice president for financial planning and analysis for LLUH, and has been with the organization for more than 10 years. She volunteers with Adventist Health International, and is dedicated to assisting Adventist mission hospitals improve their financial and business operations. Her hobbies include traveling and singing. Emily and her husband, Andy, are blessed with two daughters, Nandi, 13, and Nia, 10.

March 12

"Not only so, but we also glory in our sufferings, because we know that suffering produces perseverance; perseverance, character; and character, hope. And hope does not put us to shame, because God's love has been poured out into our hearts through the Holy Spirit, who has been given to us."

Romans 5:3-5, NIV

I didn't really want to die," he said. Mr. A had been seen in our resident clinic earlier that afternoon for a checkup on his heart. He had been sent to our ED by my coresident after he expressed thoughts concerning suicidal ideation. In the ED he had been cleared by the psychiatric nurse but was admitted to our family medicine service for a CHF exacerbation.

He explained that just a few years ago he had been a personal trainer at Gold's Gym. His congestive heart failure had worsened to the point where he could no longer walk three steps without feeling short of breath. Eventually he could no longer work his job, resulting in an inability to pay his rent. He ended up living under the 210 freeway in Sylmar and would take five buses to get to his appointments at our clinic.

"Me and God are good now. We're better than we've ever been." Mr. A recounted a story from a few years prior in which his car had spun off a narrow mountain road. He thought he was going to die, but somehow his car landed in the boughs of a tree, sparing him. That event had renewed his faith.

I was struck by the sincerity and confidence in his voice as he spoke these words. I was also reminded of a sermon Tim Keller of Redeemer Presbyterian Church preached. In it he emphasized that poor individuals are our brothers and sisters and that they understand the gospel better than we do because Jesus is all they have.

After I let Mr. A know how his faith had encouraged me, we each said a prayer for his health and for those providing health care for him. Before I left, I told him cardiology would see him in the morning to optimize his CHF meds.

As I returned to the hallways with my coresident, I felt a sense of thankfulness for the opportunity to meet this man at the intersection of mind, body, and soul. And in the twilight haze of the night shift I felt a confirmation that I was where I was supposed to be.

Cameron M. Lee, LLUSM class of 2016, completed his family medicine residency at Adventist Health Glendale in California in June 2020. Currently he practices family medicine in Long Beach, California. He enjoys hiking with his wife, playing with his nephew, and getting free samples at Costco.

March 13

"How long, LORD? Will you hide yourself forever?
How long will your wrath burn like fire?"
Psalm 89:46, NIV

Manaus, capital of Amazonas, was one of the first cities in Brazil to experience the complete collapse of its health systems and funeral services during the COVID-19 pandemic. On March 13, 2020, the first case in the city was confirmed. Then "suddenly, no, more than suddenly," "the close friend became a distant one."* When the city's hubs became potentially lethal, a crowd of people found themselves abruptly separated from their families, friends, daily routine, jobs, leisure, churches, sports, parties, and celebrations. Everything stopped. And all fell silent. As a pathologist and researcher at the referral center for serious cases of COVID-19, my job is to perform autopsies on patients authorized by their family members, to help answer what the world asks: How do these patients die?

Day by day a battalion of people moved in hospitals, without stopping, in a struggle that was without respite. It was heartbreaking to see the desperation in the eyes of doctors, social workers, nurses, and many other professionals as they witnessed the lonely death of the victims, the private mourning of family members, and the isolation of everyone. Meanwhile, the question "How long, my God?" resonated in my mind whenever I had to talk to countless families after their loved ones had been examined in the autopsy room.

Jesus experienced lonely and distressing hours in Gethsemane, in which He enlisted the support of His companions (Matthew 26:37-38). There Jesus reminds us once again of the need to turn to God the Father in times of distress. Even Jesus suffered as He faced the foreshadowing moments of death. Therefore, we sinners must take Him as an example: Humbly in the face of pain we submit to the Father's will (Matthew 26:39), so that we can be comforted by Him. The Christian is not free from suffering, and the Scriptures testify that during dark times, God does not abandon us, but consoles us (Psalm 23:4) and sends His angels for this purpose (Luke 22:43).

In these bleak moments of the pandemic in Manaus, God could be seen: in the families' resilient mourning, in the invisible and supportive hands that moved in favor of the needy, in the courage of those who worked to keep everyone with enough supplies to keep the efforts going, and in the tireless eyes and bodies of the teams that acted in the uninterrupted care for patients.

Regarding those who died, the hope of a reunion remains in eternity, in which "there will be no more death or mourning or crying or pain" (Revelation 21:4, NIV). In it death will have no victory over us anymore, for God grants it through Jesus Christ (1 Corinthians 15:55-57). For us, the first rays of the new dawns remain, cautious but better, and confident in the many mansions prepared by Him to receive us (John 14:1-3).

*Vinícius de Moraes, "Sonnet of Separation."

Monique Freire Santana was born and raised in Manaus, Amazonas (Brazil), in a family of brave and special women. She graduated with a medical degree in 2013 from the State University of Amazonas. A pathologist since 2018, she was mentored by two great and dear teachers who inspired her in her chosen profession and took her on a Christian walk through the Seventh-day Adventist Church. The verse in Ecclesiastes 9:10, NIV, inspires her daily in her work and her missionary service: "Whatever your hand finds to do, do it with all your might, for in the realm of the dead, where you are going, there is neither working nor planning."

March 14

> *"Fear not: for I have redeemed thee, I have called thee by thy name; thou art mine."*
> Isaiah 43:1, KJV

I took a deep breath before entering the room. "Breathe in grace," I told myself. This short meditation had become a practical reminder and regular practice as I walked the children's hospital units during my summer session of Clinical Pastoral Education (CPE). The meditation sprang from a desire to be more intentional with my spiritual experience.

Inside the room I was about to enter was a 5-month-old patient and his mother. Although the patient was oblivious to my coming and going, his mother valued support from all sources. What could I say to make a difference for this woman?

I posed this question to my CPE director. Her response was to the point: "Be the answer. Your influence at the bedside depends more on who you are than what you say. Be peace. Be comfort and hope. God's grace is always enough, and He always surrounds you. Just breathe Him in."

I stood outside the door and felt my chest expand. I breathed in grace. I slowly exhaled. Be peace—immersed in grace. I knocked and entered. As I had come to expect during the past three weeks, Rebecca, the mother, was sitting in her chair coloring. She was working on a series of African savannah animals for baby Erik's wall at home. Erik was hooked up to more equipment than any 5-month-old should ever have to endure. The prognosis following his first surgery was hopeful. I could see his tiny, repaired heart beating beneath the clear bandage that covered his chest. I could feel my heart beating. Breathe.

I carried my guitar. "May I share a song?" Rebecca nodded and smiled. The song on my mind was one that had resonated with my recent devotional journey. Soon the lyrics of "He Knows My Name" filled the room. "I have a Maker; He formed my Heart. Before even time began, my life was in His hands...."

There was so much hope for the future in that room. There was so much fear of an uncertain future in that room. Even though the surgeons felt good about the initial surgery, little Erik's prognosis was uncertain. Both Rebecca's and my faces were wet with tears. We breathed.

Rebecca showed me the progress on the savannah set. My personal favorites were the baby animals. Hers were the cats with their elegance and grace. She wasn't looking for answers to life's big questions that afternoon. Outside the hospital she was surrounded by people who loved and supported her. She had poured herself into her newborn's life and was at peace that everything that could be done would be done.

I continued to breathe; assured of this reality...

"He knows my name. He knows my every thought. He sees each tear that falls and He hears me when I call."

Steve McHan was born during his father's (James) senior year at CME (class of 1958). He currently works as a patient relations specialist at LLUMC. He and his wife love sharing fruit they pick from their home orchard. Tragically, the baby in this story did not survive, in spite of the heroic efforts by our medical and nursing staff, and the unwavering hope of the parents. The family's peace in the midst of grief still encourages the author.

March 15

"The LORD is my shepherd, I lack nothing. He makes me lie down in green pastures, he leads me beside quiet waters, he refreshes my soul. . . . Even though I walk through the darkest valley, I will fear no evil, for you are with me."
Psalm 23:1-4, NIV

On March 15, 2018, the evening before Match Day, my wife and I were surprised to find out we were expecting. About a month later during our first ultrasound, we were even more surprised to learn we would be having identical twins! The pregnancy was high-risk because the babies were sharing a placenta, so we had frequent appointments with both OB and MFM (maternal fetal medicine). Our friends and family were praying for us from the very beginning, and we felt such peace about everything. Upon moving to Kettering, Ohio, for residency in June, we had more frequent appointments. Our girls were growing well, and everything was going great.

Then, on July 19, at just 23 weeks and 2 days gestation, our girls were born. In a matter of one week following our last MFM appointment the girls had developed twin to twin transfusion syndrome. Twin A was no longer getting the nutrients and fluids she needed, while Twin B was getting nearly everything for both of them. Our firstborn, Georgia Ray, was stillborn. Twin B, Lyston Rose, was crying and alert when she was born at only 1 pound 2 ounces and 12 inches long. She required immediate intubation and was rushed to the NICU. Our hearts were completely broken, and we were so afraid. Our family and friends lifted us up to our Father in prayer and we were placed in God's loving embrace. The local church, which we had been able to attend only once since moving, also covered us in prayer and gave such caring support. We cannot convey the importance of those prayers, and it is impossible to say how much they meant to us. We felt the power of each request that was made on our behalf and we received the strength we needed to be there for Lyston. The next hours and days were indescribably difficult. We were overcome with such sorrow at the loss of our sweet Georgia, even as we were filled with an indescribable peace and hope for Lyston. The countless prayers spoken on behalf of our family are the only possible explanation for how any of us made it through that time. As we walked through this "valley of the shadow of death" we were comforted by our Savior and looked forward, with faith, to the green pastures and beautiful still waters that we knew only He could bring us to. God's people prayed, and He answered.

Continued on March 16 . . .

Raymond Krause, LLUSM class of 2018, completed his intern year at Kettering Medical Center in Kettering, Ohio. In November 2018 LLUSM dean Roger Hadley (LLUSM class of 1974), while visiting Kettering, presented the Krauses with silver baby cups for each of their twins, with the names of the girls engraved on them. Gifting medical students with silver baby cups is a tradition to celebrate babies born to medical students during medical school and acknowledge those who are pregnant at graduation. Raymond is now a resident in radiology at Shands Hospital in Gainesville, Florida.

March 16

"We have courage in God's presence, because we are sure that he hears us if we ask him for anything that is according to his will."
1 John 5:14, GNT

Continued from March 15 . . .

On her third day of life our premature daughter, Lyston, developed bacteremia and septic shock. Her blood pressure began to drop, her white blood cell count was nonexistent, and her lungs weakened dramatically. She was started on two antibiotics and two blood pressure medicines. Lyston was fighting hard, but by that night it did not seem possible that she would survive. She was placed on an oscillating ventilator (the most aggressive kind), and there was talk of adding a third blood pressure medication. The neonatologist knocked on our hospital room door at 3:00 a.m. to talk to us about Lyston's declining condition and at what point we might move to "comfort care." We decided, with the doctor, to continue helping Lyston fight for the next 24 hours, giving the antibiotics enough time to take effect before reevaluating. All night long we cried out to God to be with Lyston and to heal her if that was His will. We prayed for the "big picture," wanting our dear girl to have life more than anything, but wanting it to be a full life. Our family and friends prayed with us, and called on their friends and families to do the same. Truly, all around the world, prayer warriors lifted Lyston up to her heavenly Father, asking for healing for our little fighter.

The next morning we walked into the NICU as prepared as we could be to hold our precious girl for the first and possibly the last time. When we entered her room, we immediately noticed that the settings on the ventilator were less intense and the third blood pressure medicines had never been needed! Renewed hope sprung up in us as we held Lyston's tiny hands, willing every ounce of strength and love in our bodies into hers. Though we barely dared to hope, our hearts overflowed with thankfulness. By that night, almost exactly 24 hours after being started on the antibiotics, Lyston had done a complete 360 and was moved back to a conventional ventilator. Her white blood cell count, though still extremely low, was countable, and the process of weaning her blood pressure medicines had begun. We cried tears of joy and thanksgiving.

Never have we experienced the power of prayer as we did in those 24 hours. We cannot possibly identify the number of miracles that took place during that time; every decision made, touch given, and loving word spoken was divinely directed because of the prayers offered up by God's people around the world.

We could tell many stories from our 148-day NICU stay, and the common thread in each would be the power of prayer. Our worldwide church family supported us in prayer every tedious, critical step of the way, and today we have a thriving, beautiful, miracle child in our home. Her life is a testament to her heavenly Father; to His loving heart, healing hand, gracious spirit, and above all, to the power of prayer and the promise that "if we ask anything according to His will, He hears us."

Marianne Krause is a stay-at-home-mom to Lyston Rose and Matthew Carl. Her husband, Raymond, graduated from LLUSM in 2018. Raymond and Marianne met in second grade, went to school together through college at Southern Adventist University in Tennessee, and were married in 2012.

March 17

> *"But as for you, you meant evil against me; but God meant it for good."*
> Genesis 50:20, NKJV

Our perception determines how we act on God's calls to us as well as how others view our call. Eventually some perceptions about the same call clash.

From the time I was a child growing up in Trinidad, West Indies, I knew that I would someday become a graduate of CME (now LLUH). A full appreciation of what it would take escaped me for years, including the perception of race relations. When I was 19, a white man kicked me. Thinking it best to kill him to prevent repetition of his dastardly act, I considered what that would take. God stepped in: *Is this what you want?*

"No."

Then drop the hammer.

I did. Then on my first day in the USA in 1957, a young white server in Alabama refused to serve me at the restaurant counter. "Go to the back." She was simply doing her job, oblivious of my noble dreams. The earlier lesson in restraint held, but the event took my appetite away and opened my eyes to the broader realities of life.

Academic institutions were also caught up in the prevailing racial practices. Even the stellar educational goals of SDA schools appeared to be affected. I remember reading somewhere that "not many Blacks were applying to Loma Linda." Reasons were omitted. However, the possibilities of quotas, and the rumors that a Black student was held back every year affected my perception. Yet I applied.

In 1961 I was one of the first two graduates of Oakwood College in Alabama to be accepted to LLUSM. Yet I had to repeat my first year. Again, perception and reality clashed.

As a psychiatrist I have personally witnessed wonderful results of discovering how to understand ourselves and taking time to understand others. Yet my own perceptions and feelings about Loma Linda remained painful. So when invited to share my story with Oakwood students in 2019, I shuddered. I blurted sarcastically, "Who cares?" My answer shocked the inviter. Yet I went.

Just before going on stage, I introduced myself to a stranger. It turned out to be Hansel Fletcher, the LLUH recruiter on campus for the occasion. He listened to brief examples of my traumatic experiences and some of the long-harbored ill feelings. Although God had been abundantly blessing me along the way, my internal perspective persisted. "I was just a guinea pig," I told him.

He responded, "Dr. Broomes, things have changed in 58 years. You are a pioneer." With those words my perception shifted immediately. So did my grasp of the demanding administrative process required to prepare practitioners "To make man whole." Trailblazing meant sacrifices. My speech to those Oakwood students? Redemptive.

My readiness to listen to the Holy Spirit, the brief providential chat, and the standing ovation by the students that day soothed my long-carried aches. God used all of it to refine my character and mature my perception.

Lloyd Rudy Broomes, LLUSM class of 1966, is a former automobile mechanic. He is a retired psychiatrist and distinguished life fellow in the American Psychiatric Association. He is married to Lauvenia Emelia (née Alleyne), RN. God blessed their union with two daughters, one a psychiatrist and the other an attorney.

March 18

Match Day, 2022

> *"'Not by might nor by power, but by My Spirit,' says the LORD of hosts."*
> Zechariah 4:6, NKJV

I felt the blood drain from my face and my heart start pounding as I read the words on the computer screen. My thoughts were spinning. *This could not actually be happening.* I had been told I had nothing to worry about, but reality slowly started to sink in as I continued to reread the words "We are sorry; you did not match to any position."

The next few days were a blur. I knew God had led me to medical school at Loma Linda to fulfill my desire to be a missionary doctor. He had faithfully brought me through, but what was the purpose of this trial? I felt my faith failing as I let the fear of the unknown overwhelm me.

At the beginning of the school year I had scheduled an international elective at Sir Run Run Shaw Hospital in China after "The Match." It was supposed to be a time of celebration, but now it felt more like a punishment. Throughout the trip questions tumbled around in my head. I had applied to emergency medicine, but was that really what I wanted to do? Would it be the best specialty for mission work? Did I still even want to be a doctor?

Toward the end of my trip to China, I was walking through the hospital lobby when the sharp smell of tobacco smoke stung my nostrils. I had spent most of the morning feeling sorry for myself and this unwanted smell sent my mind into a bitter rant. "How can these people be so ignorant? Don't they know that smoking is bad for them? This is a hospital. Who would smoke—?" My discourse was cut short by a still, small voice, *If this bothers you so much, do something about it.* "What can I do, I don't even have a job?" I snapped back. *Loma Linda Family and Preventive Medicine combined program.* "Hold on, God; that program has only four spots, and I have done nothing in medical school that would make me a candidate. I would NEVER match there." There was no response, just a peace I had not felt in quite some time.

Back in Loma Linda, just days prior to the July 1 residency start date, I was accepted into Loma Linda's inaugural transitional year residency class, directed by Dr. Kevin Shannon. As I was preparing to start, I got a phone call from Dr. Shannon. He told me that the next year he would like me to be in the Family and Preventive Medicine combined residency program, of which he was also the program director. Tears instantly stung my eyes. God had a plan all along, and He showed me that it was not by my might or power that I got there, but His Spirit working in my life to place me where He wanted me to be.

Kelsey Cherepuschak, LLUSM class of 2015, completed her residency in family and preventive medicine in January 2020. She is a deferred mission appointee and plans to serve at Scheer Memorial Hospital in Nepal with her husband, Justin Hansen, and son, Levi. In the meantime, she is working part-time and caring for her son. Note: Match Day for all medical schools is the third Friday of March.

March 19

"Therefore, my beloved brethren, be steadfast, immovable, always abounding in the work of the Lord, knowing that your labor is not in vain in the Lord."
1 Corinthians 15:58, NKJV

It was a hot, humid day in Nigeria during the summer after first year of medical school, and we had no running water or electricity that morning. My boyfriend (now husband), Will, was scrubbed in to an orthopedic surgery where he was drilling screws into a man's broken leg, while I was in the next operating room over catching pus from a draining neck abscess. I remember the room was filled with the stench of that man who was dying of squamous cell carcinoma of the tongue because he hadn't brushed his teeth in months. He looked so emaciated. I also remember the bitterness and jealousy that was brewing within me as I thought about the "lame" surgery I was in when I could be drilling screws and practicing sutures, and how I felt frustrated at the fact that I had traveled all the way across the world to watch pus drain into a basin. I even remembered complaining to Will that afternoon about how I missed out on all the cool stuff.

The next morning during rounds, however, my same patient pointed at me with his frail fingers and called me to his bedside. He then scribbled on a piece of paper, "Thank you," and looked at me with tears in his eyes. Immediately I felt the Holy Spirit humble me in ways I had never before experienced, teaching me what it meant when Jesus Christ healed and loved the sick.

I'd like to say that the rest of the mission trip was filled with lifesaving procedures and fulfilling medical marvels, but it wasn't. I had only finished my first year of medical school and my limited biochemistry and physiology education wasn't saving anybody. I began to feel a little purposeless. Then one day Will and I were asked to help some local Nigerian students apply for scholarships to medical and nursing schools. We gladly took the opportunity to teach these young friends how to use a computer, practice typing skills, and write sponsor letters to raise funds for their education. None of it was medically related or even close to what we pictured we'd be doing on a medical mission.

Four years later, in May 2018, I received a message from one of the girls thanking Will and me for our help in seeking scholarships and letting us know that several of them had just graduated from their program. Again, I was immediately humbled at the thought that God was able to use my very limited abilities for His great glory and purpose, despite my lack of faith and complaining heart. He is able to multiply our small sacrifices in ways we could never imagine, so long as we offer them to Him.

Julia Angkadjaja, LLUSM class of 2017, completed her ophthalmology residency at LLUH in 2021 and now practices comprehensive ophthalmology at Kaiser Permanente in Redlands, California. She and classmate William Angkadjaja were married March 19, 2017, two days after the match. They had their first child in April 2020.

March 20

> *"There are different kinds of service, but the same Lord. There are different kinds of working, but in all of them and in everyone it is the same God at work."*
> 1 Corinthians 12:5-6, NIV

I'm the only one in my family who has gone to college. My fiancée just broke up with me because she said she would be humiliated to marry into a family of farmers, which we are." Matthew's posture portrayed utter defeat and deep shame. "I really don't belong here. My clerkship director said I should see you because I'm lacking confidence."

I frequently received referrals from faculty about medical trainees with the imposter syndrome. Matthew had it, but his breakup further stripped him of any sense of personal value.

"Tell me about your farm," I encouraged. "I grew up in the country too."

"Really?!" Matthew leaned forward and began to tell me about how he had grown up on land that had been in the family for four generations. They raised sheep, geese, and chickens, had an orchard, and grew alfalfa. He told me about sheep shearing, and how he and his brothers took turns tending to ewes for hours on end during lambing season. He talked about a threatening ram named Grandy, who chased anyone who didn't carry a broom or pitchfork for protection, and about Horace, the turkey, who daily threatened the mailman. Matthew had splinted up Horace's wing after he'd been hit by a car. "I slept with him in the kitchen for several nights. My mother had a fit!" he laughed. "That wing hung a little funny, but he lived a pretty decent life for another five years."

We talked about the connection between caring for farm animals and his childhood dreams to doctor people. We knew few other medical students who were as unflappable as he during OB clerkships since he had delivered hundreds of lambs. Matthew's work ethic was stellar: He was used to working 60-plus hours and managing responsibilities that involved life and death.

As we reframed the shame and "liability" of a farming background into strengths, we noticed that not everyone would appreciate his early context, but he was well on his way to becoming a physician who takes good care of patients. Thinking of physician-farmers I know, I said, "Part of you will always be comfortable on the farm. Part of you is becoming more comfortable in medicine. We're all products of where we come from, and embracing this helps us engage with patients in a more genuine way. God didn't make us all the same, and your patients will appreciate your kind of doctoring."

"Thanks, Barbara. I feel more hopeful." A pat on the back, and he was out the door.

I sat down at my desk, where a picture of Giovanni, my childhood pet rooster, stared back at me. My great-grandmother's brass school bell rests on a shelf next to framed diplomas and clinical licenses. *One part farmer, one part academic, one part provider,* I thought. The richness of our varied pasts give each of us something to contribute in the service of others. God indeed uses us all.

Barbara Couden Hernandez, PhD, LLUSBH class of 1992, LMFT, is professor of medical education and director of physician vitality at LLUSM. Barbara grew up in the rural Finger Lakes region of New York State.

March 21

> *"Be strong and courageous. Do not be afraid; do not be discouraged,
> for the LORD your God will be with you wherever you go."*
> Joshua 1:9, NIV

Calling. I typed various words for my medical school acceptance letter. I altruistically meant them. After reflecting during the past few days, I now know I didn't fully understand the meaning at that time. I still have so much to learn.

I've been contemplating my mortality and the direct relationship with this *"calling."* I know that the coronavirus is considerably more dangerous for those with chronic disease and as one ages. I also know emergency department, hospital, and first responder teams are on the absolute front lines. I hear that health care workers are three to five times more likely to contract the disease and 20 percent of U.S. admissions to the ICU are people aged 20 to 50.

Should I stay home? Absolutely not! I ride at dawn. *Calling.*

I contacted a wise physician friend and heard the following. "How could a health care clinician look a grocery store clerk, gas station employee, or a pharmacist in the eye if the professional wasn't willing to help themselves also?"

This is the moment. A crisis that hasn't happened for generations. Our Super Bowl. Our *calling.*

We put on our personal protective equipment. We wash our hands. We go virtual as much as possible. However, we will always be here in person to help our patients when they need us. It's our *calling.* We work to heal. Rich, poor, sick, guilty, innocent, worried . . . send them to us.

What would I do if I were 65 years of age? I can't be sure. But at this moment, in my mind, I'm resolute that this is my *calling.* Put me in and let me help as long as I can!

There are so many professions that take incredible risks far beyond what I experience. Thank you to each of them. Iron workers, soldiers, first responders, janitors, so much more. We don't thank you enough.

There are many who are sacrificing way more than I am. I'm so fortunate I have a job. An amazing job. My *calling.*

The risks to me are "low." Many people in our country have considerably higher obstacles. I'll stay at work to do what I can to help.

I'll stay at work, so please, if you can, stay at home.

Stay at home, but get connected with each other. Look for the good. Build one another up. Help each other. How can you contribute to the cause against this global pandemic? How do we come out of this a better people?

As a world we fight one common enemy. As a physician I'm all in. CALLING!

David Ward, LLUSM class of 2008, met the love of his life at LLUH: Sabrina (LLUSM class of 2008), a pediatric anesthesiologist. He relishes being a father, leader, and physician. He leads primary care operations for Kaiser Permanente in Washington while he lives his purpose: "to inspire optimal health."

March 22

> *"Pray one for another, that ye may be healed. The effectual fervent prayer of a righteous man availeth much."*
> James 5:16, KJV

The love and example of Christian parents is of inestimable value in conveying life values to children. As one of nine children born on the wide-open plains of North Dakota, my parents' example of hard work, economy, resourcefulness, caring, and prayer made a huge impression on my young mind. It was from observing my diligent, loving, humble, and sincere parents that I felt called to be a caregiver.

My path to health care began by completing my licensed practical nurse requirements and working in a hospital in order to be able to afford a college degree. Since several of my siblings had attended Union College in Lincoln, Nebraska, my course was set, and after four years of working hard to pay my way while going to college, I graduated with a bachelor's degree in nursing.

Over the course of several years, my nursing career led me to work in several different states, and each with increasing responsibility as I gained experience in the intensive and coronary care units. Little did I know that the care of critically ill patients would lead me to understand the power of prayer and the effect it has in the lives of our patients.

One of my patients in particular was comatose, which created unique circumstances in her care. It was during a 3:00 to 11:00 p.m. shift, and as was my custom, I enjoyed adding a little extra to a patient's experience by tucking them in with a back rub and if they wanted, would offer to pray. On this night my patient was still unresponsive, and though I wondered if it might be pointless, I decided to go ahead and pray for her. As I stood near her hospital bed I began to pray, and as I prayed, I again wondered if she could even hear me. I wondered why I was even doing this, but I finished my prayer and made sure she was comfortable and properly tucked in, then left her bedside.

Over the course of several days this woman recovered unusually well, and surprisingly, I saw her ambulating down the hall one day. She was doing great, so I approached her and told her how well she was doing and how thrilled I was for her recovery. She stopped and looked at me and said, "Your voice; I remember your voice! Weren't you the nurse who prayed with me one night when I was so sick?" I acknowledged that I had prayed with her. She thanked me for caring enough to take time to pray and that it had given her so much courage. I gave her a gentle squeeze and told her I was so glad that she had actually heard my prayer and that it had encouraged her in her recovery. I couldn't believe it! That experience reinforced to me that the power of prayer is beyond comprehension.

Caring for people involves more than just physical and mental healing. God provides spiritual blessings when we as humans might think otherwise!

Gladys Snyder Barnes, LLUSN MS class of 1982, is currently a per diem nurse in a PACU in Vancouver, Washington. This story occurred at Bryan Memorial Hospital in Lincoln, Nebraska.

March 23

> *"For this is what the Lord Almighty says: '... whoever touches you touches the apple of his eye.'"*
> Zechariah 2:8, NIV

It was 4:55 a.m., and I was running late. As I hurried from my car to the hospital, my scrubs threatening to fall to my ankles at any moment, a thought popped into my mind. It was a thought that I was ashamed of having but, because of my current circumstances, was simmering in my brain nonetheless.

Is God mad at me? Does God like me? Is God really my friend? Chances are you have had these questions pop into your mind as well. Promotions are given to someone else, a pipe in your home bursts during the winter, a car accident that was your fault, failing a year of medical school, a divorce, or a thousand other events. A seed of doubt is planted, and we selectively nourish this weed at the expense of the gratitude we know we should have.

Later that week I received some great news. God had heard my prayers for deliverance and had solved my problem in an unexpected way. *God really does care about me!* I said to myself. And then I realized I was acting like my 10- and 8-year-old children.

My kids tend to believe that their parents love them only when they get what they want. My wife spends much time washing, conditioning, detangling, drying, and combing my daughter's hair. To my daughter, however, that time is torture. She does not perceive this inconvenience as an act of love. Saying no to ice cream for dinner, making them practice the piano, telling them to clean up their rooms, have prompted my kids to doubt openly whether or not their parents love them.

I am the same way. My doubting God's love for me is a failure to see how difficulties, trials, and setbacks are shaping me into the husband, father, surgeon he wants me to be. God loves me regardless of what trials I am facing. In fact, His love is often manifested in the trials I face. *Ministry of Healing* shows the result of changing our perspective: "It is a law of nature that our thoughts and feelings are encouraged and strengthened as we give them utterance. While words express thoughts, it is also true that thoughts follow words. If we would give more expression to our faith, rejoice more in the blessings that we know we have—the great mercy and love of God—we should have more faith and greater joy. No tongue can express, no finite mind can conceive, the blessing that results from appreciating the goodness and love of God" (p. 251-253).

I hope your trials remind you that our heavenly Father wishes to see you face to face one day and tell you that you are His friend, His child, the apple of His eye.

Quince-Xhosa Gibson, LLUSM class of 2016, MBA, is currently a fifth-year general surgery resident at the University of Alabama at Birmingham Medical Center. He and his wife, Karen, have two children, Jaeden and Shiloh. March 23 is his wife's birthday.

March 24

"I am with you always, even to the end of the age."
Matthew 28:20, NKJV

Through the ICU window I witnessed my patient quietly dying. In front of my patient's face was an iPad with multiple windows of different family members expressing just how much they loved her. Her bedside nurse, fully gowned in personal protective equipment, was fighting back her own emotions as our patient slowly fell into an eternal slumber.

As a medical intensivist and being part of a dedicated team to take care of the most severe COVID-19 patients, I have witnessed firsthand the devastating effects of this virus and how it has changed our culture and the ability for loved ones to be at the bedside.

The sobering reminder of sin is our mortality, but we can find strength in our loving heavenly Father and His Son, who were both willing to pay the ultimate price so that we could look forward to never facing anything like this ever again. When confronted with health, financial, or life problems, the Bible reminds us that we should not be fearful because of the things in life, for God is with us. "So do not fear, for I am with you; do not be dismayed, for I am your God. I will strengthen you and help you; I will uphold you with my righteous right hand" (Isaiah 41:10, NIV). We shouldn't be discouraged, for He is our God. He will strengthen us and help us. He will uphold us in His victorious right hand. Peace in knowing that because Christ died, we as Christ's followers have something to look forward to. Such peace can be provided only by trusting in God. "Peace I leave with you; my peace I give you. I do not give to you as the world gives. Do not let your hearts be troubled and do not be afraid" (John 14:27, NIV). Ultimately, we can all take comfort that even when alive or with our very last breath, we are never alone.

Laren Tan, LLUSM class of 2009, is an assistant professor in LLUSM's department of medicine. He completed his internal medicine residency at LLUH in 2012 and finished his fellowship in pulmonary and critical care at the University of California, Davis. He returned to LLUH in 2015 and has since taken on various leadership roles. He is a seeker of laughter, learner of patience through fishing, running, and exercise, hobbyist, and a servant of Christ. He especially praises God for his beautiful and supportive wife, Heidi Choi (LLUSM class of 2009), and their three children.

March 25

"For you formed my inward parts; you knitted me together in my mother's womb. I praise you, for I am fearfully and wonderfully made."
Psalm 139:13-14, ESV

It was a brisk night in the early spring, and my wife, Brianna, and I were getting ready for bed. We were eagerly awaiting the birth of our second child, a girl to be named Adelyn, due in only three days. "Ugh, I feel like a whale!" Brianna muttered, turning off the light as I closed my eyes.

"Ryan. Ryan!" My eyes snapped open, and I looked over at the clock: 1:33 a.m.

"What is it?"

Brianna was sitting on the edge of the bed, holding her abdomen, appearing to be in discomfort. "Contractions. They're pretty strong. I think it's time!" She winced again.

"You're sure it's not just the burritos we ate?" I could hear her eyes rolling in the dark.

"I'm going to get ready to go to the hospital." I rolled over in bed. Our first child, a boy named Clarkston, had taken almost 12 hours of labor before arriving. There was time.

An hour later Brianna jostled me awake. "Ryan, I really think we should head over to the hospital. My contractions are coming closer together." I muttered something unintelligible and headed to the bathroom for a quick shower.

BANG! BANG! BANG! My stupor was interrupted by loud knocking on the bathroom door. My sister-in-law, visiting in anticipation of her niece's soon arrival, poked her head through the ajar bathroom door.

"Ryan, Brianna needs you downstairs!"

"Right now?" I tried to wipe some more sleep out of my eyes.

"Yes, NOW!" Something about her voice conveyed a sense of urgency. Then I heard a shout from downstairs.

"RYAN!"

I jumped out of the shower and grabbed a pair of pants, forgoing a towel. As I hurried downstairs, I could hear Brianna calling out in pain. "Ryan, I don't think we're making it to the hospital!"

I entered the small bathroom where Brianna had been putting on makeup. Breathing heavily, she was sitting on the toilet. I reached over to check.

"Don't touch me!" she yelled.

"Uhhh, honey, I kind of have to—there's a head coming out."

"What?"

Despite having performed my fair share of deliveries in medical school and residency, my hands were trembling. It's hard to describe what transpired next. It was the most beautiful and natural thing I've ever witnessed. With each contraction, Adelyn came closer to birth. I guided her rotation, checked for a nuchal cord, and with one final push, I was holding our baby girl.

She cried immediately, as did the rest of us. I handed her to Brianna, and Adelyn immediately began nursing. She was pink and healthy. Perfect.

On average, labor can take anywhere from eight to 12 hours. Brianna's short labor is called a precipitous delivery, occurring in less than three hours. I'm not sure if it was my instincts and training as a doctor, or if Someone else was guiding my hands, but things couldn't have gone more smoothly. What a blessing it has been to celebrate the birth of our daughter! God is so good!

Ryan Babienco, LLUSM class of 2015, currently practices emergency medicine in Dayton, Ohio. His wife, Brianna (LLUSN class of 2012), is an obstetrics nurse. Their daughter, Adelyn, was born March 25, 2018.

March 26

"The meaning of the Sabbath is to celebrate time rather than space. Six days a week we live under the tyranny of things of space; on the Sabbath we try to become attuned to holiness in time. It is a day on which we are called upon to share in what is eternal in time, to turn from the results of creation to the mystery of creation; from the world of creation to the creation of the world."
Abraham Heschel (1907–1972): Polish-born American rabbi
in The Sabbath: Its Meaning for Modern Man

Sabbath has been an important part of my weekly practice for many years. When I was accepted to attend medical school at Loma Linda, I knew that I would encounter circumstances in the hospital and clinical setting that would require me to consider anew how I understood and experienced Sabbath.

During the hustle and bustle of medical school, I had come to greatly appreciate Sabbath as being a day of rest, worship, and reconnecting. One Sabbath afternoon while on my psychiatry rotation, the resident on call texted me requesting that I come to the hospital to help with a patient. It was 3:00 p.m., and my wife, Andrea, and I were looking forward to attending a musical performance at La Sierra University in Riverside that evening. Needless to say, I was not excited about going to the hospital—after all, it was Sabbath.

When I arrived at the hospital, I was asked to see a patient who was having severe anxiety. I entered the room, introduced myself, and began my interview. I soon came to learn that there were many aspects of this patient's story that I could deeply relate to. The patient had recently undergone a liver transplant as a result of his past alcoholism and was now having severe anxiety because of the all-consuming guilt of what he had done to his family and his health. The time spent in the hospital had made him acutely aware of his failures.

After further conversation I came to learn that his deepest concern was that his children would never fully forgive him for failing to be the father that he should have been. His wife informed me that his children had forgiven him, but that he did not feel that he deserved their forgiveness. Her words rang in my ears. It was during my first couple years of medical school that my father had finally come to terms with his alcoholism, and we were currently working through these very same issues. Coincidentally, my father also felt he did not deserve my forgiveness, even though I freely offered it to him.

I shared with the patient a little bit of my experience of being a child of an alcoholic father, my anger and frustration with my father, and my struggle with forgiveness. I also told him about the pain and angst it caused me when, after working through many of these issues, my father did not believe that he could accept my forgiveness. I then asked my patient to please accept his children's forgiveness and not to deny them the opportunity of giving him that gift. It was a very stirring experience. At the conclusion of our visit my patient and his wife commented on how much our time together had meant to them.

After leaving the room, I took a little time to process what had just taken place. These feelings were all still very real and raw for me and talking about them was not easy. Amid the bustle of medical school, I often felt I did not have enough time to process my own emotions. I felt that my time with this patient was a gift, a space where I could talk with someone else in a similar situation about deeply personal issues, such as forgiving my father, while also offering encouragement to forgive.

I hope in the future I continue to remember the gift of Sabbath—time to process and heal.

Landon Sayler, LLUSM class of 2020, LLUSR MA Religion and Society 2019, was born and raised in central Alberta, Canada. He is now a family medicine resident at Dalhousie University in Halifax, Nova Scotia. He loves the outdoors, people, and exploring the complexities and peculiarities of life on this earth. He is married to his BFF, Andrea, and they are parents of a daughter.

March 27

> "He will bless and use in the advancement of His cause those who sincerely devote themselves and all they have to His glory."
>
> Ellen G. White (1827–1915): instrumental in the founding of Loma Linda University, one of the founders of the Seventh-day Adventist Church, and American author; in **Ministry of Healing**, p. 473

It has been commonly said that learning in medical school is like trying to drink from a fire hydrant: Complex information comes so fast, so quickly, that it can be overwhelming. As a medical student I learn the Krebs cycle, memorize the nerves of the brachial plexus, listen to the decrescendo murmur. I meet my patient, learn his story, examine his body from head to toe. I present his case, recommending the correct tests, but suggest the wrong treatments. I learn. I try. I fail. I try again. I need to know the answers, for the quiz, for the exam, for my patients.

Residency is hard, a time that shapes you, a time that truly teaches the knowledge, the skills, the art of being a physician. I am young, naive but responsible. The patient under my care is unwell, ill, unsure of this young doctor who is more afraid than she is. I learn. I grow. I develop my knowledge, my skills, my practice of medicine. My patients live; my patients thrive. I effectively and efficiently take a history, perform an exam, make a differential, devise a plan. I become confident, sure that I make a difference, confident that I know the answers my patients need, for both now and tomorrow.

I am now the attending physician. I am now the expert. There is no one listening to my patient presentations, no one reviewing my clinical notes, no one revising the orders I sign. My students look to me for knowledge, my residents ask me for guidance, my fellows think I have the answers. Frequently I do. Sometimes I don't. My patients live, my patients thrive, my patients suffer, my patients die. I study. I read. I practice. I learn. I research. I consult. And yet I do not always have the answer, do not always have the explanation, do not always know what comes next.

The practice of medicine is just that, and the art of medicine can be messy. The answer is rarely as clear cut as it appeared to be in medical school, and the expert's confidence is less certain than others may expect or hope. I have become conscious of my own insufficiency, cognizant of my own shortcomings, and all too aware of my limitations.

We are all less than what we were meant to be, in our careers, in our relationships, in our spiritual journeys. I am thankful that we have a Maker who understands the mystery, because He made it. I am thankful that we have a Teacher who knows the answer, because He created the question. And I am thankful that we are all patients of the greatest Physician, who not only cares and heals, but holds and cries with us as we live, as we thrive, as we suffer, and as we die.

Cody Chastain, LLUSM class of 2008, is an assistant professor of medicine, division of infectious diseases, department of medicine at Vanderbilt University Medical Center, Nashville, Tennessee. He and his wife, Jamie, were blessed with triplet sons (Evan, Ryan, and Jack) in 2010.

March 28

> *"Behold, I have engraved you on the palms of my hands;*
> *your walls are continually before me."*
> Isaiah 49:16, ESV

My flight had been long, coming from some international location, when I finally landed in Los Angeles. Calling home, I got no answer, despite Judy knowing my arrival time. That was strange, so I started calling others, only to discover the news. Our middle daughter, Briana, had gone into premature labor with her twins, and had delivered them at 26 weeks. I was told that they were now in a hospital in west Los Angeles and that I had better head directly there.

So a long saga began. Twin girls—2 pounds 5 ounces and 1 pound 14 ounces. With modern medical care they were immediately intubated to help their immature lungs, eyes were taped shut for protection, and life outside the womb began way too early. Cliff and Briana made the decision always to have one of them stay with the girls, now claiming the names of Emily and Abigail.

It is hard to really know someone you can only watch in an incubator, struggling for survival. Life limped from crisis to crisis, first one twin, then the other. Hope would build, then faith would be tried. Long nights were spent sleeping in the recliner by their incubators, worrying about the various beeps and sounds that could signal a turn for the worse.

During several months Emmy and Abby gradually gained strength and started having some awareness of their surroundings and visitors. My wife made frequent trips to west Los Angeles, caring for their older brother, Oliver. The day they came home, about the time they should have been born, was truly one of rejoicing and relief.

It was only three months later that Briana, while waiting for the doctor to come into the exam room, noticed that Emmy had an unusual shape to her abdomen. Things had been stable until now, but this was concerning. When the pediatrician palpated her abdomen, he found a lump on her liver. They were sent immediately to radiology where they confirmed the worst—some kind of tumor growing on her liver.

Within 24 hours a biopsy was done as we all sank back again into the world of wondering and praying. Why? How could anything else happen to this precious baby? And then the biopsy result confirmed our fears—hepatoblastoma, a unique liver cancer associated with low birth weight. The prognosis was not good, but there was hope. After resecting the tumor, a four-month protocol of chemotherapy was initiated, and the frequent doctor visits, needle sticks, blood counts, and concern about infections and side effects began.

Even at this young age, Emmy became stoical, accepting each blood draw without a whimper. As the months went by, the old routine of hope and fear, concern and faith, kicked in once again. The day finally came when the chemo was finished, and watchful waiting began. As each month, then each year, was added to her life, we all gradually relaxed.

It's been 20 years now, so Emmy is officially classified as a "survivor," and both she and Abby are sophomores in college. I never thought that could sound so good. As we compare our cancer scars, Emmy and I share a special bond, and a reassurance that God carries each of us in the palm of His hand.

Richard Hart, LLUSM class of 1970 and LLUSPH class of 1970, DrPH, has served as president of LLUH since 2008. His wife, Judy (LLUSN class of 1965), shares a lifelong passion to serve the underserved of the world. They have three children and nine grandchildren. The twins were born on March 28, 2001.

March 29

"Now may the God of peace Himself sanctify you completely; amd may your whole spirit, soul, and body be preserved blameless at the coming of our Lord Jesus Christ. He who calls you is faithful, who also will do it."
1 Thessalonians 5:23-24, NKJV

As I completed my year of postgraduate study in 1962 at Harvard University's School of Public Health, I thought back on the lessons learned. One of the most prominent came in a lecture from Dr. Edsall, a well-known microbiologist, who summarized the field of immunology and the latest science on immunization. He then asked, "What is the most important factor determining the health status of any individual?" Most of us suggested immunizations or other direct prevention. Dr. Edsall then proceeded to convince me and my fellow classmates that it was actually one's choice in daily living or lifestyle that was far more powerful than any direct preventive effort. For the first time I began to recognize how important lifestyle is.

Health workers should never be satisfied with simply helping people overcome pain or recover their previous level of health. The goal of every Christian physician should be to help everyone reach ever higher levels of health, to take steps toward increased development of body, mind, and soul—toward the restoration of God's image in humans (E. G. White, *Education*, p. 15-16). This obviously requires more than treating symptoms. It requires that we seek to identify the cause of illness and help people make lifestyle changes that can repair damage, prevent disease, and promote health.

By and large, it is in the many small choices of daily living that we begin restoration and develop sanctified characters for eternity. Sanctification is not just a theory. It's living day by day, minute by minute, in such a way that we know we are following God's will in everything. It's not easy or simple, but with God's help it is possible, and His promises are sure! "Those who wait on the LORD shall renew their strength; they shall mount up with wings like eagles, they shall run and not be weary, they shall walk and not faint" (Isaiah 40:31, NKJV). "Restoration [renewal] of all things" has been the theme of all His "prophets since the world began" (Acts 3:21, NKJV). In 1 Thessalonians 5:24 God reassures us that "He who calls you is faithful, who also will [sanctify you completely]" (NKJV). Praise God for His promise, "I can do all things through Christ who strengthens me" (Philippians 4:13, NKJV). These promises are for both our patients and us!

P. William "Bill" Dysinger, CME class of 1955, is an emeritus adjunct professor in LLUSM's department of preventive medicine and was heavily involved in starting LLUSPH and the preventive medicine residency at LLUH. At age 93, Bill and his wife live in middle Tennessee where they are active in church and community health activities. They have 4 children, 17 grandchildren, and 8 great-grandchildren.

March 30

> *"Even when the way goes through Death Valley,*
> *I'm not afraid when you walk at my side."*
> Psalm 23:4, MSG

It had arrived. In the early days we watched COVID-19 devastate regions of China and Italy in near disbelief. This unknown virus, this invisible contagion, was now in front of me. As I gowned up to see a ward full of scared patients, Psalm 23:4 repeatedly came to mind: "Yea, though I walk through the valley of the shadow of death, I will fear no evil: for thou art with me; thy rod and thy staff they comfort me" (KJV).

The fear in society and the hospital was palpable. We initially did not have reliable testing, and were designing protocols on the fly that affected thousands of people. All nonessential surgeries were cancelled. Most of the administration worked from home. As test results trickled in, taking days, a week even, the faces of the pandemic became real. Upon arrival patients were immediately quarantined, interacting only with staff who were gowned from head to toe. The only visible evidence of our humanity were our eyes behind a clear plastic mask. The primary nurse, therapists, and myself were the only people that would or could see these patients. Families were not allowed. Consultants would not see these patients in person. The medical units and hallways felt eerie. It was controlled chaos in the emergency department and ICU, but quiet everywhere else.

The shock in caring for these patients and the emotional toll it takes is unlike any disease process I have previously come across. It separates us. It erodes the very core of humanity. Each patient was alone all day, scared and struggling to breathe. I was acutely aware each moment I spent in a room with a COVID-19 patient increased the risk I may make an error and become infected.

And yet, in the midst of this great angst, the purpose of LLUH has never been clearer. We must work hard to take the entire person into account. In the case of COVID-19 the psychological, spiritual, and emotional drain is massive. It has altered the way I see the world. There are few times in life that provide more meaning than to sense a fellow human is struggling and to be there in support. In my mind there is no higher calling than to wake up each day acknowledging not only the beauty that surrounds us but also the pain so many are experiencing, and to be present.

Michael Matus, LLUSM and LLUSPH class of 2011, is an assistant professor in LLUSM's department of medicine. He trained in internal medicine at LLUH and served as chief medical resident at Riverside University Health System. He joined the division of hospitalist medicine at LLUSM in 2015 and became head of that division in 2019.

March 31

> *"But God demonstrates His own love toward us, in that while we were still sinners, Christ died for us."*
> Romans 5:8, NASB

"Am I going to die today, Remy?"

Sitting across from me in one of the ER bays is my friend Eugene. He is short of breath and is experiencing chest pain.

The personal choices that he has made in his life come into full play. End-stage chronic obstructive pulmonary disease, coronary heart disease, and congestive heart failure are taking their toll. Years of nicotine addiction have compromised his lung function, and his respiratory reserve is diminishing. Finally, after an hour of treatment, his breathing is less labored, but I still sense his angst.

"Eugene, your workup is unchanged from your baseline. I will send you home. No, you are not going to die today."

Every day the dance of life-and-death plays out in the patient's room. The following words are too common: silent ocular globes, time of death. Death is like a cosmic black hole with an event horizon. Everyone will one day approach that event horizon, and as the black maw of death comes calling there is no escape. The Creator of the universe who created everything in the cosmos could not escape the event horizon of His sacrificial death.

I am reminded of a quote by Cliff Goldstein: "I am but a pubescent version of my corpse, and we carry this on our backs, and we can never shake it off." It is ironic that my conversations with Eugene would run the gamut between end-stage COPD and troponin values, and would then slide effortlessly into a bedside Bible study. We talked about grace, life after death, the seventh-day Sabbath, and hell.

Matthew 12:29 and Mark 3:27 read, in effect: "In order to enter the house of the strong man, one must bind the strong man first." It's a puzzling verse, but after reading a book entitled *The Gospel According to Peanuts*, I had an aha moment. It's about being wise as a serpent and harmless as a dove, and to bind the strong man is to witness to people at their level of faith and understanding. The core of the verse has to do with being stealthy, and not breaking down the front door. Throwing gospel bombs over the fence as a form of witnessing is presumptuous.

The event horizon of death stalks us 24 hours a day and its inexorable pull of destruction is the reality of a fallen world. The devil puts a period at the end of our lives, but God puts a comma and the promise of eternal life. The event horizon of grace draws us in so that we can be transformed into what we were meant to be.

Only from the perspective of eternity will it be known if the conversations that we had engaged in contributed to Eugene's salvation. He passed away in 2013. What I have not told you until now is that Eugene was a Grand Dragon of the Klu Klux Klan.

Remy Sagadraca, LLUSM class of 1973-A, is an emergency medicine physician in Greeneville, Tennessee.

APRIL

∞ INTEGRITY ∞

> "Each person must live their life as a model for others."

ROSA PARKS (1913–2005)
American activist in the civil rights movement

April 1

> *"Now to Him who is able to do far more abundantly beyond all that we ask or think, according to the power that works within us."*
> Ephesians 3:20, NASB

I was performing surgery on a patient with a retinal detachment. I had seen the patient, a young man, several days ago with painless vision loss in his left eye. The patient was under general anesthesia, and I needed to identify the retinal detachment and fix the retinal tear. But where was the retinal detachment? I could not find it.

I was a young retinal surgeon, well-trained at the Mayo Clinic. I had seen hundreds of retinal detachments; they are not difficult to find. My panic worsened. What was going on? Had I started surgery on the wrong eye? I asked my surgical circulator to bring my clinic chart. Let me see my retinal drawing. Left eye. Correct. Some relief. What was going on?

Retinal detachments are almost always caused by a retinal tear. I reexamined the patient more carefully. Could I find the tear? There it was! A small superotemporal retinal tear was present. But no retinal detachment. Spontaneous resolution! Wow! I had never seen this before. What to do now? I froze the retinal tear with cryotherapy. Who knows if the retinal detachment will recur? Case over. Just not the procedure I had planned and consented for. Preop diagnosis: retinal detachment. Postop diagnosis: retinal tear.

After the surgery, before the patient had woken from surgery, I had a discussion with the family. How to explain? I started hesitantly. "I had diagnosed Timothy with a retinal detachment when I saw him in the clinic, but the retinal detachment has resolved on its own. It healed itself. I did find a retinal tear, so I treated this with a freezing probe. He should be fine. I feel bad that he was put to sleep for this procedure."

I expected a negative reaction. Surprise. Disappointment. Perhaps even anger. I received only smiles.

Said a family member, "We have been praying continually for healing since Timothy was diagnosed by you. The Lord has provided this miracle of healing."

Tears streamed down my eyes. I was filled with gratitude and humility. I could say no more; I nodded and smiled.

After Timothy awoke, I told him of this miraculous event. I asked him if his vision had changed prior to surgery. Oh, yes, he said. It had been getting better. Why had he not relayed the information to me? I had failed to ask. After all, who expects a retinal detachment to heal spontaneously? It is a rare event. Or, more likely, a miracle from God.

Michael Rauser is associate professor and chair in LLUSM's department of ophthalmology. He and his wife, Mi Ye Kim, assistant professor, LLUSM's department of internal medicine, live in Redlands, California, with their two children, Thomas (LLUSM class of 2022) and Shelly (Andrews University in Michigan).

April 2

"When I was a child, I used to speak like a child, think like a child, reason like a child; when I became a man, I did away with childish things."
1 Corinthians 13:11, NASB

The claxons blared, "Shelter in place. Active shooter on post."

April 2, 2014, was a warm day at Fort Hood, Texas. My evening shift had just started, and the residents were engaged with their first patients when the post incident commander told me there was a shooter, possibly two, on post at multiple scenes. My heart sank as I realized this would be my mass casualty to manage. I had been through the shooting on November 5, 2009, when Major Hasan killed 13 and injured 54 others. I was not anxious to repeat it.

The "MassCal" alert was sent out. Help started arriving, and the wonderful ER staff quickly started preparing the department as we assembled in the ambulance bay to prepare for triage. The first patients arrived in the back of a pickup truck. Soon ambulances followed. All were gunshot wounds of varying severity. The injuries varied from the walking wounded to life-threatening penetrating injuries. One young soldier was shot in the head, with his life ebbing away. It would be the only time I have categorized a patient as "triage category black." In the back of my mind I realized his eternal fate was sealed.

As more help arrived, they were divided into teams of four, consisting ideally of a doctor, nurse, medic, and anyone else who arrived (chaplain, X-ray technician, lab personnel, etc.). As we neared the end of the arriving injuries, I turned to look at the next team. I saw the smiling face of Heather, one of our recent graduates. She had been trained well in our program and waited confidently. My mind flashed back to five years ago.

During the Hasan shootings in 2009 I was called in early for my shift. When I arrived, I went from room to room seeing what needed to be done. When I looked into the room with our pelvic bed, Heather was there with a dying patient and had the terrified look on her face of a young, inexperienced doctor. She had been out of medical school only a few months. In her bed was a hypotensive captain with three gunshot wounds. We quickly went to work on her, and fortunately the patient lived to thank us two weeks later.

As only the military can, both events were reviewed and critiqued. However, as her attending, I reflected on the growth of Heather during those five years. It was very rewarding to see her growth from the look of terror during the 2009 incident to now a confident physician.

It also made me think of my Christian life. Each day we have patients that may be only a few heartbeats away from having their eternal destinies sealed. As I reflected on Heather's growth, I asked myself if I had grown in the Christian graces over the past five years to be an effective witness to those in crisis. Am I growing as a Christian soldier that I might more effectively share the Savior who died on the cross for them and me?

Ted Martin Kelly, LLUSM class of 1985, is an attending and teaching physician in the emergency medicine residency program at Fort Hood, Texas. He and his wife, Pam, have a passion for spreading the gospel with Maranatha Volunteers International and It Is Written.

April 3

"And I will put enmity between you and the woman,
and between your offspring and hers."
Genesis 3:15, NIV

My greatest athletic achievement consisted of completing a standing broad jump of more than six feet—backwards. Only after landing did I become conscious of the cause: a two-foot-long rattlesnake crossing the path where my foot almost landed. Thank God for enmity.

But enmity can go awry. Twenty years earlier I unexpectedly noticed that a Black friend from high school had his arm affectionately around a Caucasian girl with whom I worked in the hospital kitchen. I had not known that they even knew each other, much less that they were dating. And three thoughts hit almost simultaneously:

♦ *Doug should not be messing with our women!*
♦ *Where did THAT thought come from?*
♦ *That is the most STUPID thing you have ever thought!* because I am Chinese. And then I burst out laughing.

Enmity, unconscious or implicit bias, intrudes and makes us react, especially in emergencies. We all have it. It can save us. It can embarrass us. It can lead to tragedy.

When Jesus prepared His first followers to take God's message to everyone, He addressed their misplaced enmity against women, disabled individuals, Samaritans (2 Kings 17 and Nehemiah 13), and Gentiles. Throughout His public ministry:

1. Jesus often took His followers through Samaria (cf. John 4) and to such places as the Decapolis (cf. Mark 7:31) to increase their contact with Samaritans and Gentiles.

2. Jesus repeatedly cited such counterstereotypical narratives as "Were there not ten?" (Luke 17:17, NKJV) and "Not even in Israel" (Matthew 8:10, NKJV).

3. At the right time, Jesus made this explicit. Had Jesus responded to the lawyer by telling the parable of the good Pharisee, we would understand that good people ought to be nice to strangers. By flipping His response to the parable of the good Samaritan, I hear Jesus saying, "God's followers act contrary to their preconceived ideas of who is their neighbor."

The Master Teacher, Jesus, chose precisely the right time and the right message. Even after Peter had walked with Jesus for three and a half years, renewed his commitment to Jesus after the resurrection, and been filled with the Holy Spirit, Peter still had an aversion to Gentiles. With Cornelius' messengers only blocks away, Jesus called out Peter's visceral reaction (gut feelings) against Gentiles by using a vision of unclean foods!

Peter internalized the message. "God shows no partiality," he declared. This profoundly influenced the early church. Luke recounts the story no less than three times in Acts 10-12. But even this did not remove implicit bias from God's people. The rest of the New Testament and history continues to record the tragedy of misplaced enmity.

Today, when we follow Jesus through Samaria and listen to His words about the two Greeks; today, even when we can say with Peter, "God shows no partiality," we still have our own unconscious bias. Today, let us focus on Jesus and ask Him to help us act graciously as He would act, and not from misplaced enmity.

Daniel Giang, LLUSM class of 1983, is a professor in LLUSM's department of neurology. He completed a neurology residency and behavioral neurology fellowship at University of Rochester in New York. He currently serves as associate dean for graduate medical education in LLUSM. His wife, Sarah Roddy (LLUSM class of 1980-B), is associate dean of admissions at LLUSM. They are new grandparents.

April 4

"Let love guide your heart, let God lead the way."
Anonymous

On Thursday, April 2, 2020, I decided I needed to go to New York. I did not know how I was going to get there, where I was going to work, or even what I was going to be doing. I just knew I needed to go. In early April COVID-19 was ravaging New York, with infections and deaths reaching a record high. Hospitals were at capacity, ventilators were in short supply, and nurses and doctors were severely understaffed and overworked. Meanwhile, I was enjoying a rare break from my nurse anesthesia program, spending much-needed time with my family, when I began to learn more about the working conditions at some of the hospitals in New York. One article in particular mentioned that one nurse in the ICU could be caring for up to six critically ill, ventilator-dependent patients. Having a background in critical care, I knew I could help. But more than anything, I felt called to help.

Have you ever felt God's calling in your life? I have always tried to live my life according to where I sense God leading. But if you're anything like me, understanding God's calling has not always been straightforward. Sometimes I wish God would express His calling through an audible voice. Unfortunately I have never had the privilege of experiencing that. For me, God's calling has always been sort of a heart stirring. Something that I know to be true on a soul level. As crazy and uncertain as it seemed, my heart was telling me God wanted me in New York.

Two days later on April 4 I was on a plane headed to New York. I was placed at NYU Langone Medical Center in Manhattan. Nearly the entire hospital had turned into a COVID ICU, with units transforming overnight to accommodate the surge of COVID patients. When I arrived, I received a brief orientation of the facility and was given my PPE for the week. The very next evening I was on the unit taking care of patients. My health care background is in ICU nursing, and I have cared for very sick patients before. But what I witnessed in New York was altogether something different. To give you a sense of what it was like, 30 minutes into my first shift I had to call a code blue and perform CPR on one of my patients. Hours later I had to do it again. When my first shift had ended, two out of my three patients had passed away.

It is difficult to put my experience in New York into words. In many ways I am still processing what happened during those six weeks. But I am so thankful I had this experience. You just never know what hangs in the balance concerning your decision to listen and follow God's leading in your life. Caring for COVID patients at NYU Langone was one of the most challenging, frightening, heartbreaking, and yet rewarding experiences of my life.

Garrett Speyer, LLUSN class of 2018, lives in Fort Myers, Florida, with his wife, Cambria and two daughters. Garrett enjoys spending time at the beach and hanging out with friends. He completed a Master of Science in nurse anesthesia in June, 2021.

April 5

> *"In everything, therefore, treat people the same way you want them to treat you, for this is the Law and the Prophets."*
> Matthew 7:12, NASB

I could sense the frustration level of the resident going up as I directed him, for the second time, to take out skin stitches he had just put in and to do them over again. He took a deep breath, and I could almost hear him thinking, *Isn't this good enough?* We had been operating on an infant girl with a congenital bowel obstruction, and at the end of the case I was trying to teach him how to sew delicate skin, demonstrating the technique that I wanted him to use. Most of the sutures that he had placed were admittedly fairly good, but they were uneven in places, leaving some gaps, and had bunched the skin in others. I made him pause for a moment before he started to sew again, because I wanted to ask him if he would consider the current wound closure to be "good enough" for his own daughter. More than that, I wanted to remind him that there was a mother in the waiting room who had entrusted us with the single most important thing in her life.

For the past nine months she had looked forward to the day that she delivered her baby girl and had been dreaming and hoping for a baby that was perfect in every way. To her, despite the child's anomaly that required operative correction, her baby was perfect. For that mother to hand her most precious treasure over to us was an incredible act of faith and trust, and one that demanded that we respect that trust, and consequently do our very best to honor it. That meant striving for perfection. If it's not "good enough" for our own children, it should not be considered "good enough" for any patient. I wanted to impress upon my resident that this was a principle that should apply to every single patient entrusted to our care, young or old. The resident stood quietly for a moment, then nodded silently and went back to work, taking great care to make the wound look beautiful.

The Bible has some sage advice for those of us who are privileged to be teachers. "In everything set them an example by doing what is good. In your teaching show integrity" (Titus 2:7, NIV). In striving to do our best for this child, I was reminded of something that my mother used to tell me, specifically that any job worth doing is worth doing well. But more than that, I was reminded of how God the Father, in an act of faith, much like that of the mother of our patient, handed over His own Son, sending Him to this earth to show us the way to eternal life, and hoping to get Him back. We should do our best every day to honor that act.

Don Moores, LLUSM class of 1987, is an associate professor in LLUSM's departments of surgery and pediatrics and is head of the division of pediatric surgery. He is the son of Art Moores (CME class of 1953-B) and Verna Moores (LLUSN class of 1952) and is married to Penny (Bronsert) Moores (LLUSAHP class of 1984). They have two children, including Michael (LLUSM class of 2021). Don firmly believes that we should always do our best . . . that way we can always sleep at night with a clear conscience.

April 6

> *"He subdued peoples under us, and nations under our feet."*
> Psalm 47:3, ESV

A kind and loving spirit, the ability to listen with an open heart, a longing to learn the stories of others, appreciation of the sacred spark of creation in every living being and a sense of awe—these are the attributes of healers.

For more than a half century of medical practice, the majority at Loma Linda University Health (LLUH), I have aspired to become a healer and teach others to heal as well. I want my colleagues and students to know in their souls that their calling is to heal and that their presence, shared willingly and authentically from their hearts forms the bedrock of the healing art. Indeed, at a time when health care is overburdened with concerns of time, money, and technology, they are all that is needed for healing to occur.

I learned this from mentors and taught this at the bedside and in the clinic. I also came to appreciate this transformative lesson by joining with colleagues and students to read stories, sermons, and essays that illuminate the human condition and allow us to voice questions and share understandings of the world in which we and our patients live. We call these experiences "Story Time." Stories bring home the meaning of injustice, poverty, fear, cruelty, greed, illness, suffering, and death. Through stories we acquire an appreciation of kindness, gratitude, courage, character, faith, peace, spirituality, wholeness, and love. Through sharing questions and insights about the stories we read, we learn from one another and prepare ourselves to better care for and heal our patients.

I will let you in on a secret all healers know. Healing is a two-way street. As we work to heal others, we come to know peace and are made whole ourselves. When we reach out to embrace suffering patients, miraculously we too are comforted. Our work as healers sustains us and gives meaning to our lives. Since retiring from practice this past year, more than anything else about a fulfilling life in medicine, I miss my patients.

On the wall just down the hall from my former office is a large map of the United States. Affixed to it at appropriate geographic locations are the photos of each of the exceptional pulmonary care and critical care physicians our division trained, mentored, and nurtured over the past 40 years. We are justifiably proud of their successes and accomplishments. As I pass through the hall, I often stop to regard their images. I recall with great clarity their time with us. Their unique personalities and their ways of being are indelible in my memory. I am comforted and pleased beyond measure to know that each of them learned to bring much more than the knowledge and skill of well-trained specialists to their patients. Each of them completes a circle begun before their time at LLUH, nurtured during their time here and one that continues still by bringing comfort, hope, love, and the grace of healing to the world.

Philip M. Gold is an emeritus professor in LLUSM's department of medicine. He and his wife, Roberta, have been married for 62 years, have three children, six grandchildren, and a Labradoodle. One of his passions is monthly "Story Time" with the pulmonary/critical care fellows.

April 7

> *"Be kindly affectioned one to another with brotherly love;*
> *in honour preferring one another."*
> Romans 12:10, KJV

My high school art teacher once gave us an assignment: Paint a picture of a tree. My attempt started out strong, but as soon as I got to the branches, I began to flounder. I became frustrated as my painting looked less and less treelike. Finally the teacher walked by and noted, "You're focusing on what's there, instead of what isn't there. Focus on painting the negative space between the branches, and the shape of the tree will come together." I had no idea that this lesson would come to mind nearly 10 years later during a patient's appointment at a local off-campus, non-Loma Linda University hospital.

The day started out as so many days on the wards do: with apprehension and excitement. I stood waiting by the doctors' lounge, apprehensive about being assigned to a physician with a reputation for taking a "tough-love-without-the-love" approach to patient care. The door to the doctors' lounge burst open, and a long white coat began fluttering away down the hall. A voice yelled back, over a shoulder: "Med student from Loma Linda, right? Follow me."

Down the hall we went. A nurse held out a note with a patient's blood pressure written on it: "198/92." The doctor plucked the note from the nurse's hand: His eyes bulged as he involuntarily crumpled the little yellow square in his fist. Once again, a long white coat went sailing down the hall with me behind it, trying to keep up.

Room B neared, and in we went. A drab woman sat in the chair trying to take up as little space as humanly possible. The doctor shook her hand, introduced himself, and sat down, all in one swift motion. "I feel like I'm in trouble," a timid voice squeaked, half-laughing, half-ashamed. A whitecoat replied: "You ARE in trouble. Your kidneys are failing. You'd be a perfect candidate for a transplant, but you're wrecking your heart!" Twenty minutes later the appointment ended as quickly as it had begun. The whitecoat left the room, leaving me alone with the diminutive figure in the chair. I wished her a great day and attempted to find the man with a stethoscope in a labyrinth of beige walls and forest-green carpet. I was perturbed, as this wasn't what I had been taught to expect as a medical student.

As I walked home that day I realized I had learned a valuable lesson: I would have three more years to figure out exactly what type of doctor I wanted to be but all it took was one day to figure out what type of doctor I did NOT want to be. I had learned that I didn't want to be a physician who viewed every patient as an uncooperative vessel housing precious organ systems. So much of medical school is trying to learn what things are, how they work, and how to do things correctly. But that day my perspective flipped, just as it had back in art school: I suddenly saw the negative space, and as a result I had a much deeper understanding of the overall positive space of a metaphorical tree called medicine.

Ryan Marais, LLUSM class of 2021, is an internal medicine resident at LLUH. He enjoys traveling, fossil hunting, and sci-fi. He hopes to follow in his father's and uncle's footsteps and pursue a career in cardiology.

April 8

> *"So then, as we have opportunity, let us do good to everyone, and especially to those who are of the household of faith."*
> Galatians 6:10, ESV

Internal medicine, the final rotation of my third year of medical school, had arrived, and I was excited. After a year of struggle and persistence, I had finally become comfortable with patient care. Adding to the excitement was that I had a first-year medical student working with me. It was invigorating introducing him to clinical medicine.

Together we went to see Ms. Rodriguez. This elderly woman had come to the hospital with belly pain and skin yellow as a banana. Our workup indicated that she had something in the head of her pancreas. After the less-invasive options had been exhausted and we were still without a clear diagnosis, she was scheduled for surgery.

As I walked into her room, I noticed a small figurine of Mary, the mother of Jesus, sitting on her bedside table. With a translator present, I greeted Ms. Rodriguez. She was nervous about her surgery and with good reason. Many years ago she had suffered a gunshot wound to the head. Miraculously, she had not only survived but was still able to think, talk, and move. She did have a little trouble forming words and also had some weakness on half of her body, but other than that, she was intact. The experience, however, had left emotional scars. I could only imagine how traumatic it must have been going through brain surgery and spending weeks in and out of consciousness in the intensive care unit.

I spoke with her about the upcoming surgery. She replied that she was in God's hands and then burst into tears. Her family was a bit taken aback. I tried to comfort Ms. Rodriguez, assuring her that we would do our best to help her.

Having seen the figurine and having heard Ms. Rodriguez's reference to God, I offered to pray with her, and she accepted my invitation. Holding her hand, I asked God to help the medical teams as we cared for her. I prayed for peace for her, and thanked God for the day we would all live with Him, free of pain, disease, and suffering.

After I left, the nurse, who had been present, came over to me. "Don't lose that," she said. "Don't stop praying with patients." The first-year medical student then asked me, "So how do you know when you should pray with a patient?" which started a conversation about spiritual care.

While reaching out to people who do not know God is certainly of great importance, I have been reminded not to neglect those who already know God. A Bible sitting on a table, a family member saying, "We have to trust in Jesus," or a woman sitting outside the outpatient surgery center softly praying have all prompted me to reach out and offer prayer. It amazes me how impactful a simple prayer can be to a thirsty soul.

Ryan Rigsby, LLUSM class of 2017, is a diagnostic radiology resident at LLUH. He enjoys long-distance running and cooking with his wife, Emily. April 8 is his birthday.

April 9

"By working hard in this way we must help the weak and remember the words of the Lord Jesus, that he himself said, 'It is more blessed to give than to receive.'"
Acts 20:35, ESV

When I was a little girl, my doctor mom always handed me a dollar to put in the offering bag as it came around. Always a dollar.

Now the tables are turned. Mama is weak, and I am strong. She has no money to keep with her because it might get lost, and I look after her finances. She loses memories, and I keep them. The tables are turned; I do for her what she used to do for me.

Now when I take my parents to church each week, I hand my doctor mom a dollar or two to put in the offering plate. Always a dollar or two, because that's what she remembers giving long ago. A dollar or two held carefully in her quiet, weakening hands until the offering plate comes by. Solemnly she places the bills in the plate and then lets go and yanks her hand back as if holding on would burn her fingers.

I've realized that placing dollars in the plate is meaningful to Mama because of this: Giving is a human act. And giving is a humane act.

As long as you are capable of giving, you feel that your existence is meaningful. Mama can no longer deliver babies, no longer wield the scalpel, no longer play the piano, cook for guests, write letters, drive blind Andrew to church. A few years ago, when she was capable of verbalizing it, she lamented in quiet desperation: "I'm not useful to anyone. I'm not doing anything to help anyone anymore."

Putting a dollar in the offering is an act of defiance in face of obsolescence. It says, "I can still help." It says, "I can help this community of believers, even if it's paying for one minute of lighting or a few bulletins." It says, "If I were not here, giving my dollar, you would be a dollar short."

Putting a dollar in the offering says, "This dollar represents the investment of my time, my medical education, my years of sleep lost when babies were born at night, my faithfulness in showing up to do surgery on Wednesday mornings. This dollar represents the gifts of myself and donations to missions. And it represents my investment in my daughter, who now has a dollar to hand me because of the dollars I put into her education."

Putting her dollar in the offering also says, "This dollar represents my heart of gratitude to my Savior as I pass along in some way the gift of His goodness to me."

Mama's dollar not only symbolizes the blessing she gives away, but also the blessing she receives in the act of giving. A dollar in the offering reteaches me what she taught me long ago, that it is more blessed to give than to receive. And so each week I slip her a dollar or two and remember being a wee girl. And she participates afresh in the holy act of giving. It is a joyful and precious moment.

Ginger Ketting-Weller, PhD, is the president of the Adventist International Institute of Advanced Studies (AIIAS) in the Philippines. Her parents, Sam (CME class of 1960) and Effie Jean (CME class of 1954), were medical missionaries in Thailand and Malaysia from 1961 to 1981, serving again as relief doctors in Africa, Jamaica, and the Solomon Islands after their retirement. Her mother passed away in 2017 and her father in 2018.

April 10

"And we know that all things work together for good to them that love God, to them who are the called according to his purpose."
Romans 8:28, KJV

I have worked at Loma Linda University Health for almost 40 years and have had many moments with staff, visitors, and patients that have blessed myself and them. I am an administrative secretary for employee spiritual care and wholeness and I typically start work at 6:00 a.m. On one particular morning about five years ago, as I crossed the street from the employee parking structure, I saw a couple of employees in scrubs administering CPR to a man who was on the asphalt driveway. My heart was drawn to the life-and-death struggle that was happening right in front of me. I immediately felt God telling me to pray and intercede on behalf of this man, a child of God. I stayed there praying until I heard the Lord say it was enough. I felt as if I had joined with God in battle for this stranger's life. The wonderful part of this is that to God this man was not a stranger.

I kept thinking about this man and continued to pray for him. A few days later I was given permission to find out what had happened and was so happy to learn that he had survived and was going home soon. I then asked if he would be willing for me to visit him. He said yes, and I let him know what God had asked me to do and that it showed how much his heavenly Father loved him. He thanked me and said he was blessed to be alive! I gave all the glory to God and told him that I was the one that was blessed to pray for him. This experience has increased my boldness in praying for anyone in need.

Cheri Moreno has been an employee at LLUMC since 1981. She is married and has two daughters and one granddaughter. Her daily prayer is for God to give her divine appointments for Him.

April 11

"Get wisdom, get understanding; do not forget my words or turn away from them. Do not forsake wisdom, and she will protect you; love her, and she will watch over you."
Proverbs 4:5-6, NIV

One of my first-year medical students recently approached me with a difficult question: "What do you do when there is nothing you can do to fix a situation?" We spoke at some length about different instances of this: children who face abuse from those who are supposed to protect them, patients who face terminal illnesses, the family struggling to pay their medical bills when they make just a tiny bit too much money to qualify for aid. We commiserated and cried together, both sharing in the unfairness of the world.

We oftentimes build our lives around the element of control. For those of us who thrive with this control, to be told there is nothing you can do is shocking. We don't like feeling helpless; it makes us uncomfortable, as if we are failing. After all, we are taught from an early age that even if you don't know the answer you should take your best guess at it. This is reinforced in our medical training, when the "right" answer is always just one more journal article or lecture away. If we fail, it is because we haven't worked hard enough. The harsh reality is that we cannot fix all the problems in the world; we cannot even consistently get our patients to do what we recommend.

In the moment of the conversation I shared with my student the many people involved in medical care: the tireless social workers, case managers who know the nuances of the medical system, various community programs and support. I tried to offer some sage advice of my own, but when I went home, it hit me again exactly how much I personally struggle with this same question. As I sat down at my desk, I looked up at the cork board I have had since college. This is where memos, acquired business cards, and the rare photo all conglomerate into a collage of life. My eyes fell on a prayer pinned in the corner, placed there sometime around the beginning of medical school. It brought me some comfort, and I hope it will comfort you as well:

Dear Father, may every day I represent Your comfort, Your light, Your hope in this dark world. Give me the strength to seek after You so that I can better minister to those I touch. May I continually realize my purpose in this world and the impact I have when I walk in that purpose. Bless me so that I may bless others; may I fight the good fight when the battle appears lost. Keep me by Your side, in Your arms, carried through the struggles and joys of life so that I may be ever secure in my identity in You. Thank you, O God, for Your continual patience and love for me. May I realize that love so that I may be freed from the guilt and responsibility of a society that tells me I need to earn it. Thank you for Your continual providence, blessing, and guidance. Thank You for Your hand that I see so plainly evident in my life; may I always follow it no matter where it leads. May my purpose in You be accompanied by my obedience to Your words, always and forever, Amen.

Molly Estes, LLUSM class of 2013, is an assistant professor in LLUSM's department of emergency medicine. She works as clerkship director for emergency medicine and as a LIFE community leader for the LLUSM. She is passionate about medical education and loves cooking in her free time.

April 12

"The most beautiful people we have known are those who have known defeat, known suffering, known struggle, known loss, and have found their way out of the depths. These persons have an appreciation, a sensitivity, and an understanding of life that fills them with compassion, gentleness, and a deep loving concern."

Elisabeth Kübler-Ross (1926–2004): American psychiatrist and author

There is something special about the World War II generation, which came through the Great Depression, fireside chats, and war. Unfortunately, this generation is slowly passing away. Those who bravely wore the stars and stripes are now under the draped flag they courageously fought for. As a medical student, I had the privilege to serve them through health care.

On my first call day, the intern informed me that it was a 92-year-old male status post left hip fracture. When I met the patient, he was cordial, humorous, with a story for every question I asked. I was surprised by his jovial attitude considering the circumstances that had brought him to the hospital.

Since he was on warfarin for atrial fibrillation, his surgery was rescheduled until his INR was at the appropriate level. The patient was not perturbed by the delay. On the day of surgery his spirits were uplifted, and he served as an encouragement to me. On POD 1 I asked about pain, which he rated as a 6 out of 10. "Have your pain medications been helping?"

I was shocked by his response: "I am not taking them," not even Motrin. The nurse informed me that the patient refused his pain meds. When I returned to the patient, his answer was succinct. He understood that postsurgery he would be in pain, and accepted that reality.

Thankfully, his granddaughter convinced him to at least take Motrin prior to physical therapy. The patient recovered as expected, but his insurance coverage delayed his placement in a skilled nursing facility. Another patient would have been annoyed; he took it in stride. Following Roger Hadley's (LLUSM class of 1974) advice to our medical school class, my fellow classmate and I asked about the "World War II days." He was excited to relay his voyage in the Pacific. But one story caught him off guard. He just finished a combat mission and was coming home. Over the radio they received the devastating news that FDR had passed away on April 12. At the mention of his Commander in Chief, his eyes became misty and his voice choked. We had a moment of silence in remembrance of the thirty-second president of the United States.

As we rounded for the last time, and said our farewell, the patient remarked that he was sad. "Why?" Every patient I knew was itching to leave the hospital. His response: "I will not see you again, and you all have treated me so well." What manner of man is this? Such grace and gratitude for our simple role in his hospital experience. As we left the room, our team debriefed on the character of America's finest heroes. The consensus was simple: You don't get to be 92 without gratitude. May each of us cherish the spirit of a thankful heart, just like our fellow veteran.

Sarah Nadarajan, LLUSM class of 2019, is a resident in internal medicine at University Health System SoCal Medical Education Consortium. She has a dry sense of humor, enjoys reading, traveling, and sharing God's love either locally or globally through church programs or mission trips.

April 13

"Since then we have a great high priest who has passed through the heavens, Jesus, the Son of God, let us hold fast our confession. For we do not have a high priest who is unable to sympathize with our weaknesses, but one who in every respect has been tempted as we are, yet without sin. Let us then with confidence draw near to the throne of grace, that we may receive mercy and find grace to help in time of need."

Hebrews 4:14-16, ESV

I don't know if it's cancer or not, but it needs to come out." The first words I heard while emerging from anesthesia after my colonoscopy cut like a knife through my foggy mind. As my vision came into focus, the gastroenterologist showed me the picture of the mass that had caused my bowel rupture nearly a month before. I had known something wasn't right, but the thought of cancer had never seriously entered my consciousness.

Surgery was scheduled for the following day. Through the evening my wife and I talked, prayed, cried, and read Bible promises. I didn't fear death. I feared the prospect of chemo, of my wife and kids enduring the journey through cancer with me and then enduring the journey of life without me. Where would my wife turn for support when all her energies were spent supporting me? Who would walk my girls down the aisle? How hard it was to let go of the illusion that God needed me to stay alive to take care of things that were already in His hands and had never actually been in my control.

Hearing is supposed to be the last sense to disappear and the first to come back after anesthesia. My first post-op recollection was hearing the surgeon say, "It didn't look like cancer." After a long weekend, the path report diagnosed Crohn's rather than cancer.

Months have passed since my surgery. I am thankful for life and for family. But it has been surprising how often I've been able to talk to a patient headed for surgery, hold their hand, and let them know that I know exactly how they are feeling. I can tell them that only a few months ago I went into surgery wondering if I would hear the diagnosis of cancer when I awoke. The same questions and worries they have, I so recently had. My experience doesn't change their medical situation. They may well wake up to find they have cancer. But to have a physician who at least has been through the same mental stress they are experiencing seems to be a comfort.

Jesus knows everything. He already knew exactly how humanity felt before He came. But Jesus didn't just tell us He understands and sits and watches from a distance. Jesus took on our flesh, and He chose to face the same trials and struggles we face, except that His challenges were as exponentially greater as His Holiness is greater than ours. There is no tear that falls, no silent cry of the human heart, no moment of lonely questioning, that the Great Physician is not aware of or that He has not personally experienced.

As we struggle through the maze that is twenty-first century medicine, let's remember the original reason we entered the field. Be Jesus for your patients. Identify with them and listen to their fears. And never forget that Jesus will always do the same for you.

Brent Goodge, LLUSM class of 2000, completed his LLUH anesthesiology residency in 2004. He is happily married to his wife, Synnova, and has two beautiful daughters.

April 14

"And he said to them, 'Take care, and be on your guard against all covetousness, for one's life does not consist in the abundance of his possessions.'"
Luke 12:15, ESV

There he sat. Thick, neatly cropped silver hair set against a sun-bronzed, weathered face. Normally poised, he was uncharacteristically melancholy that day. "I've never done anything worth taking notice of, Doc," he blurted out. "If I could just have something to point to, something that I could take pride in. I'm a failure." At 80 years old, and despite nearly 60 years of contented married life, raising children and grandchildren, he was weighing his life in the balance and coming up short, baffled, and disconcerted by a problem clearly out of the reach of medication or his current worldview.

After his appointment my thoughts shifted to a colleague. Young, well-trained, with professional tenacity and seeming success—the ideal of what many physicians strive to be. However, she shared a painful regret. "If I could only talk to the younger me and tell her, 'You may not want kids now, but just wait!' I would have done things so differently. I had no idea I would ever feel this way about wanting a baby," she lamented. Above the "success" of her marriage and her professional contributions, her inability to have a baby loomed as a gaping hole. As it turns out, she couldn't actually have it all.

The prolific British journalist Malcolm Muggeridge, after coming to faith, named his autobiography *Chronicles of Wasted Time*, an affront to our mass egocentrism and certainly to his own. We might reflect incredulously, "Wasted? Surely that's going a step too far. Don't be so hard on yourself."

An eager follower in the crowd once told Jesus to use His authority to settle a family financial matter. Jesus instead made a stark warning: "Take heed and beware of covetousness." In Colossians, Paul defines covetousness as idolatry, and in Romans he gives us the insight that it was the prohibition of covetousness that alerted him to his own precarious state. We want what we want when we want it. Whatever our age, whatever our position, status, gender, or prior accomplishments, we idolize what is important to us at the moment. But idols have never been satisfactory replacements for God.

Maybe my patient made a harsh but in many ways accurate assessment. Likewise, my colleague is allowed to have regrets about prioritizing her career at the expense of motherhood. Perhaps Muggeridge was spot-on as he discovered the reasoning behind Jesus' warning: A man's life does not consist of the abundance of things that he possesses.

As physicians, how are we to deal with the unsatisfied soul? It's certainly not wrong to be successful or to have children or a rightly divided inheritance. But Jesus diagnosed His patient's ailment for what it was: covetousness and idolatry. When confronted with perceived failure or unmet expectations, we may be tempted to diffuse guilt, to soothe away and normalize uncomfortable feelings. In certain circumstances this is appropriate. But it also might be just the place where God is working to redeem our wasted time, to turn self-sufficiency to Christ-sufficiency and covetousness into completeness in Him.

Mark Warren, LLUSM class of 2010, currently practices psychiatry in Idaho. He and his wife, Brittany, have six children: Asher, Micah, Jonathan, Malachi, Anastasia, and Judah. They enjoy discovering the wonders of God's great outdoor playground and are eagerly looking forward to the Second Coming! April 14 is Jonathan's birthday.

April 15

> *"For to me to live is Christ, and to die is gain."*
> *Philippians 1:21, ESV*

As a palliative medicine physician, I have the privilege of helping my patients live as well as possible for as long as they have to live. Our patients are among the sickest, enduring the burdens associated with their advanced illness. As they confront their own mortality, many reflect on their lives and wrestle with the meaning and purpose of life. These conversations are among the most cherished and meaningful to me. I feel honored to be welcomed into their lives and the opportunity to help them through difficult times.

As I listen to my patients share about their lives, I find myself reflecting on what it means for me to live well. As a Christian, the Bible verse that helps me answer this question is Philippians 1:21, ESV, where the apostle Paul writes, "For to me to live is Christ, and to die is gain." The sentence structure in the Greek is interesting, as it lacks a verb. A more literal interpretation would be, "to live Christ, to die gain." For Paul, Christ is all-encompassing. This letter has been referred to as a letter of joy, which is striking because Paul had suffered tremendously by this time and would be executed not long after this letter was penned. By following Christ, Paul gave up many of the things that we tend to pursue and value in this life, including wealth, prestige, social acceptance, and physical comforts (2 Corinthians 11:24-28). Philippians 3:8, ESV, explains how Paul was able to have such immense joy amid tremendous loss: "Indeed, I count everything as loss because of the surpassing worth of knowing Christ Jesus my Lord." Knowing Christ is far more rewarding and valuable than anything we can gain or lose.

For the Christian, Christ is the reason we live, and this extends to eternal life, as explained in John 17:3, ESV: "And this is eternal life, that they know you, the only true God, and Jesus Christ whom you have sent." Colossians 1:16 further explains that all things were created through Christ and for Christ. To live well for the Christian means to fulfill the purpose for which we were created. We were created through Him, and our purpose is to live for Him. Remarkably, my Creator came down to die for me, so that I may live for Him (1 Thessalonians 5:10; Philippians 2:6-11; 2 Corinthians 5:21). The reason I strive to live for Christ is that I love Him, and the reason I love Him is that He first loved me (1 John 4:19). Romans 5:8, ESV, explains, "But God shows his love for us in that while we were still sinners, Christ died for us." The meaning of life should be defined by the One who created life itself. Only God has the authority to define such things, and He has revealed it through His Word. That is why for to me to live is Christ.

Practicing as a palliative medicine physician reminds me that life is both precious and fleeting. My patients have taught me many life lessons, not the least of which is never to take for granted the opportunity to live a meaningful life. As my patients confront their own mortality, I have a sacred responsibility to help them continue to find purpose in living well until their final breath. In exchange, they give me the invaluable gift of participating in their journey, reminding me to focus on that which is truly worth pursuing, and to live my own life well.

Andre Cipta, LLUSM class of 2011, currently serves as program director of the Kaiser Permanente Palliative Medicine Fellowship program in Los Angeles, California, and as assistant professor at the Kaiser Permanente Bernard J. Tyson School of Medicine. His hobbies include experiencing life to the fullest and contemplating the meaning of all things.

April 16

"None can believe how powerful prayer is, and what it is able to effect,
but those who have learned it by experience. It is a great matter
when in extreme need to take hold on prayer."
Martin Luther (1483–1546): *German theologian, professor, author, and Augustinian monk*

A low-grade fever developed in early April, and I began self-isolation despite a negative COVID-19 test. By the end of the week the fever was in the septic range, the COVID-19 test was positive, and I was a patient in the COVID unit. Despite excellent care and no preexisting conditions, my decline was unrelenting. On Thursday morning, April 16, the intensivist recommended ventilation. I consented while estimating the probability of survival was less than 10 percent, then made quick phone calls to my wife and family. By Friday my heart rate had dipped to 18, my systolic blood pressure had bottomed out at 50, and rapidly increasing inflammatory and coagulopathy markers predicted that my life was slipping away.

Saturday morning my brother Loren Hamel (LLUSM class of 1980-A) awoke with the burden of drafting a death notice, then learned that all the inflammatory markers had peaked, and clinical signs had stabilized. Five days later I was minimally aware when the endotracheal tube was exchanged for a high-flow oxygen mask. Within hours I tried to make sense of my family members' teary-eyed faces displayed over the iPad-on-a-pole beside the bed. For the next two days I suffered the greatest sense of shortness of breath.

The next Saturday I started the day with 50 percent oxygen delivered at 50 liters/minute and ended the day with discretionary use of oxygen by nasal canula at 2 liters/minute. I was discharged without oxygen and was working full-time within two weeks.

My survival may have depended on these: a superb medical team and their well-timed therapy, including prone ventilation and the earliest use of convalescent serum; the support of a skilled and loving family who, led by Loren, scoured the world literature, then met each day on Zoom, 35 to 50 people strong, to pray and ensure that no helpful therapy would be overlooked; and the power of intercessory prayer offered by thousands around the world.

My turnaround on the first Saturday may be explained by perfectly delivered health care. The unprecedented physiologic and anatomical healing on the second Saturday may best be explained as perfectly miraculous.

I could not have predicted the diversity and number of prayer warriors who knelt on my behalf. Social media carried the details of my journey to those I hold dear, those I know or serve, and countless others I will never meet. Hundreds describe hearing the voice of God compelling them to pray. From members of numerous Christian denominations, several world religions, and every ethnicity, the testimonies were the same. As numbers grew, there was no reported sense of a diminished role, rather celebration that the divine call to prayer was real and a strengthening of faith that God requests and hears our prayers.

May you this day be thankful that we can hear the voice of God and celebrate the diverse and global army He may call as He chooses.

Lowell Hamel, LLUSM class of 1981, completed a family medicine residency at Hinsdale Hospital, Illinois. He is a senior vice president at Spectrum Health Lakeland, serves as the chief operating and clinical officer, and continues to see patients at the University Medical Center near the campus of Andrews University in Michigan. He and his wife, Judy, enjoy the company of their five children and nine grandchildren.

April 17

Easter, 2022

"Knowing that Christ, having been raised from the dead, is never to die again; death no longer is master over Him." Romans 6:9, NASB

As I reflect on the many Easters I have celebrated I consider the following:
HE (Jesus, my God, Creator, Master of all but also close Friend and Guide)
IS (in the present state, not was or will be but IS)
RISEN (conquered death and sin, alive currently, came up from darkness, elevated).

The resurrection is powerful because there was death first. Without the death there could be no resurrection and therefore no victory.

This past week there was a memorial service for the men and women who had donated their bodies to the School of Medicine so that students could learn to be physicians and other health professionals. My kids saw the memorial service program and had tons of questions. "Isn't it sad, Mommy, when you work on that body in school 'cause they died?" "Why would anyone give their body to have it torn up?" "Do they bury the body afterward?" "What does the family think?" As 8- and 6-year-old minds tried to comprehend such difficult concepts, I explained that because those people chose to donate their body I got to learn how to help heal others. They made the choice to give even after they died, and the memorial service is for the students to thank the families. As I did my best to discuss death and dying, I was reminded of my first day in that anatomy lab and all the uncertainties, fears, excitement, and dreams that lay before me. We would start our career by working on a deceased person so that we could help heal and bring life.

Then I realized that it's not quite that simple. When I was a naive med student, I thought I would go into medicine to heal people, bring life, and share Christ's love. Now I realize those things are only part of the job. I also walk with patients through their process of dying, recognizing medicine's limitations. The death we have to deal with helps to make way for life. When a patient doesn't get better or a treatment fails or they just die and I don't understand why, those instances help teach me more about life and resurrection power. What did I learn? Could anything have changed that might save another life?

A long-term patient of mine died suddenly last week, but strangely, I have learned so much about life, acceptance, and hope in God's resurrection power from her untimely death. In my feelings of loss, failure, and sadness, I processed deeply my role with my patients. A great understanding and freedom came, which was a type of new life for me.

Where is there death in your life? Is there hopelessness, discouragement, feelings of uncertainty? It may be that the resurrection life will come from those dead things. When we recognize God's power to use our dead "stuff" and sometimes let things die so that much greater life can be brought forth, there can be freedom. Resurrection then to me is new life because of death. Jesus was destined to die and destined to rise; both realities were critical, and it wasn't until the two came to pass that they both made sense.

I pray the power of resurrection life: that the reality of Jesus would transform the death in your life, that new perspectives be born, healing power in your body be released, productivity and fruitfulness be brought forth, and rest and peace be transmitted to you.

Amy Hayton, LLUSM and LLUSPH class of 2004, is an assistant professor in LLUSM's department of medicine. She was LLUSM Teacher of the Year in 2018. She practices internal medicine in primary care at Jerry L. Pettis Memorial Veterans Hospital and is currently the assistant dean of student affairs and wellness at LLUSM. She is married to Andy Hayton (LLUSM class of 2004); they reside in Redlands, California, with their three children. Amy is passionate about medical student education and particularly helping students find their purpose and passion as they integrate their faith and practice.

April 18

"I can do all things through Christ who strengthens me."
Philippians 4:13, NKJV

My name is Christine, which means "follower of Christ." I always believed in God, but I didn't trust Him until recently. It's about time that I live up to my name. I am telling this story because I know there are many who may be skeptical of following Christ. Ironically, I was one of them. I used to think I could do all things through myself, that I could depend on myself for strength. I was wrong.

I need God for my strength. Jesus' life sounds like a fairy tale, but I'm convinced that Jesus Christ is God in human form. He performed miracles and died for us, so that we may have eternal life. These facts give me an amazing perspective. It breathes life in me. I don't need to see present-day show-stopping miracles to know that He is there. He is with us working behind the scenes.

Though I'm Christine, not Jesus Christ the ultimate healer, I play a small role as a healer and reflect His love. I may spend just a few moments face-to-face with each individual patient. My patients don't see the charts I read, phone calls I make, paperwork I fill out, notes I write, etc. My patients' plans could be formulated when they aren't looking. It's similar with God. We might not see all the work He is doing for our lives, but we have not been forgotten.

A misconception I had was that I just have to pray, and everything will magically be OK. That is silly, and that is false. Being a follower of Christ does not mean being lazy and waiting for God to handle everything. No, it means giving your best with what you are given and showing kindness to others. We are all given gifts and talents. We can use them for good. We can waste them. For me, having faith is about giving my best even when there is a possibility of failure.

People will notice hard work and results, especially when it's unexpected. They will wonder what makes you special. It's in those moments that you are reflecting God's love, and others will listen. Just as God doesn't need to perform big miracles all the time, we don't have to perform big acts all the time to be an influence. Take charge of your health, work hard at your job, love your family and friends, and don't take what you have for granted. Little things can make a huge impact.

I am proud to be Christine, a follower of Christ. I am amazed and humbled at how God continuously works in my life. I make mistakes, but I get chances to be a better person. Moving forward, I do my best to reflect God's love in the things I do. It's OK to ask God for help. I've learned that I can't do all things through Christine who does not strengthen me, but I can do all things through Christ who strengthens me.

Christine Tjandra, LLUSM class of 2013, currently practices neurology at Kaiser Permanente Vallejo in California. She enjoys traveling, hiking, poetry, and singing. April 18 is her birthday.

April 19

> *"Except these abide in the ship, ye cannot be saved."*
> Acts 27:31, KJV

Open racism was alive and well when we first arrived in Loma Linda. It was around 1970 that my wife and I decided to look for a new place to rent in the Loma Linda area. We found a house advertised in the *Trading Post* by an Adventist couple and made an appointment to see it.

When we arrived, however, we were told that it had already been rented in the short time between our call and arrival. This seemed suspicious to us, so we asked a white couple who were friends of ours to inquire, and yes, it was still available. This was quite common back then. There were legal remedies that had recently been passed that could have been taken, but at that time we chose not to proceed with them. Then there was the time I worked as a student worker on campus and discovered that I was being paid less than a white co-worker who was doing the same job. Obviously I felt discriminated against and quite disappointed. After all, wasn't this a Christian institution? A Seventh-day Adventist Christian institution? Not to mention the many Black applicants we knew of who were denied entrance to Loma Linda over the years because their color was more important than their intellect. What kind of Christianity was this?

Over the years I have come to believe that racism is one of the "tares" that God spoke of when He said that the "wheat would grow together with the tares." Many of us would surely lose our way if we were expecting the wheat to grow without tares, looking for the "church perfect" here and now. God, in His wisdom, warned us of the tares in advance, less we lose our way upon finding them.

Disappointments, frustrations, and difficulties will challenge us from time to time on our Christian walk, but as Paul said: "Stay on the ship, and no one will be lost." The temptation will be great to "jump ship" when we find ourselves shaking our heads in utter disbelief and disgust as various "tares" challenge our faith, but we must not. We were forewarned for that very reason. Instead, recognize and accept the fact that racism in the world and in the church has improved, but there is still work to be done. Whenever possible, we can take appropriate legal measures to remedy racial issues when legal options are available to us.

Meanwhile, we can show genuine love for one another. We can insist that the Constitution says what it means and means what it says without losing our Christianity. Resist remedies that take us to the edge of our Christianity and over. They are simply not worth it. As the late Congressman John Lewis said: Sometimes we must "get in good trouble, necessary trouble" to make a necessary difference. In this case it will be not a cure, but a difference.

Winston Richards, LLUSM class of 1974, is a retired urologist who resides in Riverside, California.

April 20

"May your unfailing love be with us, LORD, even as we put our hope in you."
Psalm 33:22, NIV

The invitation was extraordinary. In nearly three decades of work at LLUH I had been invited to take on many different assignments. But this was different. Dr. Wolff Kirsch, a neurosurgeon and one of our university's most distinguished medical scientists, called. He wanted to know if I would be willing to provide a service of blessing for a new research lab he would soon be opening. The lab, named for an accomplished Chinese researcher, would be devoted to finding an effective treatment for Alzheimer's disease.

What is the proper blessing for a research facility devoted to the study of Alzheimer's disease? In a whimsical moment I thought of the impoverished tailor in *Fiddler on the Roof* who asks the rabbi, "Is there a blessing for a sewing machine?" To which the rabbi answers, "There is a blessing for everything."

The rabbi is right, of course. There is a blessing for everything, and a uniquely special blessing for a research lab and the scientists who work there to find a cure for one of the most devastating diseases besetting humanity.

Dr. Kirsch, now in his late 80s, is one of the most hopeful people I know. He has a cheerful, contagious optimism. He believes that the research he and his colleagues are doing will lead to a breakthrough in the treatment of Alzheimer's disease. He lives, as all first-rate medical scientists must, in hope.

The text chosen for the occasion was from the prophet Jeremiah, who gave the people of God a message of hope. Even though they were living in captivity in a foreign land, the prophet delivered this promise from the Creator: "For surely I know the plans I have for you, says the LORD, plans for your welfare and not for harm, to give you a future with hope" (Jeremiah 29:11, NRSV).

Patients coping with Alzheimer's disease and their caregivers need that hope. So do we all.

As I walked away from the dedication service, through the hallways of our medical complex, past other research labs, and then patients' rooms, caregivers, and families, I thought about how much every one of us needs the hope that lives in an academic health sciences center. I thought, too, about how much brighter that hope is when such scientists as Dr. Wolff Kirsch acknowledge the gift of hope that is blessed by the God of hope.

Gerald Winslow, PhD, is professor of religion and director of the center for Christian bioethics at LLUH. He has been married to Betty Wehtje Winslow for 54 years. The Winslows have two daughters and two world-class grandsons.

April 21

> *"The good physician treats the disease; the great physician treats the patient who has the disease."*
> William Osler (1849–1919): Canadian physician and medical education pioneer

Often in this profession we come to a crossroads of mortality and spirituality. As we walk the halls of this hospital, we come to a realization that the walls of this hospital have often heard more sincere prayers than the walls of a church. But what does it mean to live and die? What does it mean to be a physician, then, when we are intimately taught of the eventual and dismal fate of all biological life?

Humans are innately social creatures, and part of it comes from being able to see the emotions written on the faces of the people around us. We see those faces and the scars embedded within, and for a brief chapter in the story of that patient's life we have a chance to intersect and learn. As the patient grapples with illness and their meaning of life, the physician grapples with health and the purpose of death. The physician garners a deeper insight into what it means to be healthy and live a purposeful life, ironically from an ailing and dying patient as the teacher. I then believe that the purpose of a physician is to serve as a guide. We serve as a guide to help them find and continue their own story, for it is not disease that we should seek to treat, but rather illness. In the face of illness and death, our devotion and gratitude to our patients should reflect our morals and principles—that we face our lives with dignity, live in honesty, and approach difficulty with grace.

What kind of legacy, then, do I want to leave? The motto of LLUH, "To make man whole," rings true with me in the sense of what legacy I want to leave. I want to become a physician that not only tends to the physical needs of my patients but also heals their heart. There is a science to medicine, and I believe there to be an art to it as well, in the form of being able to genuinely convey healing and empathy to your patients, just as a musician may convey joy and sadness through music. As a musician myself, I have a love for music and its powerful ability to express the intangible simply through combinations of chords. Just as a painter wields a brush to paint on a blank canvas and a dancer wields the body to paint on stillness, a musician wields an instrument to paint on silence. A physician is no different, with the capacity to wield his words and tools to convey emotions of empathy and compassion to patients.

So in the end, what legacy do I want to leave? As each patient composes their own story, I want to be a physician that does not regard them as merely another chart, but honors a sanctity for each person's life as it transects with mine. As each patient comes to me broken and in need, I want to continue the healing ministry of Christ to make people whole. In the end I want to be a physician who embodies both art and science in a profession that demands much, but gives even more in return.

Paul P. Kim, LLUSM class of 2022, is an avid writer who aspires to become a trauma surgeon. He enjoys music, video games, and automobiles in his free time.

April 22

> *"And he said to them, 'Go into all the world and proclaim the gospel to the whole creation.'"*
> Mark 16:15, ESV

As I looked out the window and saw the land disappearing through the clouds, my heart sank. I didn't want to return home after seven years of serving in the mission field. How could working in the U.S. bring as much fulfillment and joy as being a missionary doctor in Nigeria and Honduras? We had experienced daily miracles, both personally and with our patients. But God was calling us back to the United States to care for my mother-in-law. It was the right thing to do, but it didn't lessen the sadness of leaving.

Dr. Richard Hart (LLUSM class of 1970), had promised that he would find a job for us where we would be able to continue to serve. He arranged for me to work at SACHS (Social Action Community Health Service) in San Bernardino, California, an underserved area. He told me there was great need there and that it was Loma Linda's local mission field, but I wasn't convinced.

I had been working for only two weeks when one morning I had two patients that would change my perspective forever. The first was a Hispanic woman in her 50s with diabetes that was well-controlled. However, she was extremely preoccupied with her sugars. Curious, I probed as to why she was so concerned about her health. And that's when she opened up, sharing with me that her daughter-in-law had murdered one of her grandkids and was in jail. Now she was the caretaker for the other two grandkids since her son wasn't emotionally able to care for them. She needed to live at least another 10 to 15 years until the grandkids would turn 18 and could be on their own.

I couldn't believe what I was hearing. It was like something you would hear on the news, not from a patient in your exam room. In all my time in the mission field I had never seen such a tremendous need. I prayed with her as tears filled my eyes and encouraged her that together we would control her diabetes so she would be able to see her grandchildren well beyond 18 years.

The second patient was a young woman in her 30s. She was suffering from TMJ and had tried all kinds of treatments over many years, but nothing had seemed to help. Feeling a sense that I needed to ask more about her symptoms and when they started, she said that her husband had beaten her. She had left him and was now living alone, but the physical and emotional scars were still very evident. We prayed together for healing, and she cried. She had never shared her ordeal with anyone, and prayer seemed to be the treatment she needed the most that day.

After that morning at SACHS, I was convinced that God had brought me to another mission field, this one much closer to Loma Linda than Africa or Central America, but still with as much need.

Jason Lohr, LLUSM class of 2001, is an assistant professor in LLUSM's department of preventive medicine and the CEO of SAC Health System. He has been married to his wife, Belen (LLUSM class of 2001), for 20 years, and they have four children. They served seven years in Nigeria and Honduras.

April 23

> *"Prayer is the opening of the heart to God as to a friend."*
> Ellen G. White (1827–1915): *instrumental in the founding of Loma Linda University, one of the founders of the Seventh-day Adventist Church, and American author; in* Steps to Christ, *p. 93*

A week before Donelda's passing, a card from her appeared in our mail. I told my wife, "This may be the last letter from her," as she had just gone home on hospice, tired of dealing with progressive disability and pain. Inside it read: "Thank you for the beautiful Easter lilies—always my favorite with their beauty and perfume. Thank you for your visits and prayers. . . . Now having gout and quite painful. The devil tries to get me discouraged. . . . Stay well, and thank you for all you do. Love to all, Nelda."

I was asked to pray at Donelda's funeral. What to say? How did Donelda pray? Her sister and I talked about that. Donelda never had a dad that she remembered, so she talked to her heavenly Father like a dad. Her picture of God was that He was her trustworthy Father. She would talk to Him about tests of faith as she experienced them. Not just physical illness and pain, but also emotional tests. By nature she was fiercely independent, yet she had to deal with a progressive loss of independence. Despite tests of suffering, she remained courageous.

I decided to pray as Donelda might have, followed by the "Our Father" prayer.

Well, hello, Dad. It's so nice to talk to You. I wish I could see You as well. I'd give you a great big hug! I guess I've missed out on quite a few hugs. First it was my earthly father. I'm told he left our family when I was a toddler. I wish I could remember him hugging me, but I don't. It was such a thrill in later years to hear his voice on the phone saying "Well, hello, dear, how are you?"

You sent me a good man to be my husband. He was so thoughtful and the perfect gentleman. He was my rock. Thank You, Dad. But then he got sick and all too soon died. If it weren't for You, Dad, I couldn't have made it through. You have been my heavenly Rock, and with each trial the bond between You and me has grown stronger, because You had trials too. I can't imagine giving up a child to die in order to give life to people who mostly didn't even like me. But You did, and I'm so grateful, because that means that one day I'll see my husband again and give him a big hug. And see Jesus and give Him the biggest hug of all. I love the prayer that Jesus taught me—is it OK if we say it now?

"Our Father in heaven, hallowed be your name. Your kingdom come, your will be done, on earth, as it is in heaven. Give us this day our daily bread, and forgive us our debts, as we also have forgiven our debtors. And lead us not into temptation, but deliver us from evil" (Matthew 6:9–13, ESV). Amen.

David Bland completed his internal medicine residency at LLUH in 1981 and is an emeritus associate professor in LLUSM's department of medicine. He is retired and living in Australia with Wendy, his wife of 45 years. April 23, 2018, is the date that Donelda, LLUSM administrative assistant, passed to her rest from complications of scleroderma.

April 24

"Trust in the LORD *with all your heart, and lean not on your own understanding; in all your ways acknowledge Him, and He shall direct your paths."*
Proverb 3:5-6, NKJV

It was a Sunday night, and I went to the ER to readmit an 81-year-old patient that had been under my care for more than 30 years. To my dismay, he was highly suspicious for COVID-19. Once there, I evaluated my patient, but noticed that the staff were not following the required safety and protection protocols. Thoughts raced around in my mind as I contemplated my exposure risk to this deadly virus.

The following week I started to experience increasing fatigue and coughing with shortness of breath. My COVID swab was positive, and because I had severe oxygen desaturation, I knew I had to immediately be admitted to the hospital. Prior to leaving, I had to have the most difficult conversation with my wife and children. I promised them that I would be coming back home, but I really did not know what would happen to me with this deadly unknown virus.

I had been a patient in a hospital only once, at Bangkok Mission Hospital, when I was born. Other than that, I had never been severely ill requiring hospitalization. But suddenly I found myself in the ICU for 12 days, which gave me a lot of time to reflect on my life as a whole and all the things God had blessed me with. He had protected me from birth until now, and provided the means to accomplish many things that I know I could not have done on my own. He continued to watch over me during my stay in the ICU. I was on 70 percent oxygen @ 60L/min HFNC with d-dimer and pro-BNP continuing to rise each day. Despite these poor prognostic values, I remained quite calm, knowing God would provide wisdom to the critical care team in their daily review of my treatment. After two days of searching and delays, miraculously, my brother was able to locate the last two units of type AB convalescent plasma in California! My condition improved after receiving the plasma, and I was subsequently discharged, with recovery at home.

I recall another near brush with death experience last year when I returned home after seeing a critically ill patient. An assailant wearing a hockey mask pointed a 45-millimeter handgun at my head as I reached my driveway. My whole life suddenly flashed in front of me while I decided what to do. The assailant cocked his gun, but the bullet did not fire, and instead ejected from the side! That split second gave me the opportunity to speed away. This experience continues to strengthen my faith with God, knowing that he will continue to guide and protect me.

As a patient, knowing my family, friends, colleagues, hospital staff and others that have been praying for my recovery brings an incredibly special feeling and meaning, especially in this arduous journey. These two life-threatening events have enriched and strengthened my faith knowing God looks after and provides for me. God has never failed me nor forsaken me.

Basil Vassantachart, LLUSM class of 1979-B, has practiced as a family physician in Alhambra and Greater San Gabriel Valley for more than 40 years. He served as president of the LLUSMAA from 2016 to 2017. He also currently serves as MEC member of several local hospitals, member of the CMA CME steering committee, CME surveyor, and CME committee chair of local hospitals. He has been active in organizing several annual CME conferences, courses, and seminars for more than 30 years for medical staff and local community physicians and hospital staff. In his free time he and his wife enjoy exploring new places and having new experiences with their three grandchildren.

April 25

> *"Your kingdom come, your will be done, on earth, as it is in heaven."*
> Matthew 6:10, NIV

"I want to ride that."

Pointing to a rather formidable ride for a 2-year-old, my daughter made her desires clear for the second time that day. The miniature rocket ships twirling up around the giant pole caught her eye when we first entered the park and this time, she was insistent. So we stood in line for more than an hour and eventually strapped in for the ride. The video clip I have of her captures the joy and wonder (and a bit of apprehension) on her face as we are vaulted high in the sky with the California sunset bathing everything beneath us in a golden glow.

Disneyland truly is a fantastic place, a break from the mundane, to be enjoyed on special occasions, perhaps once a year (or every few years), or when guests come in from out of town, having heard from afar of the magical kingdom.

For most of my life I misunderstood Jesus' teachings about the kingdom of heaven to be describing some place like Disneyland. (The word "kingdom" coupled with the word "heaven" leads to all kinds of otherworldly associations—chubby angel babies strumming harps perched on clouds, wizards, or Princess Elsa). It was the good news of some other place and time, a spectacular place, that could be experienced and enjoyed one day. "Your kingdom come," I remember reciting as a child; I thought I was praying for the soon coming of the Second Coming.

It wasn't until much later in my life—relatively recently, in fact—I learned to connect those words with the ones that followed it and how it is that God's kingdom comes, God's will is done on earth as it is heaven. In praying these lines, I learned I am not praying for two things, but one thing. And this truly is good news! Life can be lived the way God intended, here and now. Each moment of the day is pregnant with this possibility and opportunity.

Sometimes, adjusting our lives to God's agenda takes a radical reorientation—a break with the past. "Repent. Follow me," Jesus said. Yet Jesus also spoke of the kingdom in other ways—a mustard seed or yeast working its way through bread dough. God's kingdom starts small, as something insignificant, and then grows to transform the world. I respond to God with this one thing in this one area, perhaps trivial in the grander scheme of things, but this can lead to responding in other areas and issues, coupled with greater insight, desire, and strength of will.

So instead of dreaming about the great things I will do for God one day or once in a while, I'm learning to look for the ways God's will can be done now—in the ways as I interact with my daughter (who is fast becoming a three-nager), respond to my spouse when I'm tired, work out a monthly family budget, prepare for my classes, deal with a difficult student, sit in traffic, surf the Internet, debate politics with friends, etc. I'm learning to surrender more now, bit by bit, and experiencing, step-by-step, more of the good life, as Jesus understood it.

Zane Yi, PhD, MA, is an associate professor in LLUSR, where he teaches courses in philosophy and theology. He also directs the MA in religion and society program. Zane and his wife, Angela, are proud parents of their daughter, Ava.

April 26

*"Let us therefore make every effort to do what leads
to peace and mutual edification."*
Romans 14:19, NIV

My father was a beloved and respected internist/endocrinologist. At one point he had in his practice a particular patient who caused greater than average puzzlement and perplexity for her caregivers.

This woman had been recently discovered to be diabetic, and as part of her overall plan she had been referred to skilled and experienced nurses who taught diabetic care classes. It was obviously important for her to learn about dietary and lifestyle issues in the management of her condition. As an integral portion of the teaching process she was also instructed in the administration of her insulin.

However, her lab values at the time of follow-up office visits demonstrated that her blood sugars were very poorly controlled. Therefore, she was sent back to the diabetic teaching classes for a refresher course, where a "small problem" was discovered.

She had been properly taught how to draw her insulin into the syringe, and the nurses had carefully instructed her in the art and science of injecting her insulin. For illustrative purposes the teachers utilized an orange as the object which to practice the act of delivering the injection. She had learned much in the classes and knew how to meticulously fill the needle with the appropriate number of units of the insulin. She then appreciatively and proudly demonstrated to the teaching nurse how she gave her injections at home. She carefully injected the insulin into an orange and would then conscientiously eat the entire orange! It was obvious to her that the insulin needed to get into her body somehow. With a "minor modification" of her medication delivery, her diabetes rapidly came under good control!

A few lessons might be gleaned from this unusual experience. Communication should be a process in which information is exchanged and absorbed. Then of course there is need for feedback and the opportunity for clarification and interchange of ideas. Did they understand what I said? Did I understand what they said? If there is breakdown at any point in the communication cycle, problems may develop which might be humorous or could be potentially disastrous. We should strive to accurately communicate the message we wish to impart to others but must also listen to what others are telling us verbally and nonverbally. Clarification and feedback are essential in a multitude of interpersonal interactions.

Second, doing the wrong thing with the best of intentions is still futile at best and dangerous at worst. Actions have consequences whether intended or unintended.

In our professional family and social interactions with others, may we accurately communicate both directly and indirectly to others that we love and are loved by an infinitely wise, loving, and caring God, who has only our best interests at heart.

Robert Rosenquist, LLUSM class of 1977-B, is an assistant clinical professor in LLUSM's department of ophthalmology. He completed his internship at LLUH in internal medicine, his ophthalmology residency at Oregon Health and Science University, his fellowship in glaucoma at Harvard Medical School, Massachusetts Eye and Ear Infirmary, and practiced at Kaiser Permanente, Redlands/Fontana, from 1993 to 2020. He has been married to Linda Drury Rosenquist for more than 46 years. He is the son of Robert Rosenquist, Sr. (CME class of 1946), former faculty in LLUSM's department of internal medicine/endocrinology.

April 27

> *"For our light and momentary affliction is producing for us*
> *an eternal glory that is far beyond comparison."*
> 2 Corinthians 4:17, BSB

April 27, 2009, was a day I will never forget. On that Monday my life changed forever. I was in my second year of medical school and had just finished taking my preventive medicine exam. I had four more days of testing left. I went to a friend's house so that we could study for the upcoming exams. True to form, I took a power nap on his couch. I was awakened by a phone call from my brother Nevin, informing me that Daddy had died.

I sat in the car with a knot in my throat trying to organize my thoughts while at the same time trying to recover from the gut punch I had just received. I knew this day would come, but it still found me unprepared. As I drove with Nevin to Riverside to inform my brother Delmont, I recall receiving multiple text messages from friends. Suddenly the 91 freeway appeared blurry as tears began to flow. The initial shock was wearing off; now I had to face my new reality.

I remember my first day returning to class after my father's funeral. It seemed as though everyone around me was fine, but I was stuck in slow motion. I felt alone, depressed, angry, confused, and stressed about medical school. I wanted to quit! A classmate of mine observed me sitting alone at the back of Alumni Hall auditorium; having lost her father in the past, she sat next to me and said, "I know how you feel." Immediately I was overcome with emotion at the compassion this person showed toward me. I was still in the slow lane, but I was not alone.

I was 23 years old when my dad closed his eyes in Christ, just 10 days prior to his 63rd birthday. I owe so much of who I am to his influence in my life. Daddy taught me to strive for excellence; 99 percent on a test was not enough when 100 percent was attainable. He taught me how to play chess, checkers, backgammon, Crazy Eights, and dominos. He taught me how to be gracious in defeat because he beat me in every chess game. He taught me how to catch crabs, dig for worms, and to fish. He bought me my motorbike, which I promptly crashed on the dirt road above my high school while wearing my brand-new, tan, Giovanni shoes. When I was thirsty, he often offered the best drink in the world, Rainbow Special, aka water. He taught me to share; he would come home with a bag of Skittles and divide it so that each of his eight sons could have some.

I can't eat digestives or bourbon biscuits* without thinking of him. He was not a perfect man and that's OK; neither am I. But his love for each of us was boundless. He was the type of father God knew I needed in order to save my soul. And God chose him just for me. I thank God for His promise that weeping may endure for a night, but joy will come in the morning. I can't wait to see my daddy again on that day.

*Digestives and bourbon biscuits are cookies popular in the United Kingdom and British Commonwealth countries and territories.

Shammah Williams, LLUSM class of 2011, was born number six of eight boys to his parents on the beautiful island of Bermuda. He was the second of three from his immediate family to graduate from LLUSM. He currently is an assistant professor in LLUSM's department of internal medicine, cardiology division.

April 28

"The LORD is good to those who wait for Him, to the soul who seeks Him. It is good that one should hope and wait quietly for the salvation of the LORD."
Lamentations 3:25-26, NKJV

It's Thursday afternoon at Loma Linda University Medical Center. I am down in the basement, "A" level, waiting for the staff elevator to carry me up several floors to a teleconference with a software vendor. The wait is long. Traffic is congested. Orderlies and transport teams are pushing a convoy of patients on gurneys from the emergency department onto the elevators. The door slides open to more patients on the ride up from being X-rayed or scanned a floor below. IVs are pumping and telemetry is beeping.

Another car arrives full of a large and complicated piece of equipment being moved from repair to service by the engineering department. Slender medical students wearing their blue scrubs as a proud fashion statement crowd in wherever they can find a space.

Patient care and medical and nursing education are the core businesses of the medical center and take precedence over negotiation with a vendor. I have no choice but to cool my heels.

Waiting is not something that I do well, and the elevator foyer of "A" level offers no incentive to linger. It is simply a bare-walled, fluorescent-lit passage for medical professionals and employees to get from here to there fast. Anything spiritual in that space has to be carried in the heart of those passing through and carried right out again. At least, that's the way it's always been for me until today.

It's been my experience that the ordinary places of our everyday lives is where we need grace. A place doesn't get more ordinary than "A" level. The walls were recently repainted an "earth" brown and the carpet replaced with a matching gray-brown pattern.

Lifting my fidgeting eyes, I am surprised to see what I first perceive to be graffiti. The "Spiritual Life and Wholeness" guys upstairs must have been at work. They've inscribed Psalm 46:10, KJV, in white calligraphy on the wall between two of the elevators—"Be still, and know that I am God."

My first reaction is to chuckle. This is a busy route to surgeries, colonoscopies, echocardiograms, angioplasties, and intensive care in the nine floors above me. Time is of the essence. Stillness is the last thing on anyone's mind when they come through here. "What's going to happen next?" is pretty much the question of the day.

No doubt prayers are prayed on the fly here. They are probably more of the "Help! Help! Help!" variety than any thoughtful reflection on the nature of the Deity. But I am a lawyer walking through on my own two feet with a briefcase full of contracts. What do I know?

I take another look. "Be still, and know that I am God" is a succinct statement of grace.

Before starting that elevator ride up for work, for diagnosis, for treatment, for surgery, for the hospital stay that has an uncertain outcome, the one essential truth to think about is that there is a God in charge of everything and that He cares about us. Other thoughts shadow us—our illness, injuries, work, budgets, what we've left back home or in the classroom—but this thought needs to stop us in our hasty, anxious tracks: "Be still, and know that I am God."

It is the absurd reality of grace that the busier the day, the greater the need for a stillness of heart; and the more responsibilities and concerns that cram into our thinking, the less we need to know anyone or anything else but God.

I make it into an elevator on the third try and go on to my teleconference, but the Lord was kind to me when He made me wait. Who knew that the elevator foyer of "A" level could be holy ground? The Word of the Lord come to life in a waiting heart made it so.

Kent Hansen is the general counsel for Loma Linda University Health, a position he has held since 2000. He is blessed to have served the institution for his entire 42-year legal career.

April 29

> *"When you judge others you reveal your inability
> to see them through God's eyes."*
> Carlos A. Rodríguez (1961–): Puerto Rican Christian author

It was late one night when my pager went off and I was called to the OR STAT! It had already been a grueling day as an anesthesiology resident at the former Riverside General Hospital. I was hoping for at least some sleep on my call night. But this was not to be. I was informed that we had a major trauma case. A person crossing the street at night had been run over by a car. The patient suffered severe internal injuries and open fractures of the lower extremities, resulting in hypovolemic shock. *Another all-nighter*, I thought, *with a "John Doe." Someone who is probably a drunk, who wandered into traffic*, I told myself, as I readied my equipment in the OR. These kinds of cases can be very demanding. Yes, this drunk would keep me busy all night, and to what end? If he makes it through these surgeries and recovers, he'll probably be back within a few weeks or months with similar problems. What a waste of time, pouring all these resources into saving a bum.

After several hours in the OR the patient started to respond to our surgical and resuscitative efforts. With the patient's vital signs stabilizing, I thought it was a good time for us to clean the bloodstained hair and upper extremities. As we wiped away the clotted blood and road debris, I noticed the patient appeared to be fairly well kept. *How odd*, I thought, *he didn't even smell of alcohol!*

Shortly thereafter, a nurse came up from the ER and announced his name. My jaw dropped. This man was a prominent pastor in Southern California! I knew him! I immediately cranked my head and took another look at my patient lying on the operating table. Sure enough, it WAS the pastor! I hadn't recognized him . . . his ghostlike appearance, along with his bloodstained clothing, hair, and face, made him unrecognizable.

What a mistake assuming this patient was a simple bum! As I was pondering this thought, I had a strong impression that it didn't matter who this patient was. All are children of God. The words, "If you have done it unto the least of these, you have done it unto me" flashed into my mind . . . as if they were blinking neon lights.

I suddenly had an overwhelming sense of guilt and shame. I had been so judgmental and unchristlike, caring more about my own needs, instead of the needs of this patient.

Now, before similar cases, I pray: "You know I certainly don't want to be up at this hour of the night. But there is a reason I am here tonight, so use me as You will. Give me clarity of mind, and the wisdom and skills I need to help this patient as best as I can."

And praise God, the pastor made a full recovery!

Jon Richards, LLUSM class of 1979-B, is a retired anesthesiologist who enjoys living near Seattle. He has a passion for making God's character of love known.

April 30

*"Realize that you are God's masterpiece created to do things
that you can't even yet imagine."*
Mark J. Musser: contemporary American Christian author

Throughout my medical school journey I have noticed that when obstacles arise, this tiny negative thought tries to take over: *Do I belong here?*

With few underrepresented minorities in medicine, and health care disparities disproportionately affecting our communities, being Black in medicine is both an accomplishment and a necessity. My path to medicine was by no means seamless, so I can confidently say that God placed me here at LLUSM.

I graduated from high school as a Gates Millennium Scholar; a successful student athlete. So why did I struggle in undergrad, and why didn't I feel that I belonged? Could it be that I didn't study as I should have? Or was it the microaggressions and discouragement from some professors whose help I sought? "Choose a different career," one said. "Medicine is not for you." Negativity defeated my confidence. I tried to replicate my high school success by making the track team, but ended the year with both hamstrings strained. I graduated unsure of the future and filled with self-doubt.

We cannot see the path ahead, but there is One who can. I decided to listen to God and God alone. I excelled in a postbaccalaureate program, and grew spiritually. Then with funding from my Gates scholarship, during my medical school application cycle I pursued a master's degree in something I loved: biomedical sciences with a focus on human anatomy.

After the first semester I still had no responses from medical schools, but every morning I played Norman Hutchins' "God's Got a Blessing (With My Name on It!)," and by February I had been accepted to a medical school in Colorado. Although not my first choice, I was very grateful, and verbally committed. Just one week later I was invited to interview at Loma Linda. Knowing how much I wanted to attend Loma Linda, my advisor encouraged me to accept. The interview went well, and the campus was warm and welcoming. I continued praying for God's guidance, and received two more interview invitations which I declined. I had faith that God would decide if I was meant to be used in California or Colorado.

Late one afternoon a letter arrived from a member of the church I had attended during undergrad. It read: "Thanking God for your admission to Loma Linda!" I explained that I had not received any news yet, but she encouraged me to stay positive even if I hadn't been accepted. That same evening I received the acceptance call from Loma Linda! I was overjoyed! It was clear. God wanted me at LLUSM!

Discouragements do arise, but with the "plague" of health care disparities more evident than ever, I am reminded why God placed me here. My life's journey has not only prepared me for medical school, but has also inspired and equipped me to mentor young Black children and to advocate for patients of various backgrounds. The enemy still sometimes whispers, "Do you belong?" But God's Word assures me that in the end, whatever the obstacle or microaggression, I do belong.

Danae Smart, LLUSM class of 2022, is the daughter of hardworking, resilient parents who immigrated from the island of Jamaica. Her goal is to impact the lives of her patients by sharing Christ's healing ministry.

MAY

☙ EXCELLENCE ❧

"The secret of joy in work is contained in one word—excellence. To know how to do something well is to enjoy it."

PEARL S. BUCK (1892–1973)
Nobel Prize Laureate in Literature, equal rights
activist, and American author

May 1

"Your body will grow feeble, your teeth will decay, and your eyesight fail. The noisy grinding of grain will be shut out by your deaf ears, but even the song of a bird will keep you awake. You will be afraid to climb up a hill or walk down a road. Your hair will turn as white as almond blossoms. You will feel lifeless and drag along like an old grasshopper."

Ecclesiastes 12:3-5, CEV

Over the years I have had the privilege of caring for several of my mentors, teachers, and their families. When I have considered these relationships with my patients, different thoughts have crossed my mind. *Who will one day be taking care of me or my family? Will they have the skills, knowledge base, and temperament to entrust our care to them? What is my role in their training? How hard should I push them? How much responsibility do I give them?* As a professor I would frequently tell the residents, "If I am hard on you, please don't take it personally. Someday I may be lying on an operating room table, and when I look up and see you, I want to know that you know what you are doing and that I can trust your judgment and skill implicitly."

In the late 1970s I enjoyed getting together with friends for a friendly game of basketball. That enjoyment ceased after sustaining a left knee injury. Over the years the range of motion gradually decreased and the discomfort increased to the point of interfering with sleep and daily activities. Climbing stairs, let alone mountains, was no longer enjoyable. Long walks became shorter, and the orthopedist's recommendation to have the knee replaced was more inviting and finally accepted.

On the day that surgery was scheduled I dutifully arrived at the hospital, signed in, had identification and insurance verified, and was ushered back to the pre-op holding area. Then the usual questions: When did I last drink fluids, eat solid food, have any symptoms of a cold or a sore throat—and the list went on and on. Having survived the cross examination and been deemed someone who was not going to ruin their statistics, I was handed a skimpy patient gown and told to undress. I donned that paper excuse for a gown and crawled onto the gurney. A "young" man opened the curtains and introduced himself as Dr. X, my anesthesiologist. His first question was: "Are you Dr. Briggs?"

"Yes." (I wondered who had spilled the beans.)

"Are you Dr. Briggs from Loma Linda?" (Now, this was getting serious!)

"Yes."

"Well, I was one of your residents back in the 1980s."

You can imagine the questions and thoughts that went racing through my mind! As he proceeded to explain the anesthetic portion of the procedure, my questions gradually dissipated under the effect of intravenous Versed and Fentanyl. After a short visit with Morpheus, I awoke from what seemed like a short catnap feeling a little thirsty but quite refreshed. Such a change from the days of ether! Dr. X proved himself to be a skilled practitioner of his craft, for which I was *very* thankful.

Yes, teaching does have its concerns and worries, but it certainly has its rewards.

Burton Briggs, LLUSM class of 1966, is an emeritus professor in LLUSM's department of anesthesiology. He and his wife, Carol, have been married 16 years and have two children, Susan and Cynthia. They are currently retired and maintain a u-pick apple orchard in Emmett, Idaho, where they reside. In the early 1970s, Burton was LLUMC's physician leader in developing the collaboration between surgeons and anesthesiology intensivists in caring for critically ill surgical patients. That model is still in use in 2021.

May 2

"There is nothing to be valued more highly than to have people praying for us; God links up His power in answer to their prayers."
Oswald Chambers (1874–1917): Scottish evangelist and teacher

Every doctor has stories that are seared in their memory forever. As a family practitioner for more than 60 years, I recall one in particular like it was yesterday.

I had just completed delivering a healthy, normal baby girl from a mother whose family was personal friends from our church. While I was tending to the baby and tying the cord, I heard the sound of running water behind me and turned around to see blood literally gushing into the splash basin! There was only one obstetrician on our medical staff, and he "happened" to be in the next room. I desperately summoned him, and he came right away. After a quick inspection, no lacerations were detected, but the blood continued to pour. He was unsuccessful in attempting to clamp the uterine arteries vaginally, and our attempt to stanch part of the flow with packs did little good.

At that time (more than 50 years ago) there were no anesthesiologists on staff. A nurse anesthetist was assigned to each delivery, and supervision of them was by an anesthesiologist in Boston who was available via a landline telephone. There was no blood bank in the hospital, and it usually took at least 30 to 45 minutes to secure blood from a nearby hospital. With such a large blood loss, the patient immediately went into shock, and we administered plasma and plasma expanders. One of the two surgeons on the medical staff "happened" to be in the hospital making rounds, and miraculously, he was of the same blood type as the patient! He donated a unit of his own blood, which was given by direct transfusion. He then assisted the obstetrician in entering the abdomen with the few surgical instruments available in the delivery room. The two physicians were eventually able to clamp the uterine arteries and perform a subtotal hysterectomy and then close the patient as quickly as possible! All this time the patient remained in shock until we were eventually able to have blood delivered by ambulance. Finally after what seemed like an eternity, we could detect a blood pressure.

My wife, Peggy, was home and knew our friend was in labor. Since the delivery was taking longer than expected, she feared something had gone seriously wrong, and she began earnestly praying. As Peggy was praying, we were anxiously checking for brain damage as the patient slowly returned to consciousness. The patient awoke, and we assessed that there was no apparent brain damage from this life-threatening episode.

The pathology report confirmed that the bleeding was from placenta accreta. Even today with all the advances in modern medicine, it may require large quantities of readily available blood to stabilize a patient in such an emergency. I have no explanation for how so many events that day unfolded: how a patient can be in shock for so long and have no brain damage. It is humbling to know that God can take over and produce a favorable outcome even when our best efforts seem so inadequate.

As a side note, this miracle patient had no negative aftereffects from that episode. Years later she was the teacher for two of my grandchildren in the nearby church school.

Robert Rittenhouse, CME class of 1949, practiced family medicine in Marlboro, Massachusetts, for 50 years. His wife of 67 years, Peggy, graduated from LLUSN class of 1955. He served in the Navy during the Korean War. His two children are graduates of his alma mater (Connie [LLUSM class of 1983] and Jerry [LLUSM class of 1985]), as is one granddaughter (Julie [LLUSM class of 2014]). Some of his interests include world travel and private aviation.

May 3

> "See what kind of love the Father has given to us,
> that we should be called children of God."
>
> 1 John 3:1, ESV

"You have value because of who you are." I have used this phrase hundreds, and maybe thousands, of times—most often with patients, but also with those in medical training. Our training is grueling, we are very hard on ourselves, and our society and system expect perfection. We are imperfect, and when we do not live up to personal and societal professional expectations, the emotional consequences can be severe.

As a residency program director, I work with trainees, and it is a privilege to play a role in their journey to become caring and competent physicians. In this position I get to rejoice with them during times of accomplishment and success and join in their sorrow during times of sadness and pain.

One time, I worked with a very nervous third-year medical student. She had significant anxiety about the volume and pressure of medical education; she was fearful she would not be successful in medicine. Adding to the stress, a parent was in poor health, and her family directed medical questions to her. Since she was in her first month of clinical medicine, she did not have the knowledge to guide them. She was concerned she was not doing as well as expected academically and was disappointing her family and not adequately serving her patients. We talked many times, and she was encouraged by hearing that she had earned her place in school and that others also struggle (but often don't share these feelings). Hearing that her feelings were normal and experiencing common and learning coping skills and guidance from the mental health professionals available for medical students led to success in medical school.

Another time a resident was doing well in training and on track to be an excellent physician. He met with me one day to relay he may need some time off work to take care of a personal matter. A story of his marriage falling apart and children needing more love and support came flooding out with tears and palpable pain. He was concerned he would let his patients down if he wasn't perfect. We talked frequently; I made an adjustment in his work schedule and checked in with him frequently to be sure he was managing well. He made it through this rough time with support from peers and others, and today is a thriving physician. He has relayed that the support of his "work family" buoyed him through.

The joy and satisfaction of helping others brings many of us to medicine. I am fulfilled by helping trainees find value in themselves and grow into compassionate physicians. These experiences, and the support I receive from colleagues during rough times, helps me be a better physician. The resiliency of humans who are devoted to caring for others is wonderful. Many trainees and physicians are hurting, and despite this, they continue to come to work and lean upon their training, compassion for others, and desire to make a difference in the lives of their patients to provide care "To make man [and woman] whole." The physician also needs compassion and support. Let's treat each other with care so we can all continue to care for our patients.

Laura Nist, LLUSM class of 1995, is an associate professor in LLUSM's department of neurology. She values time with her husband of 25 years, three children, and hiking with her dogs, as well as fulfilling her work mission of teaching neurology.

May 4

> *"Let the favor of the Lord our God be upon us, and establish the work of our hands upon us; yes, establish the work of our hands!"*
>
> Psalm 90:17, ESV

As someone who has a strong family history of coronary artery disease, I developed a nearly "fatal" attraction to it. Coupled with my fascination with the Mayo brothers as a child, I welcomed the opportunity to spend seven years at the Mayo Clinic in Rochester, Minnesota, where I first studied internal medicine, then cardiology, and finally interventional cardiology. During my time at Mayo, I met many amazing physicians and surgeons with blessed minds and hands who carefully taught me their craft.

One of my most memorable experiences, however, occurred with someone from the environmental services department whose name I never learned. She was in her 60s and her face and hands appeared weathered, consistent with one who had spent many long and hard winters on one of the surrounding farms. One night during my first year there, around 1:00 a.m., I had a break in between hospital admissions and decided to run down to the employee cafeteria, which is located on one the many mazelike corridors in the bowels of the huge Saint Marys campus, one of the two Mayo Clinic hospitals. I made a wrong turn and ended up in a hallway near the boiler room, where I happened upon this woman on her hands and knees with a toothbrush, trying to remove a black mark in a corner from an otherwise-immaculate white-tiled floor. While asking for directions to my intended location, I inquired as to why she was extending so much effort to remove the last mark on an almost immaculate floor, particularly in an area where there was very little traffic. She said, "Well, Doctor, for 30 years my job each night has been to clean these floors, and I would never leave such a mark on any floor that I clean." I was amazed. Why would someone work so diligently to remove a mark on a floor that was wandered upon mostly by accident because of a wrong turn or two?

It left a profound impact on me that remains to this day. No matter what I'm doing, even if it seems small and inconsequential, I try to do it to the best of my ability. The work done by each of us collectively exceeds the sum of the individual parts, and when done to the best of our abilities, it can create a masterpiece. The Lord has established the work of our hands to carry out His plans. My prayer for you today is my prayer every day—to approach each day with a genuine earnestness, to use your hands to continue to build the temple of God, similar to this woman from the environmental services department on her hands and knees scrubbing the little-trafficked floor at 1:00 a.m.

Anthony Hilliard, LLUSM class of 2002, is an associate professor and chief of cardiology in LLUSM's department of medicine. He is also the chief operating officer of the LLU Faculty Medical Group. He and his wife, Tammy, have two children, Sophia and Max.

May 5

> *"For what will it profit a man if he gains the whole world,
> and loses his own soul?"*
> Mark 8:36, NKJV

What does it profit a man to gain the whole world but lose his own soul? And what does it profit a man to gain 20/20 vision but not be able to "see" God? As an ophthalmologist, I perform numerous cataract surgeries every year and have done so for more than 20 years. I have helped many patients improve their eyesight, but a more significant accomplishment would be to help improve their insight into what is truly important in life.

Where I work, surgery patients are asked if they would feel comfortable if the surgeon prays with them before surgery. We don't "force" our patients to listen to our prayers, but instead would hope they recognize our dependence on the Great Physician as we perform their procedure. Most patients say yes, and we pray for God's blessing and guidance before we start their surgery. Occasionally a patient says no, so we pray for them silently. The majority of my patients are in their 70s and 80s, yet they often tell me that I was the first doctor that ever prayed with them. Some patients are very nervous before surgery, and praying for divine guidance seems to put them at ease. Even those who are not professed Christians seem to appreciate the prayers.

The Bible tells us to "pray without ceasing" (1 Thessalonians 5:17, KJV). So even during surgery, prayer helps me focus on what is important and avoid distractions. I receive many thank-you cards, and often they express appreciation for my prayer before surgery. This encourages me to pray more, especially in those situations in which we as health care providers don't have much more to offer. Prayer gives hope for the miraculous since God can do anything. Pastor Mark Finley says, "It is God's desire to heal each one of us. He desires us to be free from pain, sickness, and disease. The only question is one of timing. At times God heals us instantly. Sometimes He uses the modern miracle of science or natural means to heal us gradually, and at times He strengthens us to face death itself with the promise of healing in the resurrection. By faith we leave the timing of our healing up to God and by His strength give glory to Him in sickness and health."

While the physical healing we provide through medical and surgical care is temporary, spiritual healing is for eternity. May each of us in our own small way strive to direct our patients to Jesus, who is the true healer of all infirmities.

Paul Y. Chung, LLUSM class of 1991, is an adjunct assistant professor in LLUSM's department of ophthalmology and an ophthalmologist working at Pacific Cataract and Laser Institute in Chehalis, Washington.

May 6

> *"Children are a gift from the LORD; they are a reward from him."*
> Psalm 127:3, NLT

Parents are devoted to their children and are continually preoccupied with their well-being. Whether they are infants or adolescents, in every stage of youth parents lavish their time and energy to make sure their children are loved and cared for.

This is especially true of parents of newborn babies. They have a type of devotion that borders on obsession. Many memorize every inch of skin the baby has and mark those areas in which the hue is a decimal percentage off from what they expect it to be. Sometimes I think I may have found a new birthmark on exam, but—no, of course not—this is old news to parents. In fact, they have already counted how many hairs the baby has on its head! Parents draw up charts giving account of every feeding and wet diaper; they take note of every time the baby has a hiccup. I cannot tell you how many times parents have described and shown me—without solicitation—the subtle change in the color of their newborn's stool. Once a new mother asked me if it was OK that her baby had sneezed twice. This is love and devotion!

The love and devotion parents have for their offspring illustrate the love and devotion our heavenly Father has toward us, His children. He says, "Yea, I have loved thee with an everlasting love: therefore with lovingkindness have I drawn thee" (Jeremiah 31:3, KJV). I have often wondered what it means to be the object of everlasting love. Recently I read a statement penned by Ellen White, who was instrumental in the founding of Loma Linda University, that elaborates on this love: "Christ came to the world with the accumulated love of eternity" (*Education*, p. 76). The accumulated love of eternity. How can one begin to understand this love? The love of eternity, collected and somehow packaged all in the gift of Christ. Our omnipotent and infinite Father could not have given more. What is equally astonishing is that this everlasting and accumulated love is for all of the world, but it is, at the same time, just for you and just for me. "The relations between God and each soul are as distinct and full as though there were not another soul upon the earth to share His watchcare, not another soul for whom He gave His beloved Son" (Ellen G. White, *Steps to Christ*, p. 100).

The next time you see a mother or father coddling and admiring their newborn, pressing their noses upon their baby's cheeks, think about how God feels about you—how He cares for and infinitely loves you.

And don't even get me started on grandparents!

Daniel Calaguas, LLUSM class of 2013, is an assistant professor in LLUSM's department of pediatrics, and the associate medical director of the Pediatric Spina Bifida Team Clinic. He is married to Shannon (née Fujimoto, LLUSM 2019), who is currently an ENT resident at LLUH.

May 7

> *"Health care is an expression of the gospel, the healing and teaching ministry of Jesus Christ—to make man whole."*
>
> Richard B. Hays (1948–): American New Testament scholar

Jesus was a healer. "Many crowds followed him, and he cured all of them" (Matthew 12:15, NRSV). When He told a parable about the last judgment, he emphasized that the "sheep" on the right hand of the Son of man would be those who had cared for the sick: "I was sick and you took care of me" (Matthew 25:36, NRSV). And when he sent followers out to proclaim His message, this was His charge to them: "Cure the sick who are there, and say to them, 'The kingdom of God has come near to you'" (Luke 10:9, NRSV).

It is therefore no surprise that as the early church began to spread through the Mediterranean world, one of its distinctive hallmarks was its passion for caring for the sick and the dying. Hospitals as we know them today in Western culture had their origin in religious communities that sought to extend Christian hospitality to all in need, including strangers (cf. Romans 12:13).

The Greek verb *sozo* ("save") appears both in stories of Jesus' healings ("your faith has saved you [i.e., made you well]," as in Mark 5:34; 10:52) and in proclamations about the eschatological destiny of the faithful ("Everyone who calls on the name of the Lord shall be saved" [Romans 10:13, NRSV]).

Consequently, how are we to interpret this passage in the letter of James? "Are there any among you sick? They should call for the elders of the church and have them pray over them, anointing them with oil in the name of the Lord. The prayer of faith will save the sick, and the Lord will raise them up" (James 5:14-15, NRSV). Is this a promise of the healing of illness or of resurrection on the other side of death?

The ambiguity is perhaps deliberate, emphasizing that care for the bodies of those who are sick cannot be separated from the church's ministry of prayer and intercession. For that reason, a concern for what we have come to call "health care" is deeply embedded in the genetic code of the church.

In my time with the School of Medicine, I have more deeply experienced that what Dr. Hays says is true: Health care is an expression of the gospel, the healing and teaching ministry of Jesus Christ—to make [humanity] whole.

Susan Ranzolin is LLUSM's assistant dean for admissions and is a former OB/GYN nurse at White Memorial Medical Center (now Adventist Health White Memorial) in Los Angeles. Her husband, Leo, is the dean of LLU School of Religion. This story was originally presented as a devotional at the LLUSM dean's administrative council.

May 8

Mother's Day, 2022

> *"Can a mother forget the baby at her breast and have no compassion on the child she has borne? Though she may forget, I will not forget you!"*
> Isaiah 49:15, NIV

I was performing an obstetrical ultrasound on 26-year-old Mary. She was near the end of her second pregnancy. She was excited about bringing home a baby brother for Megan, her 2-year-old daughter.

As I moved the ultrasound transducer over Mary's pregnant uterus, I was shocked to see her fetus was severely swollen, with edematous skin and fluid collections in the chest and abdomen. The diagnosis: massive nonimmune fetal hydrops with pericardial and pleural effusions. As a maternal-fetal medicine subspecialist, I knew this condition is almost uniformly lethal. There is almost no chance of survival. How was I going to break the news to Mary?

I breathed a prayer for God to give me the sensitivity to say the appropriate words. As I gently pointed out to Mary the devastating sonogram findings and the most likely fatal outcome, she was speechless. Then came the flood of tears. And next the inevitable questions: "Are you really sure? Could the images be in error? Maybe there is a mistake."

At Mary's next prenatal visit, we discussed delivery planning: vaginal delivery versus cesarean section. Induction of labor with anticipated vaginal delivery would be less risky with more rapid recovery time for her. The downside would be that unborn son would probably not survive labor and would be stillborn. A cesarean section, however, had more risks and a longer recovery for her. Also, even though her son would be born alive, there was a 99 percent probability he would die shortly after birth anyway.

Mary listened carefully to my explanation of options, then carefully reflected, "I understand there is less than 1 percent chance my baby may survive and that surgery has more risks for me. But I want to give him that chance."

I performed the scheduled cesarean as she requested, and the surgery was uncomplicated. However, her severely hydropic baby, while born alive, tragically died within an hour after birth, as I expected. When she came to my office for the postoperative visit, I wondered how she felt about her decision for cesarean delivery. She had a long scar on her abdomen and no baby to show for her pain and discomfort. I asked if she would do it again, knowing her baby would die. I was surprised, but also inspired by Mary's response. "Do I have any regrets? None! After all, I was able to hold him for an hour, didn't I? Those are special memories."

If a mother's love and desire to spend time with her doomed baby will lead her to undergo the risks of a major surgery, how much greater is God's love and desire to spend time in relationship with each one of us. Oh, what love is this!

Elmar Sakala, LLUSM class of 1973-B, was a professor in LLUSM's department of gynecology and obstetrics and a maternal-fetal medicine specialist prior to his retirement. He was LLUSM's Teacher of the Year in 1979, 1990, and 1996. He was a LLUSM faculty member for 43 years. He is grateful to God for his wife, Darilee, to whom he has been married for 54 years.

May 9

"Excellence is never an accident; it is the result of high intention, sincere effort, intelligent direction, skillful execution and the vision to see obstacles as opportunties."

Anonymous

While boarding a recent flight out of Salt Lake City, my colleague and friend Doug Hegstad (LLUSM class of 1980-A) and I were going through the routine of balancing our carry-on bags in one hand and scanning the aircraft for our seats. As usual, there was a sluggish but inexorable flow of passengers heading toward the rear of the plane with frequent stops as bags were placed in the overhead bins and people shuffled into their seats.

In the midst of this one-way traffic there was one person who not only stopped midway on the plane, but began to make his way back against the flow of passengers. His build was slight; he was probably in his late 60s, with graying hair. As my peripheral vision caught sight of his bobbing head, my heart gave a little irritable beat of annoyance, assuming it was a passenger who forgot a bag or wanted to stow something in the front compartment. But at the same time his eyes were turned in our direction, and he continued to look at us as he weaved in and out of the aisle to let passengers by. He was smiling, which I thought was unusual, and perhaps meant that he knew us. So then I started to wonder, *Does he look familiar, and am I going to remember his name?* Finally he reached a point a few aisles away to where we could hear him.

"Excuse me," he said earnestly, leaning toward us. "I just wanted you to know that I saw your jacket."

Since I wasn't wearing a jacket, I turned to Doug, who was wearing the gray jacket we had received at our recent annual retreat, embroidered with "Loma Linda University Health" in white and red thread.

The passenger smiled and continued, "You saved my sister's life at Loma Linda, and I'll never forget it." People around us now turned their heads to follow the conversation. We were surprised and a little self-conscious to be singled out, but he continued, "She had heart failure and then needed a heart transplant. Unfortunately she eventually passed away, but she had great care at Loma Linda, and I just wanted you to know that." And then he turned back to find his seat. Those standing around us also paused, and there were more than a few smiles on their faces at this brief but poignant and unexpectedly positive encounter.

That passing moment was a reminder of the profound influence LLUH has on our patients, our providers, and our community. While each day brings a new set of challenges to health care, we should always remember that God has bestowed on us the chance to further the mission* of Loma Linda University Health in people's lives and to provide comfort and healing to those in need.

*To continue the teaching and healing ministry of Jesus Christ

---

Bryan Tsao, LLUSM class of 1996, is a professor in LLUSM's department of neurology. His wife, Juna, was a classmate and practices in LLUSM's family medicine department. They have two children, who share their passion for animals and their many pets.

May 10

"He heals the brokenhearted and binds up their wounds."
Psalm 147:3, NIV

The wrinkles on her face deepened as I walked through the door. Her face had broken into a smile—a grin, actually. I could tell she was happy to be here, in my clinic, in an exam room, to discuss her painful shoulder. It was an urgent visit; she had just called in earlier that day and scheduled it. But this was my first time seeing her.

So I smiled back and proceeded through the routine of asking her history of the shoulder pain, examining her, and discussing possible diagnoses and treatment options. But as I went through this routine, I soon realized she was there for more than just the shoulder pain. She had had this same pain for months—why schedule an urgent visit now? And she had a scheduled appointment tomorrow already—why not wait and see if it was warranted?

The answer became clear as I was wrapping up our visit and typing the last parts of my note, and I heard her voice echo behind me, "I guess I just wanted some attention."

My thoughts stopped abruptly. My focus zoomed in. My heart opened up and filled with compassion. I turned to look at her. She was smiling, her wrinkles deepened again. She had just wanted attention—she wanted reassurance that she mattered in this world, that she was loved. I admired her bravery in being vulnerable—she had opened up to me a deep desire of her heart which needed to be filled.

But that wasn't my job as a doctor, I thought . . . or was it? Was it OK that people walked into my clinic just wanting attention? The message I had gotten through my young career was *No*. That would definitely not be reimbursable; I wouldn't be able to justify it in my notes. That was the job of a psychologist or a pastor and not a doctor.

Then why was it that my heart went out to her, and something about it felt so right? My thoughts flashed back to many times in my life when I wanted attention too, and perhaps didn't get enough of it. Then I thought of all the people in this world—all of us needing reassurance that we matter, our souls needing soothing and healing. So many people don't have any place to go to get that relief, why couldn't doctors' offices—supposedly homes of healing—be one place? Yes, they should; my office will be, I told myself.

Breaking out of my reverie (all of which had probably lasted less than five seconds), I went to her and hugged her. "We all need attention sometimes," I said.

And she strode out of my office, smile still stuck on her face, having left behind an imprint on my heart.

Dipika Pandit, LLUSM class of 2009, is a family practitioner in Loma Linda, California. She was the 2009 recipient of the Wil Alexander Whole Person Care Award. Note: For Wil Alexander's bio, refer to the devotional on January 18.

May 11

> "Unless the LORD builds the house, those who build it labor in vain."
> Psalm 127:1, ESV

My wife and I had been married for four years when we decided that it was time to start our family. I was starting my chief year of urology residency, and we had a void in our lives that our cute dog could not fulfill. One of my coresidents had a young baby daughter, and we could see the joy in their lives that this young child brought. After much prayer and consideration, my wife stopped her birth control, and we thought that everything was going to proceed as planned according to our schedule.

Twelve months passed with no success. We had false alarms, but the pregnancy tests were invariably negative. As we prepared to move to the East Coast for a fellowship, our doctor told us that we would have to go through an extensive fertility evaluation since we were in the 15 percent of infertile couples. We were devastated. We started to question if God wanted us to be parents.

After we relocated in June 2010 to a new hospital, city, and state, we started to schedule a few doctor's appointments. The fertility clinic was scheduled out to October, and we would have to wait until that time to start our evaluation.

In September my wife came home from a weekend trip feeling very ill. She was nauseous and very fatigued, as if she had food poisoning. She was in bed for three days. I joked with her that maybe she was pregnant. We both knew that it was very unlikely, since her cycles had been very sporadic, and in fact, she had not been regular since stopping birth control one and a half years ago.

I was in the OR on a cold and dreary Thursday. My cell phone rang multiple times, but I ignored the calls. There were five missed calls from my wife. I called back after scrubbing out, expecting some bad news, since she rarely called me unless it was an emergency. Despite my joking, she had bought a three-pack of pregnancy tests, and all of them had come back *positive!* She was *pregnant!*

I was speechless. After 18 months of trying, we were going to be parents! How could this be? We went to the OB/GYN appointment in October, and the nursing staff and doctor could not believe it either. God had answered our prayers.

Our son was born on May 11, 2011, just six weeks before I finished my training and moved back to Loma Linda to start a new phase of our lives. Fast-forward two and a half years, and our daughter was born on October 11, 2013. Besides meeting each other, getting married, matching into residency, and getting hired, having two healthy children have been two of the best things to happen to us. I praise God for blessing us with children, as they are truly a gift from Him, according to His timing.

Ironically, my fellowship was in male infertility.

Edmund Ko, LLUSM class of 2005, is an associate professor and residency program director in LLUSM's department of urology. He completed his urology residency at Mayo Clinic in Arizona and has been with LLUSM's department of urology since 2011. He is married and has two energetic children.

May 12

*"Remember your leaders, who spoke the word of God to you.
Consider the outcome of their way of life and imitate their faith."*
Hebrews 13:7, NIV

As a junior medical student on a busy cardiothoracic surgery rotation, I had the opportunity to participate in correcting a VSD in a 7-year-old girl. The fellow and I carefully opened her little chest to expose her heart in preparation for Dr. Leonard Bailey (LLUSM class of 1969) to conduct the repair. I admit I felt somewhat starstruck as the LLU icon entered the OR. I introduced myself to him, and he invited me to stand right next to him during the operation. During the procedure we listened to a beautiful male operatic voice singing an enchanting melody. I asked Dr. Bailey who the singer was. He said it was Andrea Bocelli, the blind Italian opera singer. I explained how I loved music, since both of my parents were professional jazz musicians in New Orleans. I told him my father had recently sent me a video of an Andrea Bocelli concert. Dr. Bailey asked if I had watched it yet. When I told him "Not yet," he emphatically stated, "Son, when your dad takes the time to send you a video, you need to watch it!" As we continued the surgery and our conversation, he turned to the circulating nurse and said, "Get his dad on the phone." The nurse looked a little confused, but proceeded to carry out the order. I shared the phone number, and the phone cord was stretched across the large OR so I could remain scrubbed in and put my ear to the phone. Unfortunately, there was no answer, but I left my father a message on the answering machine. "Dad, you'll never believe where I am right now. I'm in the operating room with Dr. Leonard Bailey. I just wanted to let you know I will watch that Andrea Bocelli video. I love you, Dad." I stepped back to the OR table, and Dr. Bailey and I continued our conversation as the surgery was flawlessly completed.

A year and a half flew by, and I was at last becoming an official graduate of LLUSM. The ceremony was ending as our professors and attending physicians marched out to the beautiful recessional being played. A distinguished-looking tall figure donned in a sleek black robe and royal red sash slightly paused his step and glanced at me, simply nodding and smiling as he marched by. It was Dr. Bailey, and I felt honored but a bit startled that he would remember and acknowledge me as I stood among so many others.

The next day my father approached me as he and my stepmother were preparing for their long postgraduation drive back to New Orleans. "Son, I have a little gift for you," he said. It was nicely wrapped, and obviously a CD. I removed the paper and was excited to see an Andrea Bocelli CD. "Dad, would you please sign and date the cover?" "Already taken care of," he said with a smile. I opened the CD, and it had been signed. But I was unfamiliar with the handwriting. It read "Brett, remember that relationships are the most important thing in life. Live well! Len Bailey." I was stunned, and continue to be deeply moved by this simple message shared over 22 years ago now. How did this come about? Well, after receiving the message on the answering machine, my father contacted Dr. Bailey. And they conspired with the help of Dr. Bailey's secretary, Yvonne, and my wife, Jodie, to coordinate signing the gift that would impact my life forever. I thank God for mentors like Dr. Bailey and my father, who take time to make a difference.

Brett Quave, LLUSM class of 1999, is an anesthesiologist practicing interventional pain management in Medford, Oregon. He is also pursuing board certification in lifestyle medicine and uses a whole person care approach to help those who suffer from chronic pain. Note: Leonard Bailey died on May 12, 2019. LLUSM dean Roger Hadley (LLUSM class of 1974) read this story at Dr. Bailey's memorial service on June 23, 2019.

May 13

"When Jesus saw her weeping, . . . he was deeply moved in spirit. . . . Then Jesus said, 'Did I not tell you that if you believe, you will see the glory of God?'"
John 11:33, 40, NIV

I know you—you took care of my girl, man. You gave her a medal. I've been looking for you!" The two men stop, right there in the middle of the street—mile seven of Dexter Emoto's run. They talk about Mr. Medina's daughter Maya—who brought them together in a recovery room of Loma Linda University Children's Hospital when she went in for her port-a-cath. . . .

"She died three years ago."

This mile-seven meeting is part of the faith legacy Maya Medina's parents continue to have with God: running into a man who reminds them of the beginning—when Maya was newly diagnosed, when they were eager to believe in healing and welcomed Dexter's encouragement. He signed a medal (reminding her that she would never be alone, since Jesus was right there running the race with her), and they committed in prayer to the marathon Maya was about to start in her fight against leukemia.

Their whole story is about the kind of faith that looks for God, just as Mary and Martha did, even after their brother Lazarus died. "We have a lot of questions for God—but we believe in Him, trust in Him." Even when they were scared, even when the bone marrow (transplanted from Dad), did not work. Even when they realized they had tried everything, and still the leukemia progressed. They said, "WE BELIEVE in God—we still believe in God—to heal her!" In fact, their faith was so strong that they treated her as if she was already healed and whole.

They tell about the last few weeks, when, reading the Gospels aloud to Maya, they realized that Jesus never denied anyone healing. "Not the lame man, not the blind man, not the lepers—NO ONE is denied healing. We stood on those scriptures—we were so sure that God was going to heal her, and she was going to come out of this!"

The Word says, His ways are higher than our ways and His thoughts are higher than our thoughts (Isaiah 55:9). Well, this is one of those things that we don't understand. . . .

Maya never used her cancer as an excuse—to avoid doing homework or to misbehave, or to give up. She had faith. Her faith was the same as when she was 2 years old, and she told her mom that she saw the "Man with holes in His hands" standing outside the house, wanting to come in. Her parents admit that she had more faith than they did. "She saw Him herself—the Man with the holes in His hands. She saw Him both when she was 2 years old and all throughout her treatment."

This is truly a story of faith; the kind that lets parents believe in God even when their daughter doesn't live. And this is a story of God, the kind of God who promises life after death, but shows up in between. And this is a story about legacy, the kind that transcends understanding. "God keeps speaking to us, our faith is still here—even though we miss Maya every single day, even though it doesn't ever get easier. God reminds us that Maya isn't in our past anymore—she's in our future."

This story of Maya Medina was told via video by her parents and then written for this devotional by Jennifer Renaud Rich, who works for LLUSM. The nurse in this story is Dexter Emoto (LLUSN class of 1977), who currently works in the postanesthesia care unit at LLUMC. Dexter is an avid runner, having participated in 158 marathons and 175 half marathons. Dexter gifts his marathon medals to his patients to encourage them. He is saving lives through blood donations to the community and has currently donated 118 gallons of blood.

May 14

> *"The man who finds a wife finds a treasure,*
> *and he receives favor from the LORD."*
> Proverbs 18:22, NLT

We are dressed impeccably in black tie, driving to a charity gala, eagerly looking forward to a romantic evening together. As we stroll toward the beautifully decorated entrance, we hear that noise, yes—the beeper buzz. A few words hastily repeated from the phone tells me, as a nurse, that our evening plans are about to end. "She's lost how much blood? Take her down to the OR; type and cross for four units of blood, I'll be there in 10 minutes."

Then there was the time that I, while not on call, had planned for a very special surprise birthday overnight at a hotel. Babysitter was in place with our children; birthday balloons were tied to the headboard, Martinelli's was chilling in ice in the sink. Our favorite song softly playing on repeat—just one thing left: to go pick him up. Then my cell phone begins ringing. "Yes. . . . I understand," I say. "You promised you would be there for her delivery. . . . But she's not due for two weeks! I know, babies wait for no one." I pop the balloons, empty ice from the sink, and go downstairs to check out. Would I have it any other way? Absolutely not. My husband's love of medicine, the devotion to his craft of helping to save women's lives, makes me very proud, and happy to do my part to make sure our home is a happy place to return to at the end of his day. His love of teaching other physicians makes me truly amazed at his sphere of influence "To make [men and women] whole."

I recognize the look now from total strangers in a crowd, arms waving wildly, "Dr. Wagner, Dr. Wagner, remember me? You saved my life 30 years ago." Much hugging always follows. "Dr. Wagner, you delivered my Tommy, remember?" as she pushes her son forward. "He was breech. He's very smart, you know. He's going to be a surgeon just like you."

When you have found your effective way to serve God, whether surgeon or the spouse who holds up their arms, it makes you truly love what you do. After 48 years of ironing lab coats, getting up at 4:45 in the morning to serve breakfast, praying together every morning for all who are struggling, or kissing your spouse goodbye at the door—we are the hands and feet of Jesus. We have paraphrased Esther 4:14: When receiving every call to the hospital for help, "Who knows if you were made a surgeon for just such a time as this?" Be an effective, loving team member and thank God daily for the gifts He has given you; never stop using them.

Marian Wagner, LLUSN class of 1972, met Robert J. Wagner, Jr. (LLUSM class of 1969), on a blind date arranged by the late David Rice (LLUSM class of 1971). They married soon after, and have enjoyed the past 48 years together. They have three children, Andrea Thorp (LLUSM class of 2001), Jessica Sabo (LLUSD class of 2003), and Robert "Jake" Wagner III (LLUSD class of 2020). For 20 years she has volunteered for the University SDA Church, assisting with set building and costume design, and writing situation dramas.

May 15

"A new commandment I give to you, that you love one another; as I have loved you, that you also love one another. By this all will know that you are My disciples, if you have love for one another."

John 13:34-35, NKJV

I've grown to love almost every part of pediatrics. Yes, there are sad stories and disappointments, but my journey has been filled with overwhelming good. And when I pause to look at the enormity of the possible impact, even the small mundane interactions, I find beauty.

One experience that happened during my residency took place during a routine observation for anaphylaxis. I was on the inpatient ward services by the time I met this 14-year-old boy named Joey who had already been given lifesaving medication. I checked in on him for my prerounding early that morning and saw the excitement in his mother's eyes. I'm very familiar with that look, and it reminds me of the value of my work. Joey was Black and came from a Black family.

I am a Black doctor. It's not lost on me how showing up to work is a significant testament to how far my people have come. And the example it sets for every family who sees a Black male pediatrician taking care of them with kindness, excellence, and personability. I treated Joey as I would treat all my patients, making sure to use his name, talking directly, and explaining to his family in terms that he would understand also. They would be going home in a couple of hours. I was called by nursing after rounds were over to be told that the family wanted to speak with me. When I returned to the room, uncles, aunts, and all of Joey's siblings were present. The family wanted to show them all a Black doctor. The mother proceeded to have Joey talk to me about his dreams of going into medicine. I sat down on his bed and shared with him how valuable he would be as a doctor. How he could totally do it. How it's not easy, but if he perseveres, it will be well worth it. And that he obviously has a healthy family community to lean on to help achieve his dreams.

It's not lost on me how important representation is. And at the time of this writing (the summer of 2020), the conversation is louder than it has been in my lifetime. The blessings of the small interactions remind me of the gigantic impact of what showing up in Black excellence can look like. Through the course of Joey's time in the hospital I probably saw him for less than an hour. Three short patient encounters. But his family got to see their very first example of a Black physician. Visualization reminds us that these high goals are possible. It speaks to youth who are going through unknown difficulties and (frequently) in systems not designed to support their maximum success.

I would love to see what we each can do with our individual lives so that more Black children like Joey can achieve their dreams and beyond. What does a more perfect system look like for that to be true?

Morgan Green, LLUSM class of 2016, finished a pediatrics residency at UCSF Benioff Children's Hospital Oakland and is a pediatric hospitalist at Loma Linda University Children's Hospital. He will not forget the number of people who rallied behind him when he finally made the decision to pursue pediatrics and how accepted he felt. He and wife, Tedean (LLUSM class of 2016), both concur that having the right people in positions of authority has the power to change an entire system. They wish to carry on this excellence of character as they pursue their respective careers.

May 16

> *"Before I formed you in the womb I knew you, and before you were born I consecrated you."*
> Jeremiah 1:5, ESV

"Keep bagging and stimulating him by rubbing his back like this," the missionary nurse anesthetist instructed me as we tried to resuscitate a floppy newborn at Béré Adventist Hospital in Chad while our OB/GYN attending was performing an emergency C-section. Sadly, this baby did not survive despite our efforts. Thankfully, we were able to participate in successful newborn resuscitations. As fourth-year medical students, the three of us took turns assisting with operations, newborn cases, or rounding on the wards. Since there was limited staff, the talented clinicians had multiple roles in addition to teaching about medical care in resource-limited settings.

At Malamulo Adventist Hospital in Malawi, my coresident and I were in the operating area when a woman arrived with obstetric complications. She was transferred from another hospital for an emergency C-section. We noted that her abdomen seemed to have abnormal protrusions as she was being prepared for surgery. Once the C-section was underway, we soon found out that those protrusions were the baby's limbs pressing directly against the abdomen. The uterus had ruptured, and the baby was no longer within its confines. The obstetrician pulled out a limp baby and passed him over. While my coresident assisted with the C-section, I was on newborn duty with one of the nurses. I knew that a quiet baby was a bad sign. I immediately started suctioning and stimulating the baby as soon as the nurse set him on the warmer. From my experiences in Chad, I knew that rapid intervention could make a difference despite not having all the tools for newborn resuscitation. After a few more minutes the nurse stepped away knowing that babies in such conditions would not survive. I held on to hope and continued to stimulate the baby while praying for this new life. The entire operating room was surprised to hear a little cry emanating from what was previously a limp body. This little boy survived and was well enough to be transferred to the maternity ward with his mother after completion of the surgery.

As a family medicine resident at LLUH, I had many experiences with deliveries on the Labor and Delivery (L&D) floor. My most treasured experience was my first continuity delivery, which embodied my role as a family physician. As a resident with continuity clinic at SACHS, I saw the mother for her prenatal care and got to know her husband. They were excited first parents. Once it came time, I met them at L&D and stayed with them through labor. Following the delivery I cared for the mother and her newborn under attending supervision. I continued to see them afterward in clinic and watched their baby grow. After becoming an attending at SACHS, I saw this healthy little boy for his well-child exam. I am blessed to be in a role in which I provide longitudinal care for families.

Despite these drastically different environments—from resource-limited to rich—I am blessed to have the privilege to assist with the miracle of childbirth. As I reflect on these experiences at different stages of training, God's guidance led me to be at each place at the right time even when facing difficulties. As stated by a Malawian surgical resident I met: "Of course we believe in and worship our God. Our lives are very difficult, and God is the only hope that we have."

Mai-Linh Tran, LLUSM class of 2015, is an assistant professor in LLUSM's department of family medicine. She is passionate about teaching future physicians, working with local underserved communities and serving on mission trips abroad. She is blessed to spend time with her loving family.

May 17

"That's how we're gonna win. Not fighting what we hate, saving what we love."
Rose Tico, character from Star Wars: The Last Jedi,
created by American filmmaker George Lucas (1944–)

My father, Delmar Aitken (LLUSM class of 1973-B), was a hero. Some of his career highlights include holding a faculty position in LLUSM (1983–1997), practicing surgical oncology, and being an instrumental figure in the research and technique development of biosentinal lymph node mapping, which is now the gold standard of care in breast cancer surgeries. He may also be known for succumbing to COVID-19 in July 2020.

But my dad isn't a hero because he died. He is a HERO because he LIVED. He lived. He loved. He laughed. As a surgeon he could easily have focused on tragedy, but instead he sought the GOOD, the HOPE, the FUN, the BEAUTY, the LOVE, and STRENGTH.

According to his friend and colleague, Ted Mackett (LLUSM class of 1968): "Delmar's enthusiasm for life and surgery was contagious. He always identified with the patients in his care and even in the most hopeless of circumstances still offered hope and healing; he went out of his way to cheer those in the hospital at all times but especially on such occasions as Christmas by showing up in Santa Claus costume. He was just plain FUN for those around him—friends, medical students, residents, and colleagues."

Dad saw BEAUTY in practicing medicine. He believed that medicine was one of the many ways that God answers prayers. He took seriously the responsibility of being a servant of God through healing, teaching, and connecting with others.

More than medicine his LOVE for his family ran deep. It warmed my heart to see his eyes twinkle when my mom, Cheree—the love of his life—walked in the room or while spending time with his children. Delmar was a work hard, play hard kind of guy because he probably wanted to soak up as much of life as he could. For example, on his 70th birthday all he wanted to do was take his "kids" to Harry Potter World.

I am so thankful that during lockdown I ended up calling my parents almost every night to (somewhat) jokingly make sure they were in by curfew. During these precious months I grew closer to my dad as an adult than I ever had—those petty arguments and the busyness of life issues just melted away.

I raised my concerns about his seeing patients during the pandemic, but with his STRENGTH he assured me that he was taking all the precautions. His biggest concern was that his patients couldn't see him smiling behind his mask! So he printed off pictures of his Cheshire cat grin or his handlebar mustache, allowing his patients to connect with him better. This was my dad: compassionate and fun!

The year 2020 has been a strange one. Thus, I suggest looking for the good in your lives. FEEL the GOOD, the HOPE, the FUN, the BEAUTY, the LOVE, and the STRENGTH. I promise, that it will make the world a better place. And that is what my dad would've wanted for us all.

May the Force Be With You, Always.

April Angelique Aitken, PhD, carries her father's insatiable desire to educate, create knowledge, feel the good, and have fun! Her dad instilled the importance of being a good writer, which informed her teaching practices for special education students. She is an Institute of Education Sciences postdoctoral research fellow whose lines of inquiry include writing interventions for struggling writers and the teachers who support them. May 17 is her father's birthday.

May 18

"My son, if your heart is wise, my own heart also will be glad; and my inmost being will rejoice when your lips speak what is right."
Proverbs 23:15-16, NASB

When I was a child, I enjoyed receiving words of affirmation from my parents. Of the two of them, my mother was the one who showered my sister and me with encouragement, delight, and admiration the most. During the teen years it seemed that those words were fewer and farther between, peppered instead with words of caution in the form of proverbs she had learned from her own mother. These sayings were meant to inspire accountability and thoughtfulness as she strove to prepare us to live outside of her watchful eye. This learning was reinforced by our teachers in elementary and high school, who had us memorize scriptures and quotes, adding to the growing store of sayings that they thought would help to create an ethos of hard, honest work in our academic pursuits and life. I found this instruction restrictive and often chafed at what seemed to be profuse reminders to be prudent.

Since I had experienced the benefit of wise counsel, it was not astonishing that during my years as a teacher, I too imparted words of affirmation and certainly many words of admonition, which my students also found restrictive. As I have matured into adulthood, I realize that the deep motivation for our mother's words stemmed from her love and desire to see her children succeed. This came from her experience with her own parents. I can remember it as if it were yesterday, the look of delight on Grandpa Ehud's face when we visited their village from the city. He would comment to my grandmother how much we had grown since our last visit. Late at night, in the home where my mother and her siblings had been born, we could hear him retell something he saw one of us do or heard us say as if Grandma Hilda had not witnessed the event herself. Their hearts were glad! They had lived to see the sacrifices they had made for their child reflected in their grandchildren.

Wisdom, when applied, brings pleasure to the heart of the parent, teacher, or mentor. The value of wisdom is not readily understandable to the young or novice and may be even passively or passionately resisted. It is the patient discernment of the instructor, parent, or friend that guides the process of imparting or instilling wisdom despite the resistance to receiving it. It takes time and experience to cultivate wisdom. It takes time to appreciate and apply the wisdom that we have received. At this stage of my own life, I continue to seek out wise counselors and relish the opportunities when I learn some new wise saying. Though I live thousands of miles away from my mother and my grandparents have long since passed away, I find myself smiling when I act upon the many proverbs, scriptures, and quotes that I learned. This is a gift that I am now endeavoring to pass on to others as I have found that they are indeed words to live by.

Dilys Brooks, MDiv, MA, MS, is the campus chaplain at LLUH, where she provides spiritual care for the students, faculty, and staff. She is passionate and enthusiastic about assisting individuals of all ages to know Christ personally and accept His call to become change agents in the world for the kingdom of God. She is happiest when she is preaching, teaching, or singing about Jesus. Dilys is a partner in life and ministry with Delroy Brooks, the pastor of the Juniper Avenue Seventh-day Adventist Church in Fontana, California. They are raising their children, Micah and Matea, along with their dog, Snow, in Colton. Her life is informed by Matthew 6:33, NKJV: "Seek first the kingdom of God."

May 19

"I am the vine, you are the branches. He who abides in Me, and I in him, bears much fruit; for without Me you can do nothing."
John 15:5, NKJV

He was young, and his girlfriend was at his bedside. His hardened face told of a tough life. He had just been released from jail and would likely have to go back to court soon. He had run out of his pain medications and needed more. Why the pain? Well, as the story went, he had been threatening his girlfriend with a weapon, and someone called the police. He sustained gunshot wounds from the police in the course of their intervention and had spent several weeks recovering in the hospital. Now he was out of jail and just wanted more narcotics.

This was the beginning of my second year of residency. I was exhausted and burned-out. The conviction had come to me even before this: I needed to share God's love with my patients. But how to do so when I didn't even feel it myself?

I left his bedside with disgust. How could someone treat their loved one so horribly? But the still small voice spoke to my heart. "Go and offer to pray with him." Oh, I did not want to talk to him any more. But my feet took me back to his bedside.

"Would it be helpful if I prayed with you?"

To my shock, he accepted my offer. I took his hand and prayed that God would work in his life and that he would see hope for his future. As I opened my eyes, I saw tears in his. He and his girlfriend said thank you, and I left his bedside with a changed heart.

God had shared His love through me in spite of my burnout.

Jesus says, "Without Me you can do nothing." In medicine, where compassion seems systematically obliterated from many sides, without the love of Jesus in my heart I cannot love my patients, cannot care for them, and cannot provide compassion. "But Jesus looked at them and said to them, 'With men this is impossible, but with God all things are possible'" Matthew 19:26, NKJV.

Laurel Guthrie, LLUSM class of 2016, completed her general surgery residency at LLUH in June 2021. She is continuing at LLUH for a two-year fellowship in complex general surgical oncology. After completing her training, she plans to use her skills to provide surgical care to God's children around the world wherever He calls. In her free time she enjoys hiking in the mountains, playing classical and sacred chamber music, traveling, and sharing the good news of God's infinite love.

May 20

"Rejoice always, pray without ceasing, give thanks in all circumstances; for this is the will of God in Christ Jesus for you."
1 Thessalonians 5:16-18, ESV

He lay in bed with amputated legs, hooked up to multiple machines, and his eyes fluttered open with energy as he smiled wide when he saw us. Mr. T was a palliative care patient who had lived in the Loma Linda SICU for the past year. Though in this dreary situation, he joked about changing the outfit of his back scratcher, which was in the shape of a woman whom he had dressed with blue coban bandage. It was almost his one-year anniversary in the Loma Linda hospital, so he recounted how it all happened.

It was a Friday at home where he had sudden onset severe neck pain. He had to put his 1-year-old baby down because the pain was so severe it brought him to his knees. His wife called the ambulance which brought him to the nearby community hospital. By this time he had defecated at least three times, so the triage doctors thought he had food poisoning. But the next time he actually filled the toilet bowl with blood. So the ER doctors then decided to do a CT scan of his chest and abdomen, which showed a complete aortic dissection. He knew as a nurse and from the doctor's face that it had a very high mortality rate and that his situation was dire.

The ER doctors rushed to call all hospitals in California, looking for a cardiothoracic surgeon who would take his case. The University of Southern California was the only one who agreed, so Mr. T was flown there. He had told his wife to gather all his prayer warriors around the world and pray for him because he was going to fight it. He had his chest cut open and underwent many surgeries and complications. He had lost blood supply to his legs and had to have both of his legs amputated. Also, his heart stopped, and he needed CPR, then his liver and kidney went into failure, and he needed hemodialysis. Some of the surgeons gave up on him, thinking he was going to die, but he was extubated after two weeks. The waiting room had been filled with his prayer warriors.

He was transferred to Loma Linda University Medical Center, where he spent a year undergoing multiple other procedures and fighting for his life. Yet he had the strength to say that God had placed him there for a reason: to be an inspiration to those around him. He didn't know why God kept him alive, as most people would be dead at this stage, but he was determined to continue exploring why.

His favorite poster on his wall said, "Keep your head up. God gives His hardest battles to His strongest soldiers." I left the room thinking about his resilience and how God truly can use any person to be a blessing no matter their circumstances.

Carrie Lam, LLUSM class of 2016, is board-certified in family medicine, anti-aging, and regenerative medicine. She lives in Irvine, California, and cofounded Lam Clinic, whose vision is to provide preventive, functional, and integrative medicine to all, helping each person empower wholeness and embrace wellness.

May 21

"He will listen to the prayers of the destitute. He will not reject their pleas."
Psalm 102:17, NLT

"Lord, help me on my journey to You." That was his whole prayer. It was simple but heartfelt. Larry knew he didn't have much time left, for his liver cancer nearly had him beat. He hadn't been much of a "religious" person and wasn't one for institutionalized religion. I didn't know if in his past a "church" had truly represented God's love, but when invited to church, he would decline. On occasion he'd ask me, "What will heaven be like?" He only vaguely knew some of the Bible stories, such as Noah's flood and Daniel in the lions' den. But he did know that he wanted to go to heaven.

Larry's two favorite pastimes were fishing and smoking. Having lost his driver's license for repeated infractions of driving under the influence, he had only his old bicycle to get around. Not being able to drive greatly limited his ability to visit his choice fishing holes. It was like watching a child in a candy store when I drove him to his favorite river to fish. I wasn't much of a fisherman myself, so Larry lent me a pole, and off we went. Despite the fact that I didn't eat fish, he insisted that I take the whole catch home with me, all seven trout.

Larry loved the Chargers football team. We watched a few games together through the haze of a smoke-filled living room. Larry didn't have many friends other than a neighbor who would occasionally come over to smoke together. The only family member left was a sister who lived across the state. They would occasionally talk on the phone, but that was about it.

Knowing his own time was short, Larry asked me if I could drive him out to the ghost town where he grew up and where his family was buried. We arrived at the edge of a woods that opened up to abandoned fields. There was a disheveled barbed-wire fence that encircled a couple dozen gravestones, with some dating back to the late 1800s. He was withdrawn as we wandered through the old graveyard, undoubtedly reliving the past, wondering about his own future. As we pushed back the briers and tall grass to read the headstones, it was like clearing the cobwebs off a forgotten past. Many of the stones bore Larry's last name, marking the burial sites of his parents, grandparents, aunts, and uncles. They were the only remaining reminders of lives once lived, but now forgotten by time and covered by weeds. This was where Larry wanted his own ashes to be buried.

But this was not where Larry wanted to be left. He may never have had the opportunity to know the health message, or how the sanctuary depicted the plan of salvation. But Larry knew he was on a journey to God, and to heaven. He prayed that God would help him on that journey, and that is one prayer God will always answer! "He will listen to the prayers of the destitute. He will not reject their pleas" (Psalm 102:17, NLT).

Kenneth Rose, LLUSM class of 1988, and his family have been blessed to be living in the shadows of the beautiful Wallowa Mountains of Northeastern Oregon, often referred to as the Little Swiss Alps of America. He works there as a general surgeon in the rural critical-access hospital. May 21 is in honor of his father's birthday.

May 22

> *"This may be the day God gives me a great opportunity to serve someone who needs help from me."*
> Bill Grosz: author (from Quotes for the Journey: Wisdom for the Way, compiled by Gordon S. Jackson)

I am done! DONE! I am going home!" Dragging her IV pole, with needle, tubing, and fluids still attached, my patient sprints down the hallway. Writing notes at my computer, I receive an urgent page from the patient's nurse. Partway through listening to the nurse's frenzied explanation, I hear hurried footsteps thumping by the workroom. I open the door just in time to see my patient's back retreating down the hallway, hospital gown flapping. In pursuit, I arrive at the elevator moments behind her, but all I find is a slightly askew deserted IV pole, saline bag still swaying, and IV fluid freely flowing onto the floor. Bewildered, I whisper a prayer: "Lord, what am I supposed to do with a runaway patient?"

Moments later, with no explanation, the escapee returned to her unit and checked back into her room, chagrined. Meeting her at the bedside, I had a million thoughts flash through my mind. *So that was interesting. Is it the food? What is wrong? We should probably check your stitches.* In the end I decide to sit by the patient's bed and ask what I can do to help. Tearfully she tells me about her life and all the turns it has taken. She mentions that whenever she got upset, she would eat strawberry ice cream. I realize there may be at least one thing I can do to help as she struggles through her hospital stay.

The next morning, when her breakfast tray arrives, a cold bottle of strawberry-flavored Boost is placed next to her scrambled eggs. Weeks later, as she was wheeled out of the hospital, my patient tearfully grasped our hands one by one and said, "You are all so brilliant and beautiful. I will be sure to come back here the next time I get shot."

Transitioning from medical student to resident is tough for everyone. As a new intern starting on trauma surgery, I was especially leery. I would stay late every day rereading all the orders I had written, looking for discrepancies. Any details that I might have missed the first time around would be changed to treat the patient better. Despite these attempts to improve care, the most comforting thing I have found is knowing that with each strange or difficult thing I encounter, God is with me.

Benjamin Damazo, LLUSM class of 2017, is a fifth-year otolaryngology (ENT) resident at LLUH. He and his wife are the parents of two beautiful girls. He spends his free time laughing, cooking, and playing make-believe.

May 23

"Create in me a pure heart, O God, and renew a steadfast spirit within me."
Psalm 51:10, NIV

I first met "Mike" on an early May morning in 1982. I was starting the last rotation of my internal medicine internship at Loma Linda University Medical Center. I was a battle-hardened intern with 10 months of 80-plus-hour workweeks under my belt. I had survived Friday-to-Monday shifts on two hours of sleep. I was ready for anything except Mike.

Mike was a patient on unit 4100, cardiology. He was in his early 30s and had viral cardiomyopathy. He had reached end-stage cardiac failure with 4+ pitting edema to the thighs. Now his liver and kidneys were failing. He was on a cardiac transplant list, but things were not looking good. As we made rounds that first morning, every third patient was assigned to me. When we came to Mike's room, the resident got a knowing look on his face. "Congratulations, Andy, you get to take care of Mike." Mike was an angry young man. Not only was he dying, but every morning he was poked and prodded by a medical student and an intern, followed by a whole group of people standing around his bed discussing his deteriorating condition in medical mumbo jumbo.

With gritty determination I was going to see to it that Mike either got his transplant or at least lived long enough for me to hand his care over to the next intern on July 1. It became a daily battle, adjusting his medications and restricting his fluid intake. I knew he was cheating by drinking water from the bathroom sink. "Mike, you've got to stop drinking so much water; your weight is up again!" A polite paraphrase of his response would be: "Doc, who cares? I am dying."

Mike had a hard time sleeping at night, so he would often prowl around the central work area where I sat writing notes and orders. As the weeks wore on, Mike and I began bantering and talking. Gradually our friendship grew, and our whole relationship changed. Mike told me of his family and his dreams. We discussed his prognosis and what happens when you die. We talked about how, at the end, either you have Jesus or you have nothing. Our morning rounds changed from confrontation to collaboration.

I will never forget the morning I came in to rounds and saw his empty bed. Mike had fought the good fight. He had lost the physical battle, but I believe he had won the spiritual victory. Yes, I did learn something about how to manage end-stage heart disease with Mike, but I learned so much more than that. Mike helped me see that no matter what the circumstances, a person is first and foremost a beloved child of God and a fellow traveler on this road of life. Thank you, Mike. I am looking forward to seeing you again when Jesus returns.

Anders Engdahl, LLUSM class of 1981, is a radiologist who is enjoying semiretirement with his wife, Debbie, in beautiful northwest Montana. They enjoy hiking, mountain climbing, and sharing God's love.

May 24

6:00 a.m., and as I walk toward the automatic doors of the ICU
I look through the window of the waiting room
And there you are
With your gray hoodie and red baseball cap
It was gray for about two weeks, your lucky gray, you told me
Until you couldn't stand the smell
And you changed into a red one
Lying across the chairs with hospital pillows arranged
On your makeshift bed
Occasionally you weren't there
But in her room, on the recliner
And I would see you at 6:30 a.m.
And tiptoe inside, after I already checked her vitals and labs
And ordered platelets and fibrinogen
I would sneak around her proning bed to check for blood in her ET tube
Careful not to wake you up
And, rarely, you weren't there at all
But with your daughter at home
But you always came back,
And together we rejoiced when she opened her eyes
And moved her head
But that was it
Every day, every number,
I wrote, I circled, I debated, I treated
Every number but the one only God knows
Every day you asked me
Every day I took a breath
And I told you what I knew
I remember the last time I saw you,
The tightness of your hug
You called me doctor
But I couldn't save her
Only in His time
His number
His hand

Christine Shen, LLUSM class of 2017, is an internal medicine resident at Scripps Clinic in California. She dreams of changing the lives and hearts of people.

May 25

"Is anyone among you suffering? Then he must pray. Is anyone cheerful? He is to sing praises. Is anyone among you sick? Then he must call for the elders of the church and they are to pray over him, anointing him with oil in the name of the Lord; and the prayer of faith will restore the one who is sick, and the Lord will raise him up, and if he has committed sins, they will be forgiven him."
James 5:13-15, NASB

The charge nurse approached me with an urgent request to see a patient brought by ambulance because of her shortness of breath. I turned to see a distraught woman holding the patient's hand with a rosary in her other hand. After identifying herself as the patient's sister, she told me the patient's breast cancer had "spread everywhere." They were to start hospice, but the nursing team had not yet made their home visit or delivered any medications. The sister tearfully said, "Please, just make her comfortable. I know she is dying. I don't want her to suffer. She's been through enough. I panicked at home." Noticing how emotional she was about facing her sister's end in a hospital, I offered to pray.

This is who we are.

I noticed that a recent nurse graduate was assigned her room. I wondered quietly if she could handle this ill patient. I would later learn that this new nurse had recently been through a similar experience with her family and empathized with them. She also spoke fluent Spanish, understood their culture, and could communicate in a language familiar to all family members and the patient.

This is who we are.

After her mother and daughter arrived, the patient became more alert. She spoke to her mother, and then closed her eyes, her breathing less difficult. Her family surrounded the patient, exchanging their goodbyes. The frequency of the patient's eye contacts with her relatives slowed, as did her heart and breathing. She died at 10:30 a.m. I completed my examination and offered to pray again with her family. We held hands around the bed, and I prayed that I would see her in heaven and talk to her about her story, her walk. I thought to myself, *How sad, but how fulfilling.*

As we continued to hold hands, her family sang a song in Spanish. Her daughter, holding her left hand, wept with the rest of the family. They each kissed their daughter, sister, and mother goodbye. The sister, who accompanied her to the ER, grabbed my hands, hugged me, and thanked me for caring for her sister.

This is who we are.

Lynda Daniel-Underwood, LLUSM class of 1991, is an associate professor in LLUSM's department of emergency medicine and associate dean for curriculum evaluation and learner assessment. She loves being able to practice medicine with the integration of spirituality.

May 26

"But he was wounded for our transgressions, he was bruised for our iniquities: The chastisement of our peace was upon him, and with his stripes we are healed." Isaiah 53:5, KJV

Driving home after a full day of working at my dermatology office, I received a phone call from my primary physician that upended my life. "Steve, I am sorry to have to tell you this, but this CT scan did not turn out OK. They think they see something in your sigmoid colon and they are recommending more testing. . . . I will help you get through this," Dr. Adrian Cotton (LLUSM class of 1996) said. I had had multiple abdominal CT scans in the past for various forms of abdominal discomfort and pain; they had never shown anything to worry about. But in that moment, my life changed from that of doctor to patient.

I was 56 years old, and cancer was the furthest diagnosis from my mind. I felt in the best shape I'd ever been. I hardly ever got a cold! No family history of cancer, life-long vegetarian, nonsmoker, SDA lifestyle—why I practically live in the Blue Zone!* I thought to myself, I have been working hard most of my life, have been happily married to my beautiful and wonderful wife, Sheila, for 23 years, have four great children aged 16-22 years old, have the best parents, siblings, numerous extended family members and friends—how could this be happening to me?

A diagnosis of Stage 4 sigmoid adenocarcinoma set me on a whirlwind of multiple procedures, tests, and visits to the hospital during the midst of COVID-19 lockdown. Tumor Board reviewed my case, and I was placed on chemotherapy every two weeks. I barely had time to breathe, and I had already lost 25 pounds. I couldn't believe that was my name on the chart and on all those orders. My wife sought out prayer warriors and wasted no time in calling our pastors for anointing. We prayed, read the Bible, and recited scriptures daily. Each time we claimed Isaiah 53:5, NKJV—"And by His stripes we are healed."

The physician in me knew that my physical prognosis looked bleak, but as I received my first chemotherapy infusion, I was ready for a major spiritual infusion as well. I prayed for God to guide the nurses and for me to tolerate and respond to the treatment. So many family, friends, medical staff, and others who didn't even know me joined in prayer for my healing. This collective outpouring of care brought healing in ways I didn't expect. I have a renewed appreciation for the Bible and so many scriptures that are full of important messages and promises for healing.

I also gained a new sense of empathy for my own patients as I became a patient. Many of my friends shared their own cancer journeys. Although I would have preferred to have never received this cancer diagnosis, I have seen the hugeness of God's heart for me. I realize that God is bigger than any diagnosis or prognosis. Over the past 11 months, I have been feeling better and have been able to work and do more things with my wife and children. My CEA level has gone down immensely. I am so grateful to God, my wife, my children, my family, my friends, my pastors, and my medical team. The transition from doctor to patient is not easy, but I count myself blessed to know that my true identity is in Christ, and by His stripes I am healed!

*Blue Zones are regions of the world in which people live much longer than average, mainly because of their diet.

Steven E. Hodgkin, LLUSM class of 1990, is a board-certified dermatologist with office practices in Victorville and Redlands, California. He is the husband to "the best wife in the whole world," Sheila, and the father of "the most wonderful children," Savannah (LLUSM class of 2024), Sophia, Alex, and Summer. May 26 is his birthday.

May 27 — Consecration and Hooding Ceremony, LLUSM class of 2022

"Before they call I will answer; while they are still speaking I will hear."
Isaiah 65:24, NIV

What an adorable couple! I said to myself as the wife was being rolled up to the OR for an appendectomy. They were newlyweds—he was finishing his MBA and had a job lined up. Both were active in their church, and madly in love. The well-dressed and articulate husband stopped me in the hall. He asked if I remembered him. I had to admit that I didn't and hid behind the number of patients I see every shift in the ER. He described our previous meeting—and it all came back to me....

I was called to a patient's room as the patient had been spitting at the nurses and sneaking into the bathroom to shoot heroin into his IV. As I sat by his bed, he turned his back to me. I sat quietly, taking in the situation and waiting for his response. The odor in the room evidenced his need for a shower. His hair and beard were long and matted. When he finally peeked over his shoulder to see if I was still there, I asked how I could help, and he responded with a string of expletives. He told me about his love affair with heroin and that he had no other reason to live. No one loved or cared about him. His only friends were drug dealers.

I paused and said, "God cares." He responded with another string of expletives. He said the nurse had called a hospital chaplain to pray with him, but that was the chaplain's job. It didn't mean anything. I responded again that God loves him and that Jesus died for him. He visibly calmed and turned to face me. I offered to pray. He shrugged, but didn't decline my offer. I prayed a brief prayer asking God to bless his life and for him to feel God's love. There was no response. I left the room to plan his transfer to a psychiatric rehab facility. Typical case. A wasted life. The whole situation made me feel sad and helpless.

Tonight, however, he told me that my prayer had made all the difference. He thought about the prayer while he was in detox and placed on a medication to stabilize people addicted to narcotics. He stayed the course—and was still following up outpatient for treatment. Here he was 10 months later—a changed person.

He said he trusted my prayer "because everyone knows that doctors don't get paid to pray."

I asked if I could pray with him again—both for his wife in the OR and to thank God for the patient's new life. He didn't have any reluctance for this prayer as he joined me in praising God.

Kathleen Clem, LLUSM class of 1989, is a graduate of LLUH's emergency medicine residency and the first female department chair at LLUSM. She is currently serving at Dartmouth's Geisel School of Medicine in New Hampshire as professor of medicine and emergency medicine faculty. This devotional was read by former LLUSM dean Roger Hadley (LLUSM class of 1974) at the consecration and hooding graduation ceremony for the LLUSM class of 2019.

Baccalaureate, LLUSM class of 2022 — May 28

Our most gracious heavenly Father,

On this weekend of high celebration, we come to You full of gratitude for each graduate in this class. Thank You not only for them and their heeding Your call to service, but thank You for each person in their lives, who has loved them, encouraged them, mentored them, and prayed for them along this journey.

We pray that You will be with them as they disperse to continue their medical education. May they be filled with a sense of wonder and be reminded of You with each new life they see take their first breath and may they cling to Your promises as they witness those who draw their last.

Thank You for the visions and tenacity of our founder, Ellen White, who more than 100 years ago said: "This is the very place"*—a place where medical missionaries of the highest order will be educated to treat not only their patients' physical diseases, but to address ailments of their minds and feed their spiritually hungry souls.

We ask that the reason these graduates chose to come to a Christian medical school be what keeps them focused throughout all their professional days. And when You come in the clouds of glory to take them home, may they hear the words "Well done, good and faithful servant. . . . Enter into the joy of your lord" (Matthew 25:21, NKJV).

We ask all these things and Your richest blessing on these, Your graduates.

Amen.

---

*Ellen G. White, *Testimonies and Experiences Connected With the Loma Linda Sanitarium and College of Medical Evangelists*, p. 38.

Roger Hadley, LLUSM class of 1974, is dean emeritus and professor in LLUSM's department of urology. He wrote and offered this prayer at the baccalaureate services during the years he had the privilege to serve as dean of LLUSM (2003–2019). He is married to Donna and they have three sons, two of whom are LLUSM graduates, and nine grandchildren.

May 29

Commencement, LLUSM class of 2022

Strangers

To my classmates:

You were a stranger to me,
Blank slate with blank short coat
With no name until you took the seat next to me.
Nudging me awake, sharing your grapes,
You sat with me through the longest hours
From 5:00 a.m. in our corner of Centennial
To 10:00 p.m. eating popcorn while "studying,"
Though we both knew we just wanted company.
Lying with a hospital gown, shirtless in clinical skills lab,
With my hand to your chest, abdomen, knees, and feet.
You were my first patient,
And you let me see your heart dance on a screen.
On the wards, you picked up the patient I feared,
And stayed to admit while I ran down to eat.
You saw my tired eyes
And gave me your last granola bar.
Whispering answers, saving seats at grand rounds,
Watching movies on night call,
You filled my days with laughter.
With you there, I didn't feel lonely.
As we marched, you fixed my graduation hood.
You took pictures with my family,
And you loved them.
You loved me,
And I can never repay your kindness.

Eunice Marpaung, LLUSM class of 2019, is a resident at Tacoma Family Medicine in Washington. She is a Southern California native with Indonesian heritage and still keeps in touch with friends from LLU. The poem above was published in the summer 2019 issue of the Alumni Journal LLUSMAA.

Memorial Day, 2022 **May 30**

"Forgiveness does not change the past, but it does enlarge the future."
Paul Boese (1923–1976): American author
from the February 19, 1967, issue of Quote: The Weekly Digest

He was a medical resident at a hospital in Los Angeles, where he was realizing his dream of becoming a doctor. Twelve years earlier he had moved from his home in Hiroshima, Japan, where it was rare to find a devout Christian in a society in which the main religion was Shinto. He attended a private college in the Napa Valley, California, and was accepted to a private medical school in 1933. He was widely accepted by his classmates and teachers, as he was a kind and caring person.

After finishing his residency, he and his wife had to return to Japan in 1939 on important family business. Both feared the Japanese army could draft him. That fateful letter came in 1940 from the Imperial Army.

Half a world away a strapping 16-year-old worked in the Appalachian coal mines. The life of a coal miner was brutally hard and dangerous, so in his 17th year he joined the U.S. Army, even though he was not old enough, but at six feet tall he looked older than he was. He was convinced that the army would be easier than coal mining.

The lives of these two men, Dr. Paul Tatsugushi (CME class of 1938) and Dick Laird, would intersect on a tiny island called Attu, the westernmost island of the Aleutian chain of Alaska and was known by the natives as the "cradle of storms." It snowed 8 months of the year; the rest of the year was rainy and foggy, with only 10 days of the sun breaking though. There were only 42 natives on this island and 2 missionaries.

On June 7, 1942, the Japanese Imperial Army landed on Attu with a force of 2,500 soldiers; they expected great resistance but got none. The American forces landed on Attu on April 30, 1943, with a force of 15,000 troops. What was to be a three-day battle turned into a three-week battle. The Japanese soldiers had been indoctrinated for centuries in the Samurai code of "bushido"—death before surrender. Of the 2,500 soldiers that landed on Attu, all were killed or committed suicide.

Paul Tatsugushi knew that when the Americans landed it would be a short period of time before all 2,500 Japanese soldiers would be killed, so he began a diary to say goodbye to his wife and two daughters. On that fateful day of his death, it was Dick Laird's grenade that ended the life of this promising physician. Attached to the young doctor was a satchel with two items: his 18-day diary and his Bible.

From the diary Laird realized he had killed a doctor of faith and a husband and father. The war and so many deaths caused Laird to have sleepless nights for four agonizing decades. Finally, through a Japanese correspondent, he was able to find Paul's family and meet Paul's daughter, Laura Davis. At the end of their initial, awkward meeting, Dick Laird blurted out that he was the one who had killed Laura's father, whom she had never met—and then drove away leaving Laura stunned, sickened, and reeling in confusion. It was only after having time to process everything and after several more visits that Laura was finally able to forgive Laird. And for the first time in decades, Laird was able to sleep without nightmares.

Reference: Mark Obmascik, *The Storm on Our Shores: One Island, Two Soldiers, and the Forgotten Battle of World War II*, (2019).

Paul Kozik is a 1976 graduate of La Sierra University in Riverside, California, and a retired principal/teacher living in Hayden, Idaho. His son, James, graduated from LLUSD in 2007. His father-in-law, Rolland Olson (CME class of 1946), was drafted three times and served in the U.S. Army as a physician, including more than a year in Japan (1946–1947). Note: This story of the Battle of Attu was featured on CBS's 60 Minutes on April 5, 2019.

May 31

> *"Simon Peter answered him, 'Lord, to whom shall we go? You have the words of eternal life.'"*
>
> John 6:68, NKJV

It was the last day of May 2017. I came home to an empty house, dropped my bags on the floor, and listened to the messages on the beeping machine. "Hey, guys, they're going to release me today. So I'm coming home. I should be there in a couple of days, so I'll see you soon. Love ya. Bye."

I sat down, stunned, a lump in my throat. After 11 years my son was being released from prison, unexpectedly. I closed my eyes. A weight had lifted from my shoulders, a weight that until that moment I didn't realize I carried.

When his mother arrived home an hour later, I took her by the hand, and together we listened. She gasped. I held her trembling body in my arms, and together we wept. During the days that followed, I had the chance to work on the old house we purchased for our son in Spokane. It was what he wanted, something to work on, something to make beautiful. I saw it as a chance to restore his humanity. As we hung sheetrock in his kitchen one afternoon, I looked up at him, and I was suddenly overwhelmed by how good it was to see him there, and how much I had missed him. Then, 70 days later, four U.S. marshals showed up at his probation appointment and took him back into custody. It broke our hearts and devastated our son's spirit. They decided they weren't done punishing him yet, though he had gone to every appointment, every urine test was clean, he went to work every day, and went to every evaluation required.

It's been hard, and I hate watching my son and my wife suffer. I wake up nights in tears, unable to sleep. But in those dark hours my prayer is "Thank You, God, for waking me tonight. I needed to have a conversation with You about my son. Could You watch over him tonight? Could You be there for him, as You are here for me?" What He reveals to me in those moments about Himself, about His own suffering, about His own Son, and about His deep love for me is beyond words.

A friend stopped me on the street and asked me, "How can you keep your faith after what you have gone through?"

I puzzled at her question. "He's the One who is holding us up," I replied. "Where else would I go?"

We don't know what the end of this nightmare will be. We keep waiting for the "happily ever after" part of our story to show up. It's just not the way life is. But the truth is that I have found Him to be an eternal Friend who loves my son more than life itself. He will walk through fire, to the gates of hell itself, for my son, and I have put my full confidence in Him. This story is not over yet.

Note: On December 19, 2020, Patrick was found unresponsive in his prison cell in Illinois. CPR was not successful, and tragically, Patrick passed away. Barry and Shelley (Patrick's parents) have set up a memorial to honor Patrick. It is called Patrick's Place, a home for the homeless (patricksmemorial@gmail.com).

Barry Bacon, LLUSM class of 1984, practices family medicine in northeast Washington. He is developing a medical school in Gambella, Ethiopia, and initiating a project to address homelessness called Hope Street Colville in Colville, Washington. He has four children, and his oldest daughter, Allison, is an LLUSM alumna (class of 2008).

JUNE

ॐ HUMILITY ॐ

"I have been driven many times upon my knees by the conviction that I had nowhere else to go. My own wisdom and that of all about me seemed insufficient for that day."

ABRAHAM LINCOLN (1809–1865)
Sixteenth president of the United States

June 1

"I am the light of the world: he that followeth me shall not walk in darkness, but shall have the light of life."
John 8:12, KJV

I had just come from an internal medicine residency at a Harvard hospital and a research fellowship at Washington University, and was already board-certified and on the clinical faculty of CME (to become LLUH). At age 31 I was a hotshot. It was 1960.

Dressed in a white shirt and tie and new business suit, I would lead teaching rounds this morning while we walked from patient to patient at the old Glendale Sanitarium (now Adventist Health Glendale) in California. Following me would be the head nurse in a white starched uniform and striped cap pushing a stainless steel cart with a stack of patient charts and a vase of white carnations. Then, in various styles of white, a resident, a medical student, and finally two student nurses.

To start and end the rounds, we would visit two very old terminally ill men in rooms at opposite ends of the long straight hall. In an expansive jauntily professorial mood, I led our white-clad retinue to the first room. Waiting for us outside the door was a large family, agitated, angry, hard-faced. Before I could open my mouth, the old man's eldest son started haranguing, his fist clinched. Quickly the others joined in, all shouting at once. "You doctors aren't doing enough for our dad! Do everything, everything, anything! Spare no expense! You can't just let him die! He needs more blood. More oxygen, turn it up; antibiotics, more antibiotics. Why hasn't the lab tech been here yet? Why doesn't he have another special nurse? Call consultants. When is the kidney specialist coming? You simply must not let him die! That's malpractice. He's used to a fast life, and you're snuffing it out! We're going to the administrator; the state medical board will hear about this. And you'll hear from our lawyer!"

Now less buoyant, and followed by the cursing son's dark aura, we silently labored down the long hall to the last room. Waiting there was another large family, this one weeping, holding hands or hugging, heads down, hushed. A graying lady, her hands still covering her wet eyes, finally pleaded, sobbingly, "Doctors, please, we beg you, have mercy! My husband is in misery, such awful misery, and you're torturing him! Why are you piling up expenses? He doesn't need all that oxygen. That mask is suffocating him. He can't stand all that blood. Why was a kidney doctor here? He doesn't need all those blood tests. He doesn't need those antibiotics. So many medicines. He doesn't need that special-duty nurse when we're all here. It's inhuman. Please let him have peace. He's had a beautiful life, and he's ready and wants to go. We all agree; so does the chaplain. Maybe you'll listen to our pastor," she managed to say before subsiding into sobs.

Pushing 90 now and white-haired, I have often thought of how my teaching rounds that day left me speechless, deflated, and bewildered. Finally I have begun to comprehend LLUH's unique message. Only Christ, though unseen, can lead with us in His footsteps. He teaches, comforts, calms, and heals in ways we alone cannot.

Wesley Kime, CME class of 1953-A, *"is an artist who was sidetracked by medicine."* After retiring from pathology at Kettering Medical Center in 1994, Dr. Kime proceeded with serious painting. *"My second career requires as much study, intense thought, and practice as medicine. I am now very old and realize that the physician's true goal is Christ-centered healing and, yes, evangelism."*

June 2

"Most of what I really need to know about how to live and what to do and how to be I learned in kindergarten. Wisdom was not at the top of the graduate school mountain, but there in the sandpile at Sunday School."
Robert Fulghum (1937–): American author

During college and medical school, I had a poster on my wall entitled "All I Really Need to Know I Learned in Kindergarten"—a lot of you have read that credo written by Robert Fulghum. I liked it, no, actually I loved it—here I was in graduate school—reaching the "top of my graduate school mountain", and this was what still inspired me.

Medical school and residency are all about learning as much as you can about anatomy, physiology, pharmacology, and taking care of patients. There are countless hours of lectures and tests, interviewing patients and being asked questions on rounds—all designed to make us better doctors so that we can do what we have been trained to do: Treat the disease and make people well again. Sometimes we are successful, sometimes we are not and sometimes we do not know why things turned out the way they did. We can all think back to our professors during the first two years of medical school, the residents, and the attending physicians with whom we spent so many hours on the wards and the impact they made on us. Upon reflection of those years, I have realized that the most important thing I ever learned was not taught in the traditional sense of the word. It didn't come from a lecture in the preclinical years, and it didn't come from interviewing a patient and presenting that information on rounds. It came from a simple walk down the hallway between units 4200 and 4700 at Loma Linda University Medical Center.

I was a second-year resident in internal medicine rotating on a very busy cardiac care unit. I had the privilege of being on Ken Jutzy's (LLUSM class of 1977-A) service. As we walked down the hall, me just a pace or two behind him, I watched in awe as Dr. Jutzy said a personal hello to everyone we passed: doctors, nurses, respiratory therapists and janitors–he knew them all by name and greeted them as such.

Here I was, rotating with the chair of cardiology, an interventional cardiologist, someone with the knowledge and skill set that set him apart from even the best of the doctors, and what made the biggest impression on my life was how kind he was to everyone. He understood (as I do now) that the health care team is truly that–a team (it's not just "us doctors")–and it takes all of us working together to give patients the best outcomes.

As Ephesians 4:32, NIV, states "Be kind and compassionate to one another," I have tried to model that behavior since—somedays I succeed, most days I fail—but I will continue to keep trying.

Adrian Cotton, LLUSM class of 1996, was born in England and grew up in Canada. He completed an internal medicine residency at LLUH and served as chief resident in internal medicine at LLUH and later as a hospitalist. Currently, he is chief of medical operations for LLUH. He is married to Maggie (LLUSN class of 1995). They have three boys: Luke (born 2002) and twins, Bruce and Alex (born 2007).

June 3

"When he had washed their feet and put on his outer garments and resumed his place, he said to them, 'Do you understand what I have done to you? You call me Teacher and Lord, and you are right, for so I am. If I then, your Lord and Teacher, have washed your feet, you also ought to wash one another's feet. For I have given you an example, that you also should do just as I have done to you.'"

John 13:12-15, ESV

In the summer of 1995 I unexpectedly found myself on a plane to Hangzhou, China, to serve as a medical missionary in the new Sir Run Run Shaw Hospital. At the time I had recently completed my residency in internal medicine at LLUH and was unsure of what the future would look like for my life and young family. In the midst of uncertainty I embarked on this three-month medical missionary trip.

I'll never forget my first impression of Gordon Hadley (CME class of 1944-B), who was the president of the hospital. The newly built hospital had just opened, but the sanitation standards were so poor that dirt lined the corridors of the hospital. Instead of harshly reprimanding the cleaning staff, Dr. Hadley picked up a sponge and quietly began to clean the floors himself. I watched him in astonishment! The legendary Dr. Gordon Hadley—renowned pathologist and previous dean of the Loma Linda University School of Medicine—was on his hands and knees scrubbing the floor of a dirty hospital in the middle of developing China!

As I picked up a sponge to help him clean, the story of Christ washing His disciples' feet came to mind. Foot washing can be a repulsive task. Yet Christ—the Lord and Savior of the universe—stooped down to wipe the grime and stench off of His disciples' smelly, muddy, and blistered feet. Humility is not easy—it demands that one lay aside all titles and accolades in service of love. Up to this point I had spent my entire life chasing after degrees, but as I watched Dr. Hadley clean, my focus shifted. A person's status should never come in the way of showing love. This is what Christ demanded of us, especially as physicians.

I was supposed to stay in China for only three months, but I ended up staying for what I consider to be the best three and a half years of my life. The experiences that I encountered and the lifelong friendships that I made have had a profound impact on my family and life. In those short years Dr. Hadley taught me what it truly meant to "dedicate my life to the furtherance of Jesus Christ's healing and teaching ministry." I had spoken those words in the physician's oath at my graduation, but those words came alive under Dr. Hadley's tutelage. There was never a patient too poor or too sick for Dr. Hadley to admit for treatment. There was also never a task too small or lowly for Dr. Hadley to address. Dr. Hadley led with humility and was a servant of Christ through and through.

Ten years prior to our first meeting in China, Dr. Hadley had admitted me into the Loma Linda University School of Medicine class of 1990—the last class he admitted before "retirement." I owe Dr. Hadley my career, both because he ushered me into becoming a physician and because he instilled in me my mission as a Christian physician: to carry out the Great Commision of Christ with humility.

Daniel Choo, LLUSM class of 1990, currently practices interventional cardiology in Hacienda Heights, California. He served at the Sir Run Run Shaw Hospital in China from 1995 to 1999 as acting chief of internal medicine.

June 4

> *"Jesus looked straight at them and answered, 'This is impossible for human beings, but for God everything is possible.'"*
> Matthew 19:26, GNT

My phone woke me up about 11:00 p.m. I was not on call, so this was curious. It was Dr. Palomero, the visiting pediatric resident, calling me.

Residents frequently come for a month or two rotation at Malamulo Adventist Hospital, a mission hospital in rural Malawi. There happened to be an OB/GYN resident visiting at the same time. She had been called to do a C-section around 8:00 p.m. Thinking she may need help after the delivery, the pediatric resident went along to lend a hand. Dr. Palomero told me the baby had come out limp, blue, and not breathing. They had started ventilating the baby with a bag and mask. For more than two hours the two residents had taken turns squeezing that bag every couple of seconds, holding the mask tight to the baby's tiny face. He was still totally limp. She had called me to see if I had any suggestions. "According to Malawi protocols," I explained to her, "you bag a baby for 20 minutes. Then, if there is no improvement, you stop." There are not many ventilators in Malawi, and babies needing hand-bagging for more than 20 minutes generally do not have good outcomes. Most will die, and the few that survive have permanent brain damage and very hard, short lives.

She told me the mother had received magnesium for pre-eclampsia. Magnesium frequently makes babies deliver with poor muscle tone and poor respiratory effort. We discussed what this could mean for the baby. The heart rate was good, but the baby was totally limp and not breathing, zero spontaneous movement. We debated whether to continue artificially breathing for the baby, and for how long. As we discussed, she interrupted, "Wait, he's moving his legs a little." We discussed some more. We decided to give him a few more minutes to see what happened.

I called her back about 30 minutes later. The baby was slightly better. He had become a little wigglier, and even taken a few breaths on his own. However, he was still heavily dependent on the doctors pushing air into his lungs every couple of seconds. As he had improved some, Dr. Palomero wanted to continue. Thirty minutes later, another call, same news. Some improvement, but not fully breathing on his own yet.

The next morning I came in to see if the baby was still there. He was on oxygen, but was breathing on his own and looking great! We turned off the oxygen, and he continued to look great. By the following day he was ready to be discharged. He looked perfect, breathing well, breastfeeding well, normal physical exam, normal neurologic exam—we couldn't find anything wrong with him.

All in all, the residents squeezed that bag for more than three and a half hours, but today he is a normal, healthy baby. Had he been born in almost any other hospital in Malawi, he certainly would have died. Thanks to their hard work, that baby boy received a new chance at a long and meaningful life, not just 20 minutes.

Wilson Thomas, LLUSM class of 2013, is an assistant professor in LLUSM's department of pediatrics and is currently a pediatrician and medical director at Malamulo Adventist Hospital in Malawi. Along with his amazing wife and two children, he has served at Malamulo Hospital since 2017.

June 5

> *"And so we know and rely on the love God has for us. God is love. Whoever lives in love lives in God, and God in them."*
> 1 John 4:16, NIV

This morning I read the disturbing news about our country ablaze in race riots. I was struck by the disquieting irony of civil unrest today on Pentecost Sunday. In my church I look forward each year to the celebration of this special day on the seventh Sunday after Easter. On this day our church celebrates the spirit arriving in a mighty wind, giving Jesus' earthly disciples words to speak to all nations. Pentecost Sunday is the annual celebration of the Holy Spirit's calling of all people from all nations to participate in the inclusive love of Jesus Christ. It is particularly poignant that this day clearly reminds us that the love of Christ is for all people of all colors and all languages. After all, Christ, who came and walked among us, remains among us through His Spirit.

The story of Pentecost, as recorded in Acts, leads me to reflect on what the incarnational love of Christ means in America today. I asked myself: How would Americans open their hearts to His Spirit and act today? What would be a Spirit-filled response to watching Ahmaud Arbery jogging in the neighborhood? In fact, what would Christ do if He were in that position? I believe He would have come out to the sidewalk and said, "Hi," jogged a block alongside Ahmaud, and commented on the spring flowers. What would Christ have done when He saw Breonna Taylor? I believe He would have laid a hand of protection on her. What would Christ have done if Christian Cooper had asked Him to leash His dog in an area where unleashed dogs were illegal? I believe Christ would have humbly called the dog over, leashed him, and then engaged in conversation about birdwatching. If George Floyd had tried to buy a sandwich with an unusual bill in the midst of a pandemic and record-breaking unemployment rates, I believe Christ would have asked him if everything was OK.

At the end of church today I took virtual communion with my church family and heard the words "The body of Christ given for you, the blood of Christ shed for you. Through Christ's sacrifice, you are forgiven." As a white person, I have much to be forgiven, and I believe many of us have much to be forgiven. There are numerous times that I have looked at my fellow Brown or Black neighbor with suspicion instead of through the eyes of Christ. I pray that Christ will continue to forgive me and give me His eyes. And may I remember that Christ loves us all.

"For by one Spirit we were all baptized into one body—whether Jews or Greeks, whether slaves or free—and have been made to drink into one Spirit" (1 Corinthians 12:13, NKJV).

Jennifer Veltman is an associate professor in LLUSM's department of medicine and head of the division of infectious disease. She completed her med/peds residency at Wayne State University/Detroit Medical Center, and infectious diseases fellowship at David Geffen School of Medicine at UCLA. Following fellowship, she joined the faculty at Wayne State University, where she supported community-based projects to improve access to care for patients living with HIV, she increased minority representation in clinical trials, and she prioritized medical education. She continues with these three goals in her role at LLUSM.

June 6

> *"If the Son therefore shall make you free, ye shall be free indeed."*
> John 8:36, KJV

She is a 54-year-old female with stage 4 breast cancer with metastasis to the lungs and brain, and we are being consulted for management of chronic, malignant pleural effusions," the resident casually informed me. As she went through her presentation, I peeked in to see the consumed figure that was my patient. Eyes closed; every breath labored with the intensity of someone who clings to her fleeting existence. Her coarse, thin hair revealed every inch of her bony, fleshless facial structures. I did not want to wake her. I gently placed my stethoscope on her emaciated chest and heard the agonizing sounds of death—you soon learn to recognize the rattles of life's end. I mechanically continue with my examination, but the routine act came to a halt. She was handcuffed to the bed. I had somehow overlooked the two guards at the entrance. In my brief time working with inmates I have become aware that the more dangerous the criminal, the more guards you see at the door. I wanted to talk to her, to share the comfort of instant freedom in Jesus, but she was in a deep stupor. A conversation wouldn't be possible. She was dying in chains.

The option of a "compassionate release" just before her death was discussed with the primary team. This is a process by which inmates in criminal justice systems may be eligible for immediate early release on grounds of "particularly extraordinary or compelling circumstances which could not reasonably have been foreseen by the court at the time of sentencing." This was, no doubt, the ultimate compelling circumstance. The thought of her being reunited with her family for the last time added the only dose of excitement possible in this condition. We were told she had an aging mother who was anxious to come. The release was granted by the court late that same night, a few hours before the patient finally rested for good. I believe that her "compassionate release" was symbolic of a more infinite, benevolent deliverance granted by God, not only to her, but to any prisoner of sin.

We are also chained. Some chains have nothing to do with the legal system. We actually choose them. We link them to our hearts and carry them around with pride and/or shame. Sometimes we become aware of their weight, and we ask for liberty. Freedom is guaranteed with each claim in the spiritual realm, but not in a criminal court. In the spiritual system we are not half innocent or partially condemned. We are all uniformly guilty, and on death row. However, a "compassionate release" from sin, suffering, and death is available. Let this good news penetrate each patient's soul. As you start your day today, choose freedom for yourself and for those who are under the shadow of your doctoring. Today's—actually, every day's—commission is found in Isaiah 58:6, KJV. Says the Lord: "Is this not the fast that I have chosen? . . . to let the oppressed go free?"

Dafne Moretta, LLUSM class of 2011, is an assistant professor in LLUSM's department of medicine and a pulmonary and critical care specialist. She is passionate about sharing her faith, especially when medicine offers no hope in the critical care setting. One thing that has kept her motivated throughout the years: the soon coming of Jesus.

June 7

"But we do not want you to be uninformed, brothers, about those who are asleep, that you may not grieve as others do who have no hope. For since we believe that Jesus died and rose again, even so, through Jesus, God will bring with him those who have fallen asleep."

1 Thessalonians 4:13-14, ESV

My first rotation as an internal medicine resident in 1979 was on unit 9200, the oncology ward, at LLUMC. It was a busy unit with many admissions each day. Many of the patients were at the end stages of their battle with cancer. As a young, impressionable resident, I was exposed to much death and sadness. I was called on numerous occasions to pronounce patients that had expired. I was also tasked with contacting the family to give them the sad news as well as trying to comfort them. I particularly remember caring for a young 17-year-old girl with end-stage melanoma with metastasis to her brain. There was little treatment available at that time for metastatic melanoma. I felt helpless as she lapsed into a coma and passed away. I remember how upset I felt about the unfairness of my patient contracting this lethal disease at such a young age.

None of this, however, prepared me for the tragedy of my precious daughter Brittany being diagnosed with advanced high-grade urothelial cancer. Brittany was a graduate of LLUSM class of 2010. She had completed a family medicine residency and was practicing in Reno, Nevada, at the time the diagnosis was made. She loved and had a passion for family medicine. She emphasized preventive medicine in her practice and encouraged her patients to adopt a healthier lifestyle. She had a kind, gentle, and unassuming nature that connected well with her patients. There were many glowing reviews for Brittany on her medical group web page. One patient wrote that Brittany was the best doctor she ever had. She felt as though she had found the North Star when she found Dr. Brittany Penner. She knew that everything would now be OK because Dr. Penner would look out for her. I had a very difficult time understanding and accepting why a young, dedicated, God-fearing physician like Brittany would be stricken with such a deadly disease in the prime of her career. She had so much more to give.

I learned a great deal from Brittany as she faced so much pain and suffering. She underwent multiple courses of chemotherapy, immunotherapy, radiation therapy, and even spinal decompression surgery for metastasis. She met each diagnostic test and treatment with hope and courage. Her faith in Jesus never wavered even as our constant prayers for healing went unanswered. She clung to the promise that all things work together for good to those that love God, even though she did not understand why this was happening to her. Unfortunately, the aggressive cancer slowly strangled the life from her, and she lost her battle with cancer on June 7, 2020. We are sustained by the many memories of Brittany and the promise of being reunited with her as we wait "for our blessed hope, the appearing of the glory of our great God and Savior Jesus Christ" (Titus 2:13, ESV).

Doug Brockmann, LLUSM class of 1978-B, is Brittany Brockmann Penner's father. To turn this tragedy into something of lasting benefit, the family, along with the help of the Office of Philanthropy of LLUSM, created the Brittany Brockmann Penner Scholarship Fund to honor her life and legacy. This scholarship is to benefit worthy medical students with Christian values pursuing a career in family medicine.

June 8

> *"But whoever would be great among you must be your servant,*
> *and whoever would be first among you must be your slave."*
> Matthew 20:26-27, ESV

After denying symptoms of coronary artery disease for months, the angiogram results gave me no other option than to be admitted to the hospital for coronary bypass surgery. There are many things I learned through this ordeal, but one stands apart from the rest—the "patient gown!"

I was the first to arrive in the surgery suite for pre-op preparation at 6:00 a.m. And the very first thing I did was to shed my clothes, all my clothes, and put on the dreaded patient gown. Before I knew it the IVs were in, the surgical site was prepped, and I was out for the next 10 hours. When I awakened, nothing was the same. My body certainly did not feel the same. The pain was beyond description. But there was one constant: my patient gown!

I learned to embrace this gown because it identified me as a patient, someone in need. There are many people who go through a hospital on a given day. There are doctors and nurses, physical therapists and occupational therapists, respiratory technicians, and medical assistants, to name a few. And then there are the administrators and all the visitors. Everyone has a role to play. There is an unspoken hierarchy based upon the title of each individual. This is true even of the visitors. But the patient, every patient, is simply a person in need of healing.

There is no patient hierarchy. We are all sick. We are all in need of medical care. We all need to humble ourselves before those who will help us while donning our patient gowns. Prior to this experience, I have identified myself as a doctor, a surgeon, a pastor, a father, a husband, a follower of Jesus. I donned these titles with pride. But that Wednesday when I entered the pre-op arena, my titles didn't matter. The patient gown was a constant reminder that I was not a doctor or a pastor, but rather a person in need of care. That's when I realized we all need to put on our "patient gowns" as we walk through life and interact with one another.

As I consider this experience, I remember the words of Jesus that "whoever would be first among you must be your slave." In other words, put on your patient gown! When we embrace our patient gowns by identifying and admitting not only our weaknesses but also our shortcomings in loving and serving others, we experience the healing ministry of Christ. It is only by donning our patient gowns, which lets it "all hang out," that we fully embrace the healing power of the gospel through transparency, self-awareness, and submission to the Healer. By becoming a servant, we not only receive the healing ministry of Christ, but extend it to others.

Eric Shadle, Sr., LLUSM class of 1982, is currently the Group VP for Mission Integration at Centura Health in Denver, Colorado. He has a passion to make whole person care available to every community, every neighborhood, every life, and works to do this every day.

June 9

"And whatever you do, in word or deed, do everything in the name of the Lord Jesus, giving thanks to God the Father through him."
Colossians 3:17, ESV

The ambition to become a physician can consume a student's identity. A view of oneself defined by one's own achievements, however, can be indicative of erroneously placed confidence. The LLUH spiritual care practicum challenged us to be aware of where we place our confidence by asking us whether we will be a doctor who happens to be a Christian or a Christian who happens to be a doctor?

Through contemplating this question, I was reminded of some difficult times I had experienced. In high school, my family was separated soon after Thanksgiving because we were evicted from our house and we had to live with different family friends. We eventually were able to come back together as a family under the same roof before Christmas that year, but my awareness of the uncertainty that surrounded my family increased: *Will I be able to afford college? Will I have to give up my dream of becoming a doctor to start working? I don't see my life going the way that I planned at all, so will God still lead me to where I am supposed to be? Who am I going to be?*

Through this consideration I was struck by how many ways I can use my talents to bring glory to God outside of medicine. Glorifying God and acting out my Christian faith is not restricted to a specific profession, even if I feel called to the point of conviction; following Him can be done in all aspects of life wherever I find myself. My life may be completely different than what I planned, but wherever I find myself and whatever I do I can have confidence that I am defined as a loved child of God seeking to honor Him in whatever way I am able.

Daniel Ryan Day's book *Intentional Christian: What to Do When You Don't Know What to Do* talks about his struggle to determine what he should do with his life. In the end, he concluded that if it is not directly against God's commandments, then he can go and do whatever he is able, to God's glory.

Pursuing a specific call may be a wonderful way to bring glory to God after discernment through prayer. However, following that calling should not narrow a broad view of ways in which we can bring God glory. He calls us to walk with Him in every aspect of our life and wherever we may go.

In what ways can you glorify God in where you find yourself today? How will you dedicate it to God? How many things can I find today to thank Him for?

Andrew Folkerts, LLUSM class of 2022, has hopes to serve God as a missionary surgeon. If God has other plans, however, then let His will be done.

June 10

"Behold, I am the Lord, the God of all flesh; is there any thing too hard for me?"
Jeremiah 32:27, KJV

When I first came across this verse, I had little idea how much these words would come to mean to me, and how tightly I would soon have to cling to them as I went through one of the most trying times in my life. I was struck by the directness of it—here was the Creator of the universe declaring His own omnipotence, without exception and without reserve. I tried to imagine just how much the word "anything" encompassed; the possibilities, as you can imagine, are endless. Perhaps I knew it then, perhaps I didn't, but the more I thought about the verse, the stronger my conviction grew to take Him up on His words—to believe that the One who promised "anything" could make "impossible" things possible for me.

When I completed my undergraduate studies at Andrews University in Michigan and received my acceptance letter to the Loma Linda University School of Medicine, I was overjoyed. I don't have the words now to describe what I felt when I received the call from the dean's office, any more than I did then. My joy, however, was tainted with fear. I didn't have the faintest idea how, as an international student, I could afford the tuition for medical school. In fact, a small part of me had thought, *At least I know that I can get into medical school. Perhaps simply knowing this will have to be enough.* In the weeks and months that followed, I prayed to God and pleaded for Him to make a way for me to attend. Up until that point I had counted on financial support from family members, which, much to my dismay, did not come through. We spent days praying and asking for a miracle.

During this time, as I grew through this experience, I simultaneously started on a new spiritual journey and began studying the entire Old Testament. This was easily one of the most remarkable, thrilling, and pivotal moments of my life, one that culminated in a decision to be rebaptized and to renew my commitment to Christ. As I journeyed through the Old Testament and followed the children of Israel, I saw myself in them in a lot of ways. I saw how time and again God bent even the rules of nature on their behalf and how time and again they doubted Him, rebelled against Him, and broke His heart.

To put in a few words: God moved mountains before my eyes to make it possible for me to come to Loma Linda; but as far as I could see, the provision had been only for the first two years of this four-year program. I had to take a leap of faith, not knowing how I would ever finish medical school. But I trusted God, and I came regardless. Now, having completed my second year of medical school and starting my last two clinical years that God miraculously provided for with no effort on my part, I can confidently say in the words of Ellen White: "We have nothing to fear for the future, except as we shall forget the way the Lord has led us, and His teaching in our past history" (*Life Sketches*, p. 196).

When we walk in the path that God has purposed for us, we have no need to fear or be anxious for what we will eat or drink, or what our future will hold. If God can part seas, restore the sight to the blind, heal maladies of body, mind, and spirit, and has power over life and death, what, truly, is impossible for this God to do?

Hazel Ezeribe, LLUSM class of 2022, is currently obtaining a dual degree master's in the bioethics, MA program. She is passionate about God, people, and mentorship. She enjoys good conversation, and loves learning about people and other cultures. In her spare time she enjoys immersing herself in literature, writing, being outdoors, photography, and enjoying good Afro-beats music. She aspires to practice medicine both nationally and internationally as a general surgeon in the near future.

June 11

> *"For everyone who exalts himself will be humbled,*
> *and he who humbles himself will be exalted."*
> Luke 14:11, NASB

The day had finally come! I was heading to Toronto. Growing up in Egypt, I had envisioned immigrating to the United States. I had dreams of practicing medicine in the world's most advanced health care system. I knew that my opportunities as a Christian living in Egypt would be either to choose a remote area in Egypt to practice medicine or to work in the pharmaceutical industry. To be able to travel and seek a career in the U.S. was very fortunate and I knew it, but I was not yet thankful for it.

I had a grand plan. My aunt was a physician, practicing medicine in Niagara Falls, 15 minutes north of the American border. She had chosen to send her two daughters to Buffalo to receive their high school education. My plan was to live with my aunt and save on rent; I would drive my nieces every day to school and save my aunt from paying a driver. In the meantime I would study for my United States Medical License Examinations (USMLE) in a local library until it was time to pick them up and drive back to my aunt's house. It was a great plan! I thought that I had covered all of my bases.

For a while the plan worked just fine. I crossed the border daily, and no one asked any questions. On weekends I would drive to Toronto and meet with friends, go to church, then quickly go out for some fun. As a young man away from his parents for the first time, I loved my new independence! I made new friends and enjoyed my North American way of life. I slowly but ever so surely began to feel overconfident, proud, and perhaps a little arrogant.

Then one day as I was crossing the border, driving my nieces to school, the agent at the border asked to search the car, and I obliged. The agent then asked me about my medical books and if I was studying in the U.S. I answered that I was in fact studying in preparation for the USMLE. He became very angry and told me that I was breaking the law. He indicated that since I had no student visa, I had no right to study in the U.S. Assuming I would enter the U.S. illegally and stay there permanently, the agent stamped my passport with a declination to enter the U.S. I was forced to return to Canada!

I remember how I felt that night. My future was ruined, my dreams were shattered, and I was an utter failure. I prayed out of desperation and confessed how proud I had become. I was made to understand the fragility of my own plans. Then God spoke, and I was reminded by His Word: "Trust in the LORD with all your heart, and lean not on your understanding; in all your ways acknowledge Him, and He shall direct your paths" (Proverbs 3:5-6, NKJV). I understood and appreciated the promise, and in the process learned a valuable lesson: I would never again trust myself and my plans. I promised to depend on the Lord wholeheartedly.

My circumstances did not change; I was not able to enter the U.S. However, I already had peace. I did not know what was to happen, nor how. I simply trusted that the Lord would direct my path, and He did. First, I passed my USMLE, not knowing if I would ever practice medicine in the U.S. Second, I opened my mail one day to find out that I had been awarded a green card and permanent status. Third, I met my future wife at church, and what a blessing that was! A beautiful woman who was willing to cast her lot on a young man with an unknown future! Last, I received an offer for residency at the Cleveland Clinic Foundation in Ohio, which was given *before* the match! I did not even have to use the match system to find employment!

Now, as I practice medicine every day, I remain humble and trust the Lord in all that I do. The Lord honors those who depend on Him; I am a living testimony of that!

Ihab Dorotta is an associate professor in LLUSM's department of anesthesiology and critical care. He is the director of the critical care center and the chief of quality and patient safety at LLUMC.

June 12

"Cast your bread upon the waters, For you will find it after many days."
Ecclesiastes 11:1, NKJV

Are you working or in school?" I asked the young man sitting next to me with our paper plates on our laps enjoying a Sabbath lunch at a friend's house in the Philippines. What he told me I tried to push out of my mind for the next 40-plus hours. This was his final quarter in pursuing a BS degree in theology at the local university, but he was not allowed to finish unless he could come up with $200 by the following Monday morning. He had worked overtime, borrowed funds up to this final quarter. But still he lacked that $200 to register for the final quarter. He promised that if the university would allow him to graduate, he would work through the summer to pay back the $200. After much negotiating with the university, their final answer was no.

Early Monday morning I felt a strong urge to help this young man whom I had just met two days ago. Not knowing his last name, nor a contact phone number, I took a bus to the local mission office with a check for $200. The receptionist gratefully promised that she'd contact this young man right away so that he could pay the tuition before the deadline at 12:00 noon that very day.

Fast-forward 25 years. I was looking through the *Potpourri* (the student directory) for the incoming class I'd be teaching in medical microbiology, and a name jumped out among the class of 170 students. Could this be the daughter of the young man I had met so many years ago? Flipping a few more pages in the *Potpourri*, I saw a picture of another young woman with the same last name two classes behind. Perhaps that young man had two daughters attending the Loma Linda University School of Medicine?

Immediately following the class, I rushed over to this woman with a familiar name. Yes, her father did graduate from the university in the Philippines, and had served as a pastor in the Philippines. Now he was pastoring a church in Tennessee. And yes, she had a sister just two classes behind her! That evening she called her father and was told the story of that $200 graciously given to him by a professor from Loma Linda University Health whose daughters are now his students. Indeed, cast your bread upon the waters, for you will find it after many days.

Praise the Lord.

Benjamin H. Lau, LLUSM class of 1980-A, PhD, is an emeritus professor in LLUSM's department of microbiology and immunology. He was LLUSM's Teacher of the Year in 1980, 1987, and 1990. For three decades he and his associates have conducted cancer research using phytochemicals (plant chemicals) to overcome cancer. He has authored 200-plus scientific publications and eight books. The latest book is Stop Cancer With Phytotherapy. June 12 is his wedding anniversary.

June 13

> *"Behold, God is my helper; the Lord is the upholder of my life."*
> Psalm 54:4, ESV

"Everyone has their limits. Everyone has a breaking point," stated the Marine Corps veteran in a sober voice as he sat on the exam table. It had been four decades since he had served in the military, but his downcast eyes and quiet tone communicated how clearly these memories were still etched in his mind.

The older I get, the more I have come to see and understand that part of being human is being limited. Limited by my need for sleep, limited by my need for food, limited by the number of hours in the day and what I can accomplish in any given hour, limited by the amount of wisdom and strength I possess within myself. I have limits to my patience, limits to my generosity, limits to my love, limits to my kindness, limits to my happiness, limits to my self-control, limits to my sense of peace and well-being, and most of all, limits to my mortal existence.

It is not by accident or chance that we experience limitations as humans, but by design. I have come to learn that my limitations as a human actually serve a divine purpose to help me understand my humble state as a created being and cause me to turn to my Maker for whatever I lack. To turn to the One who has no limitations, who Himself is the source of all wisdom, strength, peace, love, joy, and life.

Again and again in the Scriptures, God communicates to us both His desire and power to provide supernatural heavenly help to those who would simply ask Him. I have come to learn that a humble heart is the avenue through which one is able to see their need and then turn to this great God for help.

"God is my helper." What an amazing and glorious truth that the all-powerful God of the universe would care to help me in my daily struggles. Yet the greatest help He offers me is salvation through His Son, Jesus Christ; that when my mortal body reaches its ultimate limit and passes into death, I will then be raised again to eternal life and immortality through the forgiveness and righteousness that is in Christ Jesus.

Shawna McCarty Langley, LLUSM class of 2007, is an assistant professor in LLUSM's department of dermatology. She practices at the Jerry L. Pettis Memorial Veterans Medical Center in Loma Linda, California.

June 14

> *"You, LORD, give perfect peace to those who keep their purpose firm and put their trust in you."*
> Isaiah 26:3, GNT

"Daddy, I'm scared. I don't want to do this."

Sarah did not need to tell me. I could see it in her face. I could sense it in her quivering 6-year-old body.

"I know, sweetie, but you are going to be OK. Daddy's here," I said, trying to sound calmer than I felt. "All these people are here to take care of you."

Sarah was looking up at me from her hospital bed at the Outpatient Surgery Center, trying bravely to hold back tears. But the tears of little girls are no match for fear. I held her hand and stroked her cheek, hoping that she would find comfort in my touch because the tightness in my throat would not let me speak.

Sarah understood why she was there. Sarah has never hesitated to ask questions, and she did not hold back when talking to her doctor. At the end of the informed consent discussion a week before the date of surgery, Sarah's doctor turned to her and asked, "Well, Sarah, do you have any questions for me?"

"Yes!" exclaimed Sarah.

Somewhat surprised by the abruptness of this little patient, the doctor responded, "Well, OK, what questions do you have?"

Sarah paused, then looked up at her doctor and said, "This surgery—what's it all about, anyway?" Sarah and her doctor then engaged in a rather mature back-and-forth discussion. Sarah questioned her doctor with a number of open-ended questions that made her lawyer-father proud.

It was now time for surgery. I wanted more than anything to hold my little girl and comfort her, or even pick her up and run out of the building! Instead, as the surgeon distracted Sarah in conversation, my wife and I hurried back toward the waiting room, hoping Sarah would not notice we had left. My wife sat down in the waiting room, but I kept walking until I was outside.

In the crisp morning air I found myself standing under a tall pine tree. It was there that I wept. Sometimes Daddies cry too. I closed my eyes hard and cried to my heavenly Father. I prayed a prayer of pleading. I asked Jesus to give the anesthesiologist not only extra skill but also compassion. I begged Jesus to guide the hands of the surgeon. But I pleaded most of all that Jesus would comfort Sarah and heal her, and that she would feel His comfort. I asked Jesus to hold my little girl in His arms when I could not hold her in mine. I prayed for peace—the godly peace that transcends human understanding and fear.

And it was there, under that tall pine tree, that Jesus gave me His peace. The calm came over me as suddenly as I had asked for it. I knew that Jesus would care for my little girl more than I ever could, and I knew that He would care for her through her doctors and nurses.

There is holy ground on the campus of Loma Linda University Health. It is located under a tall pine tree just outside the Outpatient Surgery Center. I know because I saw Jesus there.

Chris Johnston, JD, serves as associate general counsel for LLUH. He and his wife, Zina, have two daughters, Sarah and Natalie.

June 15

"As thou knowest not what is the way of the spirit, nor how the bones do grow in the womb of her that is with child: even so thou knowest not the works of God who maketh all. In the morning sow thy seed, and in the evening withhold not thine hand: for thou knowest not whether shall prosper, either this or that, or whether they both shall be alike good."

Ecclesiastes 11:5-6, KJV

A 30-something-year-old Caucasian male named James stepped into my office a couple of years ago for a consultation for biopsy-proven psoriasis. As an uninsured patient, I was limited as to what I could prescribe him, and so his disease would wax and wane as he tried samples of varying ointments and injections. A rebiopsy confirmed a diagnosis of psoriasis, yet his disease did not seem to respond very well to any of the treatments we tried. During one particular office visit he expressed his frustration with his skin condition, as well as his mounting stress levels. He was working as a personal trainer, attending college courses to fulfill his prerequisites to apply to nursing school; he drank and smoked heavily to escape from memories of a very difficult childhood (he shared this information later in a letter).

Because stress can play a role in psoriasis, I knew he needed more support than what medications could offer him. I thought, *This guy needs Jesus, but he doesn't look like the type to respond positively to such a question.* I took a deep breath and asked him if he believed in a higher power and prayer, and offered to pray for him. He looked nervous, and his response shocked me. He said, "I grew up in an atheist home, and I've never prayed before. I don't even know how to pray."

I told him, "You pray to God like you talk to a friend," and we said a simple prayer. James later told me that his first thought at the time was *This woman is a Jesus freak; I came for professional medical treatment, and this woman wants to treat me with prayer.* Nevertheless, prayer happened several more times in subsequent visits—at James's request. He came to a health event at our Adventist church.

Eventually he began praying on his own, praise the Lord; and said that his favorite place to pray was in his car. Before he turned the car stereo on, he made it part of his daily routine to pray. James said, "Without realizing it, I started noticing changes not only to my spiritual well-being, but I was experiencing mental and physical changes as well. I began to notice the blessings all around me, one right after another. Accepting God brought faith, hope, and love into my life. Each day my life improves. Before finding God, my life was in crisis mode, and now with the love of God in my heart, I am enjoying a new beginning."

I learned an important lesson: You never know who will respond to an invitation to know Jesus.

Jane Clark, LLUSM class of 2005, works in the fields of internal medicine/dermatology. She is married to Georgia-Cumberland Conference vice president Chester Van Clark III, and has three daughters: Ella and twins, Mabel and Marilee.

June 16

*"Be faithful to me, even if it means death,
and I will give you life as your prize of victory."*
Revelation 2:10, GNT

For the past several years it has been my privilege to serve as the Loma Linda University Health (LLUH) representative to the Pan-African Academy of Christian Surgeons (PAACS). PAACS runs Western-style surgical residency programs in Africa to train and disciple Africans to be Christian surgeons. LLUH has been accrediting these surgical residency programs for 20 years. As part of that, I recently went on an accreditation trip to the 12 PAACS surgical training programs throughout Africa.

While on this trip, I met countless missionary surgeons who have given their lives in service to God. Through their selfless work they are creating sustainable surgical care in rural Africa while sharing the gospel. I also met many African people who have also given selflessly to spread God's Word through PAACS. One particular story stood out—the story of Rosa.

I met Rosa at Harpur Memorial Hospital (HMH) in Menouf, Egypt. HMH is a Christian hospital in a rural town that is 99.9 percent Muslim. The people of Menouf are proud to have HMH in their town even though it is a Christian hospital. The hospital has provided outstanding medical care to the Muslim community for more than 100 years. While the hospital is a welcome part of the town, there is, however, a strict prohibition on Muslims converting to Christianity.

Rosa had previously been a patient at HMH and was incredibly impressed not only by the medical care that she received, but even more by the Christian caring that she felt from all of the hospital workers. She was so impressed that she decided to become a Christian and work at the hospital. I asked her what this meant for her in a small Muslim town like this. She matter-of-factly told me that her father had already disowned her, and that he would try to kill her. I asked her if there was a safer way forward for her. She told me that Jesus had called her to help her people, and there was no turning back.

During the time that I was at HMH, I could see that Rosa had an amazing impact on the people of her town. She was an effective liaison with them, because she had been one of them. As the time came for our team to leave to go to the next PAACS hospital, I said goodbye to Rosa. She told me how much our visit had meant to them, and I told her how much her stand for Jesus had inspired me. To her it was no big deal. She loved Jesus and was willing to do anything for Him. As we left, she told me that she would see me in heaven.

I have not heard from Rosa since then. I was told that Muslims in that town who convert to Christianity are often murdered. They told me that it was likely that Rosa's father did kill her.

I am looking forward to seeing Rosa in heaven.

Mark Reeves, LLUSM class of 1992, PhD, is a professor in LLUSM's department of basic sciences, division of biochemistry, and is the director of the Cancer Center, the VP for Institutes, and practices surgical oncology, all at LLUH. He has a passion for training surgeons around the world and spreading the good news about God. He has been married for 36 years to Michelle Reeves (LLUSM class of 1986).

June 17

> *"Should you not also have had mercy on your fellow slave, in the same way that I had mercy on you?"*
> Matthew 18:33, NASB

Don't worry. It will last only a few seconds, and then the worst will be over."

With a glare she responded with a particularly virulent "That's what they always say, and it always hurts!" It was late on a Friday, and it had been an extraordinary busy day on the general surgery service. The sun had started to set, and all I wanted to do was to be at home with my wife to celebrate the Sabbath's arrival. All the tasks from the day had been accomplished save one— the one that I least wanted to do.

She was middle aged, chronically ill on hemodialysis, with a problems list longer then my arm. Many of those problems were caused by a lifetime of poor choices. Simply put, late on a Friday afternoon as a burned-out intern, I lacked compassion. I gave a hefty dose of Dilaudid, but that isn't a substitute for compassion.

As the smell of infected tissue filled the room and my nostrils, I began to think, *This is taking way too long.* Thoughts filled my mind of how annoying the whole situation was, how maybe she really wasn't having that much pain and was only seeking more drugs, and how this was the one thing standing between me and leaving the hospital. Worst of all, I began to think that she didn't deserve my compassion. After all, wasn't her kidney failure and all her medical problems the result of a lifetime of bad choices? If this was all self-inflicted, why should I expend the emotional energy needed to have compassion and empathy for her?

Then I looked into her eyes. I saw an existential suffering that far exceeded the pain of a dressing change. I heard an audible voice say, *Stephen, did you deserve My dying on the cross for your sins—sins that you willfully committed?*

The conviction hit me like a ton of bricks. Did she not deserve my compassion? If she didn't deserve my compassion, how could I be deserving of Christ's compassion, salvation, or healing? Yet because I had experienced Christ's love, compassion, healing, and the benefits of salvation—all of which were wholly unmerited—I was compelled to give the same to her. I was compelled to show her Christ through my actions. To do otherwise would be to forsake the gifts Christ had given me.

While I couldn't do more to alleviate her pain from a medical standpoint, I could give her my compassion and time. So I did. I sat and took five minutes to listen to her story. Her husband had left her because of her chronic medical problems, her son was a juvenile delinquent, and her mother was dying in a different hospital in the same town. Talk about a bad day and a sad situation! In the process of treating her as a person, child of God, and sister in Christ, I became changed.

I ought to have mercy and compassion for all my patients and everyone I interact with, because that is what Christ did for me.

Stephen Thorp, LLUSM class of 2016, completed a general surgery residency in June, 2021, at Michigan State University in Grand Rapids, Michigan. He is married to Cherilyn, a nurse, and they plan on long-term, cross-cultural mission service through the deferred mission appointee program.

June 18

"If my people who are called by my name humble themselves, and pray and seek my face and turn from their wicked ways, then I will hear from heaven and will forgive their sin and heal their land. Now my eyes will be open and my ears attentive to the prayer that is made in this place."
2 Chronicles 7:14-15, ESV

I wanted to be a doctor because medicine can bring healing when the world has turned its back. I struggled through science classes waiting for the day I could be a part of this healing process. My time came during a summer preceptorship that taught the art of emotional and spiritual care for patients. I was really excited to be a part of this preceptorship because it felt tailor-made for me and that I would shine with my theological training. Medicine will humble you.

After receiving my initial training to work from, I went to my assigned floor and said a quick prayer before starting. I prayed that God would lead me to the right patient to make a difference; this is the scariest medical prayer to voice to a listening Father.

After praying, I spotted my patient. He was a physically imposing man of different ethnicity and tattoos covering every square inch of his body. He had a sour look on his face, and I could feel his hostility. I was silently thinking, *Man, what a rotten first experience; lets get this over with as soon as possible.* I had written this man off before saying a word; my bias, pride, and ego had blinded me.

With a quavering voice I started my script and asked if I could speak with him about his emotional and spiritual journey. At this his face slowly transformed. The snarling lips softened into a smile, piercing eyes mellowed, and tense shoulders relaxed. He looked at me and said, "Nobody has been to see me in a long time; I'd love to tell you my story." So began the most remarkable 45 minutes of my life. This ex-gang member bared his soul, telling of his life through gangs, prison, work problems, divorce, and finding love again. He finished his story telling me how he's working in a ministry to help gang members experience Christ.

I was left speechless. I had written off this lost cause and he was showing me how to be a healer. My patient had tears running down his face, relieved at getting his story off his chest. He took my hand and prayed for me on the spot.

Leaving, I wasn't the same person walking out. Something profound had changed within me; it was love for the unloved. Unconditional love had been missing from my heart, and it took a tough, muscular ex-gang member to help me find it. Medicine is a privileged profession because it gives us a front-row seat to the most intimate struggles of humanity and the human heart. We are there when the world comes crashing down in the lives of our patients, when all hope is taken from a trembling soul. We have to have the opportunity to love our patients unconditionally as they begin to put their life back together. We can be the listening heart, the helping hand, and the calm assurance that they are not alone and are loved.

Thomas Flynn, LLUSM class of 2020, matched to the family medicine residency through Florida State University in Fort Myers. Combining his degree in theology with medicine, he plans on practicing broad spectrum primary care in a rural setting, with medical mission trips as vacations. He is driven to follow in the footsteps of Christ as a healer, and his goal is to one day hear the words "Well done, good and faithful servant."

June 19

Father's Day, 2022
Juneteenth

> "But while he was still a long way off, his father saw him and felt compassion, and ran and embraced him and kissed him. And the son said to him, 'Father, I have sinned against heaven and before you. I am no longer worthy to be called your son.' But the father said to his servants, 'Bring quickly the best robe, and put it on him, and put a ring on his hand, and shoes on his feet. And bring the fattened calf and kill it, and let us eat and celebrate. For this my son was dead, and is alive again; he was lost, and is found.'"
>
> Luke 15:20-24, ESV

"Mr. X is back again, Doc. What are we doing this time?" the nurse asked. The intoxicated Mr. X had seemingly become my personal patient, as I'd been unfortunate enough to be there for each of his three recent ED visits.

The shadowing medical student asked for my permission to see the patient. "No need; I know this guy," I replied. "He's been here numerous times for intoxication, so there's nothing really to do. Paramedics bring him in, and he ends up sleeping it off. You'll know he's ready for discharge when he starts cussing everyone out. Sometimes despite your best efforts you realize that some people are just unwilling to accept any grace."

As I hurriedly rushed to see my next several patients, I continued to replay the conversation with the med student. Did I actually just say that? My sense of remorse grew as I further realized that despite satisfying my professional obligation, I really hadn't done anything that would constitute as a genuine effort to promote Mr. X's well-being. I hadn't even had a real dialogue with him other than to satisfy that he was sober enough to walk out of the ED. Perhaps there was a reason Mr. X and I continued to cross paths.

Praying for a more generous spirit, I returned to Mr. X's room and actually listened while he told his story. He had been the victim of a major accident years prior, it turns out, and had sustained a disabling traumatic injury, leaving him in chronic pain. His problems with alcohol and prescription drugs had developed as a result of his attempts to cope with the pain and depression associated with his injury, and the loss of his physical independence.

I asked if he would like me to pray for him, which he accepted. We discussed rehabilitation programs in the area and discharge advice. I then asked if there was anything else that would be helpful to him. He paused before reticently asking, "Can you call my dad?"

I dialed the phone number he provided, expecting to reach a disconnected number or an indifferent party unwilling to help which is the common response in my experience. "Hello," the voice on the other end of the line answered.

"Hi, I'm an ER doctor taking care of a Mr. X. He asked if I could call this number to—"

"He's there? Doctor, please don't let him go; we've been looking for him. My son's been missing for a long time. Please let him know I'm coming to get him."

I still reflect on what prevented Mr. X from simply picking up a phone and calling what appeared to be a loving family in desperate pursuit of him. I also like to imagine that the reunion of Mr. X with his family that day might have represented the opportunity for restoration and a new beginning.

How cherished we are by God. Grace is so much bigger than we could ever imagine, and God is desperately in pursuit of all of His children.

James S. Kim, LLUSM class of 2000, practices emergency medicine and serves as chairman and medical director of the department of emergency medicine at Pomona Valley Hospital Medical Center in Pomona, California. He and his spouse are blessed with four wonderful children.

June 20

> *"Love does no harm to a neighbor. Therefore love is the fulfillment of the law."*
> Romans 13:10, NIV

It was a warm, sunny day in Loma Linda, California. I had just received my dragon fruit smoothie at the Loma Linda Market when I noticed my former organic chemistry professor and close friend, Dr. Glenn Phillips, enter the store with his two daughters, ages 5 and 7. I had not seen them since before quarantine began, so I decided to join them in the checkout line to catch up.

I had just stooped down to speak with his younger daughter when suddenly an older white woman being rung up in front of us stormed over to our group. "Excuse me!" she exclaimed loudly. "I just want you to know that my husband was a police officer! And he died in the line of duty!"

Let me pause the story here and provide some context. Recent events in the news concerning police brutally murdering unarmed Black individuals had led to weeks of unrest and protests all over America. But as mentioned before, neither my companions nor I were currently protesting; we were simply buying groceries with and for our loved ones. After her sharp and sudden remarks, I managed to reply flatly, "Oh . . . OK." She then marched back to the register while I glanced around at the other patrons in the store, confirming my suspicion that we were, indeed, the only Black patrons in the establishment.

I attempted to continue my conversation with the 5-year-old, hoping to distract her from the incident that had just occurred. Meanwhile, my professor and I exchanged worried glances over our masks as we continued to listen to the loud, ongoing rant happening at the cash register. The woman proclaimed her annoyance with protests and protestors before exclaiming, "Not all cops are bad! Just because one cop did something wrong doesn't mean they're all bad! . . . My husband was a good man, and he saved a lot of lives!"

I stood up, clearly uncomfortable, as she continued. "*Those* people are racist!" she jeered. "They're the real racists, and they don't care about anyone but themselves!"

My professor and I tried, unsuccessfully, to keep the children distracted from the active disturbance. We had just begun a new conversation about football (what Americans call soccer) when we heard the cashier announce, "Register 4 is open." When we showed no sign of moving, she repeated a bit more emphatically, "Register 4 is *also* open." We realized she was giving us an opportunity to switch lanes and to spare ourselves the proximity to the unending tirade.

We switched lanes.

By the time our transactions were complete, the unruly woman had disappeared from the store. My professor sighed and with a heavy heart told me how he now had to explain to his young daughters what had taken place. I wondered how that conversation would go, thankful that I did not yet hold that same responsibility. I wondered if he would mention Romans 13:10 when explaining to them that instead of approaching others in an obtuse manner, as the woman in the store had, they should instead demonstrate love, which "does no harm to a neighbor," no matter their age, race, orientation, or religion. Just as police are expected to uphold the law, we, too, as Christians are expected to love. Because that is the fulfillment of God's law.

Va Shon Williams, LLUSM class of 2020, was born and raised on the island of Bermuda. He is the youngest of eight sons, and the third to pursue a career in medicine. He is a proud graduate of Oakwood University (2016) in Alabama and is currently an anesthesiology resident at LLUH.

June 21

> *"For God so loved the world, that he gave his only begotten Son."*
> John 3:16, KJV

On June 21, 1983, our lives stopped when the phone rang and the voice on the other end said, "Mrs. Raines? Please sit down; this is the park ranger from Yosemite National Park. Your son Steffan was lost on the trail to Half Dome. We called off the search after sundown."

When the call ended, we checked to see if there were flights from Southern California to Fresno. There were none, so my husband, Gary, and I decided to drive to Yosemite immediately. As we drove toward the Yosemite ranger station, we both began to process and prepare for the loss of our 8-year-old son, Steffan. Visions of every danger filled our minds.

The local church had invited our two boys, Jonathan, 11, and Steffan, to participate in a youth outing that would have as many children as leaders. Yosemite National Park was the destination, and the boys begged to go. After reassurances from those in charge that the children would be well supervised, we agreed.

The children began the nine-mile hike up to Half Dome in the morning. Sometime in the early afternoon the bigger kids raced ahead with the teenage leaders, while the youngest, ages 5 to 7, brought up the rear with the adults. Our boys were by themselves in the middle and followed what they thought was the trail, but was not. Jonathan begged his brother to follow him, but Steffan wanted to find his own way. Jonathan made it to camp and was frantic when he realized his brother was nowhere to be found. As the sun lowered and darkness fell, our son was alone and lost. It was then that the park ranger made the phone call.

As we drove, I was wide awake. Energy surged through my body as we sped through the mountains. Already my mind was preparing for the possibility of never seeing Steff again.

In the early morning we arrived at the main entrance of the park and were guided to the ranger station. Jonathan had been brought there to try to identify where he and Steff had separated. We were thrilled to see him and hold him close—and saw how drained and worn he was. As the search commenced, I remember being speechless as Gary and Jonathan boarded the provided helicopter. When asked to join them, I responded that I preferred to stay at the station "in case any news came in."

Three long hours followed. At 9:15 a.m. word came that a volunteer dog search team had spotted a blond head in a clearing. It was our son, and he was alive! When I received this news, my tears were unstoppable. I was driven to the heliport where they had brought Steff for this miraculous family reunion. Arms outstretched, I ran toward him as he and my family exited the helicopter.

The ranger confided that Steff had acted with amazing self-preservation instincts. I was so touched as Steff told them, "It was dark. I was scared. It was cold. I sat by a big rock. I grabbed my legs and made my body into a ball and prayed: 'Dear Jesus, this is my last prayer. I am freezing to death.'"

We felt so humbled yet blessed as we realized our family was part of an amazing miracle that day. And then we thought of the gift of God's Son freely given to humanity—only love understands love.

R. Marina Raines, LLUSD DH class of 1970, is married to Gary Raines (LLUSM class of 1972). They live in Glendale, California, and are the parents of three children: Jonathan (LLUSM class of 2000), Steffan, and Jacqueline. They are the joyous grandparents of one grandchild. This story was written in 2020 for this book, 37 years after this frightening experience took place.

June 22

"Jesus went through all the towns and villages, teaching in their synagogues, proclaiming the good news of the kingdom and healing every disease and sickness."
Matthew 9:35, NIV

"How much longer does she have?" asked a young man whose mother had been hospitalized for terminal colon cancer at the hospice ward of Tokyo Adventist Hospital. "Maybe a week or two," I answered as an attending physician. His face turned gloomy.

"Is there any way to help her attend my wedding three weeks from today?" he continued. Knowing his mother's poor prognosis, he had hastened his wedding plan, but it appeared that she would not live that long. "Medically, no. If you hope for any chance, you should do it ASAP, even as early as tomorrow!" I suggested.

He immediately got on his phone and started calling around, trying to secure his wedding site for the coming weekend. Unfortunately, not a single place was available.

Then a nurse at the hospice came up with a bright idea. "Let's have the wedding on our ward!"

There is, at the hospice, a small chapel that seats about 15 people. It is a cozy place well decorated with stained glass and a cross. Our chaplain uses it for consultation and prayer.

The young man and the patient (mother) looked at the place, and they liked it. Then the plan was on. We found a wedding coordinator, a florist, and whoever was willing to help. Many of our nursing staff were involved. Our chaplain would serve as a minister. Everything was prepared in a couple of days.

On the wedding day at the hospice a handsome bridegroom in a black tuxedo, a beautiful bride in white wedding dress, their close friends and relatives, and the hospital staff were all present. At the center was the patient, the groom's mother who had been given a morphine injection for pain, was on oxygen for dyspnea, and on the verge of liver failure from metastases. She sat in a wheelchair, wore a nice dress, and put makeup on her face to hide jaundice. But most of all, there was the greatest smile on the patient's face, enriching the audience with deep feeling of happiness and joy. She appeared to be a totally different person free of her terminal symptoms. Definitely that was one of the happiest moments of her life.

That night she quietly passed away with a smile on her face, watched by the newly wedded couple at her side.

Even with the great advancement of modern medicine, there still exist situations that we as physicians cannot cure. Our best efforts may not produce the best medical results on many occasions.

But I believe that what God wants us to do is to serve humbly for others with all our heart and knowledge, always seeking their health and peace. When we do so, God will intervene and make the impossible possible beyond our imaginations.

Jesus is our ultimate example. Let us be like Him in our practice.

Toshihiro Nishino, LLUSM class of 1988, currently serves as the president and CEO of Tokyo Adventist Hospital in Japan, while continuing his practice in general surgery. His son, Kevin, graduated from LLUSM class of 2019, and his daughter, Melissa, is in LLUSM's class of 2022.

June 23

> "God is not unjust; he will not forget your work and the love you have shown him as you have helped his people and continue to help them."
>
> Hebrews 6:10, NIV

Almost anything that could go wrong did go wrong. My first flight was already behind schedule, and the pilots hadn't yet arrived. During their startup routine they discovered the right engine wasn't working. Mechanics were called in, but then they needed to retrieve a special tool. Finally they decided that all passengers would have to deplane. Since I had multiple connecting flights (Vancouver-Toronto-Istanbul-Nairobi), this was a poor start to traveling alone to join my Kenya mission trip group.

I was rebooked on another set of flights (Vancouver-London-Dubai-Nairobi), but that first flight was also delayed. Coupled with unusual passenger volume at Heathrow because of weather delays, I missed my connection. Waiting in a line for so long that I picked up some local vocabulary, I was rebooked again for a direct flight to Nairobi scheduled to arrive only two and a half hours behind my group. Unfortunately, when I arrived for that flight, I was denied boarding because my rebooked ticket had not been issued properly and they were about to close.

I experienced an overwhelming feeling of defeat. The airline counters that could help me were closed, I had no idea how to catch up to my group, and my luggage was lost because of the multiple rebookings. Despite all my determination, I was now stranded. While riding the train toward the terminal where I could have my ticket reissued for the next day, I neared a breaking point. A British woman riding the same train must have sensed my devastation and offered a mint after hearing about my ordeal. I don't typically accept candy from complete strangers, but I did that time and appreciated the small gesture.

I had been fortunate with air travel before that point in my life, never losing luggage or experiencing anything beyond minor inconsequential delays. I was long overdue to have that finally even out. Now I had experienced nearly every possible complication that could arise while flying, all on the same trip. I'm not sure if what promised to be a memorable mission trip really needed that precursory drama to make it even more memorable, but I am certain that the opportunity was appreciated that much more after enduring the challenges of just making it there. When I stepped out of the chaotic world of international air travel and onto the doorstep of the Maasai Mara, I found myself the furthest away from home that I had ever been and eager to serve.

Lost among the masses and in the flurry of everyday life, we can find it easy to forget that God never stops watching over our lives and cares about the details. As we dedicate ourselves to His service as physicians and more, we can lean on His promise always to remember the work that we do and the love that we show on His behalf. And mint woman: Keep on doing what you do. What would the world do without people like you to look out for and help lift the discouraged?"

David A. Ngan, LLUSM class of 2023, had the tremendous opportunity to help serve in a mobile medical clinic, help with construction of a secondary school building, and develop music and sport activities for primary schoolchildren. June 23 was the date of this unforgettable travel misadventure.

June 24

"Prayer is not a convenient device for imposing our will upon God, or bending his will to ours, but the prescribed way of subordinating our will to his."

John Stott (1921–2011): English Anglican theologian

Our son, Greg, was born in Hong Kong during our mission term there in the 1970s. During breastfeeding at 10 days old, his mother noticed he was turning blue. She called me in a panic. I tried to reassure her that it was probably just the effect of the fluorescent lighting. But I too was both puzzled and fearful when normal lighting made no difference. He quickly went into respiratory distress. I ran down two floors to the nursery and placed him in an intensive-care incubator with the oxygen at 100 percent. It gave very temporary relief. His pulse was 250-plus. Cardiac failure and death threatened. I called Dr. Fung by "randomly" opening the huge phone book. Despite the congested traffic of that city, he arrived promptly.

He gave expert care, but to little avail. In those days we believed that no one could run those high pulse rates and survive much beyond 40 minutes. Greg's condition deteriorated. His blood backed up within his liver as well as his lungs, and the former grew so large that it entered his pelvis. When he surprisingly did make it through 24 hours, we felt time was running out. How long could his tiny heart survive the physical stress before it would succumb to total exhaustion and ultimate collapse? What to do? Chinese friends made phone calls to about 15 churches in Hong Kong and Taiwan, asking that all their members pray for Greg at the same hour. They did so, and he converted immediately at that very hour. It was, I truly believe, a direct answer to fervent prayer—a miracle of divine origin.

Greg did fairly well after that on medication, but would periodically revert to a fast and dangerous heart rate. This was triggered by hiking at high elevations in the mountains behind our home in Canada, or when he received a blow to the chest, which was usually when he was "boarded" in hockey games. However, he grew up to be a very strong and aggressive player in college, often getting the most goals because of his size, strength, and tenacity—but he also often chalked up the most penalty minutes because of those same qualities!

Later his condition, diagnosed as Wolff-Parkinson-White syndrome, was corrected with ablation. During that procedure Greg was awake, and when the doctors had to periodically stop his heart in order to "fry those wires," he would remind them politely but emphatically that he'd like to have it started again and "pronto, if you please!"

He has never really looked back since. His heart is stable and strong. We love you, Greg! And we love You, God, for giving him to us and then saving his life as a mere infant.

Sid Kettner, LLUSM class of 1969, has spent seven years of mission service in Hong Kong and Arctic Canada. He has been in family practice in Creston, British Columbia, for 30 years. Over the years, he has traveled to four continents while conducting one-month medical evangelism seminars. June 24 is his birthday.

June 25

"The LORD himself goes before you and will be with you; he will never leave you nor forsake you. Do not be afraid; do not be discouraged."

Deuteronomy 31:8, NIV

Have you heard of FOMO? "Fear of missing out" is something that millennials know all too well. FOMO is the idea that other people are enjoying awesome life experiences without you. You might miss out on an opportunity for a social connection or update!

This is something I deal with regularly. Who wouldn't want to be included? In the same way, as doctors we strive to keep up-to-date on the constantly developing field of medicine. The responsibility can become crippling. What if I miss an abnormal lab result or drug interaction, and my patient experiences a negative outcome?

A lesson I'm still learning is that FOMO is really a lack of trust in God's sovereignty. He prepares my way and path—nothing surprises Him! As a believer, I have been promised the companionship of the Holy Spirit. He goes before me into my patient encounters, walks with me on my journey, and resides in my heart.

Here's another struggle for young doctors, including myself: imposter syndrome. This is an unfounded sense of inadequacy and self-doubt, despite proof of competence and skill. I easily slip into this mentality when busy with multitasking and overwhelming responsibilities.

I began residency at a younger age than my peers, and I often worried that my knowledge base or experience was not enough. To broaden my learning, I spent my spare time working after-hours at a community clinic in downtown Orlando, Florida, that provided free medical care to vulnerable uninsured populations, including immigrants, ex-convicts, the homeless, and refugees.

Because of lapses in access to health care, these patients were a challenge, both medically and emotionally. We had limited state-allocated resources, and only specific cases met criteria for hospital charity. I had to trim down my "by the book" workups and settle for what was cost-effective. Many patients were lost to follow-up. In what seemed like hopeless situations, I often felt that all I had to offer my patients was prayer.

However, one day toward the end of my residency, I was delightfully surprised to see a familiar name on my schedule. Newly blessed with insurance, a patient from the community clinic had chosen to establish primary care with me!

While wrapping up her appointment, I summarized my plan for her: bloodwork, new medications, and referrals. I was excited that she would finally get the care that she deserved! But as I turned to leave, she exclaimed, "Dr. Fitch, aren't you going to pray with me, as you always do? That's the reason I wanted you to be my doctor." As you can imagine, that stopped me in my tracks. Humbling as that moment was, that's when it clicked for me: Patients are not just a collection of problems to solve or fix. They are spiritual beings in need of God's love and healing.

As a Christian, I am an ambassador—not an imposter—and I represent Jesus Christ. As long as I can share the compassion and grace of God, I don't ever need to fear that I'm inadequate or "missing out."

Klaireece Fitch, LLUSM class of 2015, is a board-certified family medicine physician. In 2011 she served as junior faculty for the whole person care preceptorship at LLUMC and was president of the Christian Medical & Dental Association, Loma Linda chapter, from 2012 to 2014.

June 26

"Don't let anyone look down on you because you are young, but set an example for the believers in speech, in conduct, in love, in faith and in purity."
1 Timothy 4:12, NIV

In light of the dismal data on physician well-being, my charge to you is this: Make curing physician burnout be the cause of your generation.

How do you start? Start by asking good questions. In his 2016 commencement speech at Harvard, Dean James Ryan outlined essential questions for finding the best answers and solutions to any problem.

The first question is "Wait, what?" The wait part reminds us to pause; the what part reminds us to ask ourselves if we have asked all the right questions. So when we hear that the physician burnout rate is more than 50 percent, we need to stop and ask, "Wait, what?"

The second question begins with "I wonder," which is usually followed by why or if. "I wonder why" shows you are seeking further understanding. "I wonder if" shows you are searching for better solutions.

The "I wonder why" question may be something like: "I wonder why the burnout rate among physicians is so high?" The why questions then can be followed by "I wonder if" questions, such as: "I wonder if faculty modeled discussions about burnout, would that facilitate more open discussions among medical students, and lead to improved well-being during residency and beyond?"

The third question is: "How can I help?" By asking "How can I help?" you are asking with humility, while acknowledging the other person's sense of self-determination. Just hearing this question is incredibly therapeutic. It empowers the receiver to reflect on whether he or she needs help in some way. Even if the answer is no, the receiver feels cared for, that someone is looking after them.

The final question is: "What truly matters?" As you progress in your careers, there will be more and more demands on your time. Because life is limited, in the solitude of your minds and hearts, and with guidance from family and God, you must define what truly matters to you. Once defined, peg all investments of your time on these things.

Why is your generation uniquely qualified to cure physician burnout more so than any of us in the older generation? If you look back in history to individuals who led generation-defining causes and discoveries, such as Ellen White, Einstein, Gandhi, and Steve Jobs, what do they have in common? The common denominator is that the work leading to their accomplishments began when they were in their 20s—the age many of you are now.

The explanation for this is best encapsulated by President Obama, who said: "Most big change, most human progress, is driven by young people who don't know any better and figure 'Why can't we do something different?' Old people get comfortable, or protective of status, or get set in their ways."

So, future physicians . . .

Let your ignorance of what is impossible guide your vision;

let your stubbornness refuse to accept no for an answer;

and let your courage lead you to do what is best for yourself and your families.

Khiet Ngo is assistant professor in LLUSM's department of medical education and assistant dean of curricular innovation. He was LLUSM's Teacher of the Year in 2015. He enjoys washing dishes, exploring the outdoors with his family, and continually learning from students. Note: Above is an excerpt from his clinical commencement address for LLUSM's class of 2020.

June 27

> *"Everyone should be quick to listen, slow to speak and slow to become angry."*
> James 1:19, NIV

As a new fellow in infectious diseases at Mayo Clinic in Rochester, Minnesota, I would be caring for patients with HIV. In preparation for my first appointment with KJ, I read over his chart and grew increasingly nervous. Although one physician had developed a therapeutic relationship with him, subsequent physicians had not. One had confronted him for having multiple sexual partners without using condoms. KJ had responded with profanity-laced letters. He stopped coming to the clinic, but still did labs and demanded prescriptions.

Things started off well after our first meeting, though I did hear repeatedly about perceived unjust abuse he had suffered at the hands of prior physicians. Armed with a desire to help and determination to succeed, I listened a lot and talked less. My goals were simple: Persuade him to stay on his antiretroviral medications so that his HIV would be controlled. His likelihood of passing HIV infection to anyone else would then be minimized, and his own health would be improved.

Our relationship was tested early on. He asked for controlled substances, mainly anxiolytics. As a trainee learning how to treat his HIV, I did not feel it my place to prescribe him psychotropic medications, because his primary physician was already doing so. I referred him to psychiatry, whom he very reluctantly agreed to see, but after the visit he proceeded to angrily tell me it was a waste of time. Though discouraged, I persisted in listening to him. Another year passed. I tested our relationship further by challenging some of his ideas of hatred toward other physicians, suggesting that perhaps his view wasn't accurate. The instant backlash and string of profanities was fierce, leaving me temporarily fearful for my own safety. I continued listening.

Despite setbacks and challenges, after three years I slowly built up a rapport. KJ ranted to me less and looked to me more as a trusted ally. One major turning point involved me practicing humility. I had challenged one of his rantings, commenting that perhaps he needed to try to see the situation from the other side. He accused me of not listening to him. I realized he was right, and I simply said, "You're right. I'm sorry. I wasn't listening to you. I was focused on trying to get my point across. I'll try to listen better next time." This completely surprised him, and he grew calm. Though we still had rocky times ahead, I sensed a complete change in his attitude toward me that day, and I had a more therapeutic alliance going forward.

When I left Mayo Clinic to come to Loma Linda, KJ voiced deep regret that I was leaving, and he didn't know what he would do. He doubted that any other physician would listen to him the way I did. I surprised myself by also feeling regret about not seeing him again. I learned so much about being slow to speak and slow to anger; about listening and not preparing the next comeback; about trying to hear what someone is actually communicating; about not letting someone else's deep psychological hurt make me hurt too. I thank the Lord for what He taught me through my relationship with KJ.

Daniel Rogstad, LLUSM class of 2009, PhD, is an assistant professor in LLUSM's department of medicine and an assistant dean for basic science education at LLUSM. He continues to teach biochemistry to medical students, is helping to lead the curriculum renewal at LLUSM, and is an infectious diseases attending physician at LLUMC. He has been married to his wife, Katie, for 18 years, and they have five children.

June 28

> *"His strength is perfect when our strength is gone.*
> *He'll carry us when we can't carry on."*
>
> *"His Strength is Perfect," Steven Curtis Chapman and Jerry Salley: contemporary American singers and songwriters*

Tired and weary after a long day, I see an earnest and worried mother hovering over her 1.76-pound premature infant. I have just entered the small crowded room with a sink, counter, and five incubators that houses the premature or sick infants on the maternity ward at the Kanye Adventist Hospital in Southern Botswana. It is important to note that most babies born below two pounds do not survive at our hospital. The "tertiary care center" with a neonatal intensive care unit that is one and a half hours away from our village does not accept infants less than 2.2 pounds because of their high risk or mortality. I have been called by the medical officer to consult on the baby because of signs of necrotizing enterocolitis. It is with this knowledge that I enter the room.

I see the baby ill-looking and mildly struggling to breathe. I see the mother with a blank stare. I begin to exam the baby and gather further history from the mother. Blood is collected, antibiotics and IV fluids are started, supplemental oxygen given, and the feedings are stopped. The abdominal X-ray confirms necrotizing enterocolitis, stage 2. As I explain to the mother the disease process and the prognosis, a tear trickles down her cheek. Two babies born with the same weight have recently died, and the mother realizes that she may also lose her baby.

It is at this time that I ask the mother if it is OK for me to pray with her. She gladly agrees. We know that medicine always has limitations and those limitations are more pronounced in resource-limited settings. I am also not a neonatologist, and many times I feel ill-equipped to manage many of the infants that I am asked to consult. Here I have realized that despite my weaknesses God can work miracles. Every time I come to see this infant, the mother and I cover her child with prayer.

Seven weeks after the initial consult I saw the mother take her baby home.

In our setting, a miracle.

Jasmine Turner Walker, LLUSM class of 2013, specialized in pediatrics and is currently living and serving in Guam as an outpatient pediatrician along with her husband, Ronald (LLUSD class of 2014), who works as a dentist in the dental clinic. She feels motivated by the desire to be the doctor that she wants to have for their son.

June 29

> *"The angel of the LORD encampeth round about them that fear him, and delivereth them."*
> Psalm 34:7, KJV

Have you ever had days when nothing seemed to go right, and you asked yourself the questions "Does anyone care? Why is this happening to me?" During the 70 years I have lived, I have asked myself these questions on multiple occasions. As I move toward the end of my medical career, I have begun to reflect on my relationship with God, especially on those days when nothing seemed to go right. Where was God?

When I looked objectively at just a few of those days, I realized I didn't have a clue who God was, even though I thought I did. Because I've been a Christian all my life, that seems hard to believe. However, in truth, ask yourself the question, "Do I realize who God is?" Our reference to who God is comes from Scripture, the Word of God. Elijah prayed to God and saw fire come down out of heaven and consume the sacrifice and the altar. He had the 450 prophets of Baal killed, and he ran in the blinding rain in front of King Ahab's chariot. After all this, he ran for his life at the threats of Jezebel. He was awakened from his exhausted sleep by the angel of the Lord and given food to eat (1 Kings 18-19).

As a surgeon, I have always found myself in a hurry. Perhaps the only time I had not hurried was when I would find myself in a very difficult situation and had to pause and ask God for help when I finally realized there was nothing I could do. Just as with Elijah, God is present when we are not asking or looking for Him.

Early one morning I was coming home from work on Interstate 40. I was driving my sports car at 145 miles per hour. I know this sounds bad, and it is. I am not writing this to tell you to drive 145 miles per hour, but to help you realize who God is. As I was approaching a curve in the interstate in the left lane, the road divided, and I could not see the oncoming traffic. The angel of the Lord said to me, *Slow down to 70 miles per hour and move to the right lane.* I instantly obeyed. Immediately a large semitruck rounded the blind curve on the wrong side of Interstate 40 in the very lane I had just moved from. "The angel of the Lord encampeth round about them that fear him, and delivereth them" (Psalm 34:7, KJV). The preservation of my life was based, not on my knowledge, but on listening to and obeying the voice of God. Do you realize who God is? He is omniscient and omnipresent. Do you understand why He is offering something different and better from what we think we have in this world? He is our Savior, Redeemer, Protector, Defender, and closest Friend. He is the Lord God omnipotent. He reigns (Revelation 19:6). His goal is salvation for all His children no matter the cost. He demonstrated this by dying for all of us.

Lloyd Ruff, LLUSM class of 1976-A, decided at the age of 6 to become a physician and surgeon. He is amazed how God can take a child's desires and make them reality to serve Him. He is now a retired general surgeon and gastroenterologist, currently working in emergency medicine and preaching the gospel message.

June 30

"Even there your hand shall lead me, and your right hand shall hold me."
Psalm 139:10, ESV

In our clinic the women's health department refers out our mammograms to a breast center three miles away. It is a straight bus ride down Vanowen Street, and easy for our patients to reach. From the breast center about three women each month receive a report of an abnormal result, breast sono, or mammogram result requiring a biopsy. Our office would receive the report too, and we'd call these women to be sure that they were scheduled and would be seen for follow-up. Many of these women wanted to come back to see us in GYN as well, just to talk, even though, if needed, all of their follow-up would be with the surgeon and the oncologist who had offices on the same hallway. A few months ago my personal story paralleled that of these women.

I had a routine mammogram. There was no lump, but suspicious calcifications were seen. My biopsy was positive for breast cancer. I got the phone call at work at the end of the day. Within three days I had arranged for time off for chemo and surgery after that. Once those things were taken care of, it was time to get started on the unknown of chemotherapy.

I'll admit that my first thought as I considered chemo was that it was like wading into a watery, dark tunnel. This tunnel, as I imagined it, had ledges along the sides, with friendly people holding lanterns and waving them. The lights and encouragement from the providers and care coordination team were there to get me along the way to the next ledge and light. They did an excellent job. My primary provider has a small patient panel and limited office hours because of teaching residents, but she kept me in her panel in spite of my new diagnosis. The care coordinators answered all kinds of questions, and my surgeon kept the links of communication strong.

As the cycles of chemo went by, I shifted my thoughts. Instead of a tunnel, I began to think of it as a book chapter that would unfold. It was a brighter metaphor, and one that I, as a book collector who had read my way through chemo days when I was too tired to do much else, liked better.

However, there was one more way to think about the journey. I gradually told my friends about my cancer diagnosis. As I did, a large group of people promised to pray for me, not just for a week or two, but for the months ahead. This added my third and favorite view: a sense of being in the palm of God's hand, not out on the edge. This view did not come quicky, but it came with a deeper hold. Their prayers, as well as my own, gave me a sense of hope and perspective and my future being in God's plan. It was much different from what I had when the news had first arrived, and it will be something I can share with my patients when I return to work as well.

Jill Hughes, LLUSM class of 1986, currently practices OB/GYN in Southern California. She and her husband have two young adult daughters. June 30 is her birthday.

JULY

෬ SERVICE ෧

"At the end of life we will not be judged by how many diplomas we have received, how much money we have made, how many great things we have done. We will be judged by 'I was hungry, and you gave me something to eat. I was naked, and you clothed me. I was homeless, and you took me in.'"

MOTHER TERESA (1910–1997)
Albanian-Indian missionary to the poor in India and
Nobel Peace Prize Laureate

July 1

> "From noon on, darkness came over the whole land until three in the afternoon. And about three o'clock Jesus cried with a loud voice, 'Eli, Eli, lema sabachthani?' that is, 'My God, my God, why have you forsaken me?' ... Then Jesus cried again with a loud voice and breathed his last."
>
> Matthew 27:45-46, 50, NRSV

July 1. Any year. At academic medical centers doctors in training get a promotion on that day. On June 30 I was an intern training in internal medicine. The next day I was a senior resident overseeing interns in the medical intensive care unit (MICU), a training rotation known for its difficulty. I was prepared for the technical challenges—managing septic shock with potent drugs, recognizing respiratory failure, and initiating mechanical ventilation.

I was training at Loma Linda because its mission resonated with my ideals: "To continue the teaching and healing ministry of Jesus Christ—To make man whole." I was about to embark on a journey that would test the limits of that mission.

The COVID-19 pandemic struck our hospital in the middle of March 2020. Initially a trickle of patients, then a manageable peak in the middle of April and early May. With the onset of summer I hoped that the illness might recede.

I was wrong. In July the intensive care unit filled with patients. Some patients were my age. Some doctors I knew had become infected taking care of their patients. I tried to push away my own recurring fear of becoming ill.

On July 1 the hospital issued an updated visitor restriction policy: "Visitors are not allowed in any of our adult hospitals. No visitors are allowed for patients under investigation for COVID-19 or patients who test positive for COVID-19 at any time. We will make every effort to connect the patients with their family/caregiver virtually (by phone or video) when possible." No visitors. Loved ones wanting to hold a hand, share a memory, caress a forehead. Not allowed. A journey to darkness or recovery would be alone.

A few days into my MICU rotation, Salvador Rodriguez, 40, was transferred to the ICU. His breaths came quickly; the oxygen in his blood was falling. Between gasps he told me about himself. He and Gabrielle married 16 years ago. His calloused hands testified to hard work in the construction industry. He and Gabrielle had two children. Their boy, an avid soccer player, was 12; their daughter, 10, had musical talent. Gabrielle kept things organized and oversaw Zoom school.

I dialed Gabrielle for Salvador. "I miss you, Gab. I love you. I'll be strong. The doctors are going to put me on a breathing machine. I won't be able to talk. Dr. Bailey will update you." Salvador was connected to a ventilator. An endotracheal tube enabled him to breathe but made him mute. His messages came via scrawled notes, nods, and facial expressions.

The COVID-19 visitor restriction policy barred Gabrielle from the hospital. She awaited my daily calls, seeking hope. Three weeks into our shared journey, she confided, "I'm 28 weeks pregnant. It's a boy. His name will be Salvador."

As I did each day, I became Salvador's and Gabrielle's voices. I shared his love and his hope for recovery, and sometimes his loneliness. Over the phone, I prayed for Gabrielle, for her children, for her pregnancy, and for her husband's recovery.

Continued on July 2...

Josianne Bailey, LLUSM class of 2019, MBA, is a fourth-generation LLUSM graduate. She is in her third year of an internal medicine residency program at LLUH, pursuing a future as a hospitalist and clinician. She is indebted to her God-fearing family for always pointing her toward her heavenly Father, whom she has personally seen guide her through experiences with patients, as noted in this devotional. She would like to say a special thank you to Douglas Hegstad (LLUSM class of 1980-A) for guiding her through the process of how to pen such a personal story.

July 2

Continued from July 1...

The next day Salvador's health took an ominous turn. A crescendoing cacophony of change—speeding pulse and falling blood pressure, urine output and oxygen levels, then agitation and confusion—heralded danger. Late on a hot July afternoon, as I sat in the ICU workstation, the code blue pager interrupted my reverie. Someone had suddenly taken a turn for the worse. Immediate action was required. It was Salvador. The heart showed a slowing pattern. Blood oxygen levels plummeted. The electrical complexes signaling heart contractions diminished in size and ceased. Asystole.

Technical interventions—drugs to stimulate the heart, adjustments to the ventilator, chest compressions. The pulse returned, but Salvador no longer blinked yes or no to my questions. His unseeing eyes stared blankly. A few days later the neurologist confirmed my fears. Sometime during the cardiac arrest, perhaps for as little as three or four minutes, too little oxygen had reached Salvador's brain. He had anoxic brain injury. He would never speak or perhaps think again.

I knew no words to grasp the sadness of the situation. My brain reeled. Should I cry? Should I push forward? I didn't learn about this in medical school!

I dreaded calling Gabrielle. Two children. Baby Salvador coming in 10 weeks. Financial and personal uncertainty. I expected her to ask as usual, "Isn't there anything else you can do?"

I reported the somber news to Gabrielle. Instead of her usual queries, she concluded the conversation with a simple "Thank you, Dr. Bailey."

The following day Gabrielle wasn't crying. Instead, her tone conveyed resignation. "I must be strong. Strong for me. Strong for Salvador. Strong for our children."

When Salvador died, I lost a part of my voice—maybe it was his voice and Gabrielle's voice. Salvador wasn't the first patient to die under my care, but he was the first barred, in illness and death, from comforting closeness.

We weren't the first to feel the pain of separation and darkness. Our feelings echoed Jesus' plaintive Friday afternoon cry to His Father, "Why hast thou forsaken me?" (Matthew 27:46, KJV).

The Gospel of Luke records the same crucifixion darkness reported by Matthew, but adds final words of resignation and acceptance: "Father, into thy hands I commend my spirit" (Luke 23:46, KJV).

I pray for the day when with touch, voice, and proximity patients and families can again journey together. They may be powerless, but they will be present. I pray for a resurrection of spirit and a return to wholeness.

Doug Hegstad, LLUSM class of 1980-A, is an associate professor and chair in LLUSM's department of medicine. He was awarded LLUSM's Teacher of the Year in 1998. He loves good stories—hearing them and telling them. He and his wife, Alane, and youngest daughter, Chloe, live on the redundancy of a beautiful hill in Loma Linda. (In Spanish, loma linda literally translates to "hill beautiful.")

July 3

"When you are in the service of your fellow beings you are in the service of God."
Anonymous

Some patients leave a never-to-be-forgotten impression. Though I have been retired for many years, I last saw a patient decades ago whom I will never forget. I will call her Rose. She first appeared in my office in the early 1970s. Her face radiated cheerfulness and optimism. She came because she needed a new physician and, in retrospect, was probably seeking another opinion regarding her care. To behold her face and to hear her talk, one would think she was the picture of health. There was little in the way of complaining, just seeking a possible alternative to her treatment regimen. If one could see her only from the neck up, she would appear to be in optimal health. Sadly, from the neck down, her body told another story. She arrived in her wheelchair with hands, arms, feet, and ankles hopelessly distorted from the ravages of severe rheumatoid arthritis. This was in an era with limited therapeutic options for treating her disease, which had been present since her teen years. To all appearances she seemed to be absolutely and totally disabled. We had a lengthy discussion, and finally I approached her with the question about how she spent her days, what she did with her time.

"Oh," she replied, "I work full-time."

I am sure I had a rather shocked expression on my face, and I finally asked, "What sort of work do you do?"

She answered, "I work for the Social Security Disability Determination Unit, evaluating people when they come in to apply for disability benefits."

I questioned, "You mean if anyone wants to seek disability benefits, they have to have a personal interview with you in order to apply?"

"That's correct," she said.

Can you imagine what must go through the minds of her co-workers and many others who come to her office and see someone with this degree of disability working full-time? What an inspiration!

We cannot always prevent adversity from striking, but we can choose to have control over our response—showing peace, courage, and an attitude of gratitude, even when everything in our lives seems to be going wrong. We are not promised a life free of storms, but we are offered the knowledge that there is a God who cares, and that He will help us no matter our circumstance. What a better place this world would be if we all, like Rose, possessed peace, courage, and an attitude of gratitude.

Robert Bond, LLUSM class of 1964, is a retired nephrologist residing in Salt Lake City, Utah.

USA's Independence Day

July 4

> "He will cover you with his feathers. He will shelter you with his wings. His faithful promises are your armor and protection."
> Psalm 91:4, NLT

The year was 1966, and the Vietnam War was escalating. It was the first year of my internal medicine residency, at Loma Linda Sanitarium (now Loma Linda University Medical Center), and I was ordered to report for duty in the U.S. Army on May 1. After basic training I joined the medical staff of Ireland Army Hospital at Fort Knox, Kentucky. That experience ended abruptly when I was ordered to fly to South Vietnam on January 10, 1967, where I was to serve as a battalion surgeon with the 1st Infantry Division.

When I met with the chief physician in Vietnam, he informed me that there was an urgent need for a physician for the 62nd Engineer Battalion, and asked if I would consider switching my assignment. The 1st Infantry Division was, at that time, involved in fierce fighting with the Viet Cong. I gratefully agreed to make the change—the first of many times during my year in Vietnam when I felt God's protection.

When I joined my battalion in Long Binh, 18 miles north of Saigon, my medics informed me that a major in our battalion, who was known to be an alcoholic, had become unhappy with the prior doctor for the battalion and arranged for him to be transferred to the 25th Infantry Division. I felt that God had opened this unique opportunity for me to be there as a Christian witness to the approximately 1,000 men in our battalion.

Another time, one of our companies, with 200 men, was deployed about 20 miles south of Saigon. The chaplain and I were required to travel by jeep down to the Mekong Delta, monthly, to check on the safety and morale of these men. Our battalion commander instructed us to travel in a jeep with the engineer symbol, a castle, on the side. He said the Viet Cong would more likely attack us if we were in the medic's jeep, with a cross on the side, since they would try to wound or kill anyone with medical training. He also instructed us to travel alone, rather than in a convoy. I feel that the wisdom of our battalion commander, along with God's protection, saved our lives on several occasions, as every time we made the trip to visit our company we would pass a convoy that had been ambushed.

Nearly once a month many of the Seventh-day Adventist soldiers had the opportunity to spend a Sabbath at the Adventist compound in Saigon. The opportunity to worship together and eat delicious food was an enormous morale booster. My non-SDA medics were always happy to come along on these Sabbath trips!

The devastating effects of the war did not end when the peace treaty was signed, as many of our Vietnam veterans came home with serious medical problems, including head injuries, loss of extremities, drug addiction, alcoholism, PTSD, and suicidal thoughts. The continued despair felt by these individuals begs us to share Jesus' love for them even these many years after the war.

John E. Hodgkin, LLUSM class of 1964, attended LLUSM after being inspired by his father's (Williard "Bill" Hodgkin [CME class of 1934]) ability as a Christian physician to help people. His two sons, Steven (LLUSM class of 1990) and Jonathan (LLUSM class of 2018), and granddaughter Savannah (LLUSM class of 2024), continue this legacy.

July 5

"And thine ears shall hear a word behind thee, saying, This is the way, walk ye in it, when ye turn to the right hand, and when ye turn to the left."
Isaiah 30:21, KJV

There was no celebration that Fourth of July in 1985. Along with my husband and three sons, I watched the mission vehicle leave the hospital compound and disappear down the dusty road. I had been assigned to Gimbi Hospital in Ethiopia for six months as a General Conference medical volunteer for the SDA Church, and there was no physician replacement in sight. The departing surgeon had painted a grim picture—danger and political uncertainty under the current Communist regime, the hospital in shambles, and widespread discontent among the hospital workers. The Adventist church had been closed, and the church members were meeting in a crude tin structure near the hospital morgue. The doctor advised that we leave without delay.

Surveying the scene, I saw that the hospital matched the doctor's description. The wards were bare and cheerless, with few patients. Hospital linens had taken on the color of the red Gimbi soil. The TB ward, located below the main hospital, was dark and cavelike. I imagined that one could contract tuberculosis from just being there. Available medications were mostly outdated vials and bottles of uncertain vintage. Surgical instruments and other essential equipment were either nonfunctional or nonexistent. The staff were reserved and had hung out no welcome signs. I questioned the Lord: Just what was I doing there? With no other options available, I decided, by God's grace, to make the best of a bleak situation. As the days went by, we settled into a mostly untroubled routine.

Then one morning, in the midst of a busy clinic schedule, the hospital chaplain announced that the clinic would be closed for a mandatory staff meeting. My suggestion to reschedule the meeting was disregarded. When I asked if my attendance was also required, the answer was a resounding no! I soon discovered this was a government meeting purposely held in the large, closed Adventist church. I incredulously thought: How could God revive this failing institution while its workers were united with a godless organization? Then I recalled seeing some Spirit of Prophecy books relating to medical missionary work in the abandoned X-ray room. Perhaps I could find some guiding principles for this situation.

As I studied these books, I found pertinent counsel for the hospital staff. But more important, I heard the Holy Spirit speaking to me personally: *Mary Ann, your new calling is to train gospel workers in the simple, effective ways of disease prevention and treatment that you are reading about.*

Our mission at Gimbi finished on a positive note. Shortly before our departure God miraculously arranged for two young Ethiopian Adventist physicians to replace me. And we were blessed with warm, lasting friendships among the hospital staff. But most significantly, my defining moment occurred when I accepted the Holy Spirit's calling.

Mary Ann Kimmel-McNeilus, LLUSM class of 1972, is a retired family practitioner in southeastern Minnesota. She served as a medical volunteer with SAWS (now ADRA) in Cambodian refugee camps along the Thai/Cambodian border (1980–1982); Juba, South Sudan (1983–1984); and Gimbi Mission Hospital (1985). She received training in lifestyle medicine and natural remedies at Uchee Pines Institute in Alabama. She has authored several books and taught healthful lifestyle and natural remedies, both overseas and in her Amish neighborhood.

July 6

> *"Then you will call, and Yahweh will answer.*
> *You will cry for help, and he will say, 'Here I am.'"*
> Isaiah 58:9, WEB

It was July, and it was hot. It was the kind of day that makes you wonder why you bothered to leave the house at all. We were fishing on the Columbia River near Umatilla, Oregon. My wife and I had met up with my parents, brother, and sister-in-law for a weekend of camping and fishing. Though we had not had much luck fishing, we were enjoying some much-needed rest away from our busy lives. My wife and I were expecting our first child and the first grandchild for both of our families. We had always wanted to be parents, and when that little + sign appeared on our home pregnancy test in May, we were ecstatic. What a blessing God had given us. Then came July.

It started the first day of camping when my wife noticed a little blood. Both of us being in medicine (I'm a family medicine resident, and my wife is an RN in the NICU) knew that bleeding could be normal at times during pregnancy. Nevertheless, as you can imagine, we prayed, and we prayed hard. As the weekend progressed, she began to experience cramping pains as well. We eventually shared with my family what was happening, and they joined us with prayers. However, by Sunday, a disgustingly hot July day, we experienced a miscarriage just shy of 10 weeks.

This was undoubtedly one of the toughest moments of my life. I had no idea that it was possible to feel this level of heartache. To see my wife's beautiful soul aching was suffocating. It was as if my entire body were being crushed by an enormous invisible weight. We shared hugs with my family, quietly packed up our campsite, and then left for home. I remember vividly the three-hour drive home. My thoughts were racing. *Why had this happened? Had we done something wrong? Where was God, and did He even understand this level of pain?* Then, my beautiful wife played a song entitled "Even If," by MercyMe. I encourage each of you reading this today to listen to that song when you are done with my story. There is simply nothing I can write that could capture my emotions from that time.

I share this story as a reminder that we worship a God who not only witnesses our personal sufferings but who is intimately familiar with suffering. A God who desired a relationship with us so much that He Himself suffered and died not only to save us from sin but also to be able to relate to us when we hurt. Because God experienced suffering Himself, we can truly trust that God understands. What an utterly clear demonstration that God Himself is love!

The story does not end here. I am happy to write that by the grace of God we are expecting once again.

Ryan Manns, LLUSM class of 2016, currently practices family medicine in Oregon. His wife, Rachael, graduated from LLUSN in 2012. On May 7, 2019, they welcomed their beautiful baby girl, Jade, into the world.

July 7

> *"Jesus looked at them intently and said, 'Humanly speaking, it is impossible. But with God everything is possible.'"*
> Matthew 19:26, NLT

For Loma Linda University Health, miracles explain its raison d'être and continue to propel its 116-year-old mission. God's leading since the founding of the institution is unmistakable, and with humility we recognize the limits of human efforts and marvel at His greatness.

It has been my privilege to experience one of God's displays of impeccable timing and sure provision during LLUH's journey in building the new hospital towers to comply with the state's unfunded mandate. Funding had to be secured through bond financing, Proposition 61/3 CHFFA grant dollars, philanthropy, and operating cash flow. God's omnipresence in LLUH has been evident—during the 2014, 2016, and 2018 bond issues, the CHFFA grant approval in 2016, the three-year funding delay and consequential receipt of CHFFA funds in 2020, and tremendous support from donors. On multiple occasions, after employing everything humanly possible, we found ourselves in situations where only divine intervention could have cleared the barriers. The past several years have been a lesson in humility and faith for me. I could hear God saying, "You have done a lot to build the hospitals; now step aside, and watch Me press the execute button."

Completion of the new towers and preparation for occupancy was set for 2020. However, as transition planning commenced, the curveball hit in the form of the COVID-19 pandemic. In mid-March elective surgeries were mandated for suspension. Consequently, patient encounters and revenue dropped by at least 40 percent, resulting in devastating losses from March through May. Palpable anxiety and pending threat over the hospitals' compliance with its debt covenant by the June 30, 2020, year-end curbed our enthusiasm.

Through teamwork and collaboration, performance improvement and austerity measures were implemented across LLUH to prevent further financial disaster. Stimulus funding received was insufficient to compensate for the COVID-19-induced losses. Morale began to dip, but LLUH's legacy and God's miraculous, mighty hand were too formidable for this challenge. In His infinite wisdom and His unending provisions, additional government funding came in June. On July 7, in what seemed to be God's reminder of His miraculous provision for the $5,000 funding our pioneers needed to purchase the Loma Linda property on July 26, 1905, we were notified of an unexpected $15 million supplemental funding the state had withheld from 2013 to 2019—enabling LLUH to comply with the debt covenant! Coincidence, human effort, or genius? Those of us with faith anchored in God recognize these as testaments to God's watchful care over LLUH.

As of this writing, we are still months away from project completion, and COVID-19 continues to pose uncertainty. However, remembering God's providences and faithfulness prods us toward the finish line—to continue Jesus' teaching and healing ministry.

Angela Manalo Lalas, MBA, CPA, currently serves as LLUH chief financial officer and has held various finance leadership roles in LLUH since 2006. A product of Seventh-day Adventist education, she shares, with her husband, Serafin (child and adolescent psychiatrist at LLUH), a passion for sponsoring and supporting students in pursuit of SDA education. They are happy parents to two children, Anna Sophia, age 14, and Serafin Alexander III, age 6.

July 8

"If the foot says, 'I am not a part of the body because I am not a hand,' that does not make it any less a part of the body. And if the ear says, 'I am not part of the body because I am not an eye,' would that make it any less a part of the body? If the whole body were an eye, how would you hear? Or if your whole body were an ear, how would you smell anything? But our bodies have many parts, and God has put each part just where he wants it. How strange a body would be if it had only one part!"

1 Corinthians 12:15-19, NLT

Uncomfortable. It was a feeling I was learning to ignore as I began to embrace the fact that this was my new reality. For the most part having attended a Historically Black College or University and a predominantly Black high school, I had grown very comfortable in my previous surroundings. In my postgraduate training I was in a new demographic. I was immensely blessed to make many lifelong friends in medical school and residency. Some looked like me, and some did not.

However, a sliver of discomfort remained when I would go to conferences, grand rounds, fellowship interviews, and realize I was the only African American in the room. There was an elation I would feel to see someone else in the room who was also Black. I see that same glimmer of excitement in many of my minority patients when I greet them. Only 2.5 percent of ophthalmologists are African American compared to the 13.4 percent of Blacks living in the U.S. In ophthalmology, a disproportionate number have diabetes and glaucoma. Many are reluctant to seek or receive medical treatment. I am thankful many programs are attempting to diversify their trainees and faculty. However, there is still a long way to go.

God made us diverse because there is so much beauty and richness in our differences. Just because we are different does not mean that we are not equals. It is instead a reflection of our Maker's limitless creativity in crafting us for our mission. We each have a kingdom assignment to fulfill. We should embrace our differences and use them to reach those with whom we have commonalities. Each of our skills, heritage, and perspectives meld together to form the beautiful tapestry that is gospel ministry.

It's time medicine reflected that.

Nichelle Warren, LLUSM class of 2015, is currently in private practice as a cornea specialist in Atlanta, Georgia.

July 9

> *"It is through self-forgetting service to others that the highest self-fulfillment is realized."*
> V. Norskov Olsen (1916–1999): *president of Loma Linda University (1974–1984) and Norwegian-American author*

Since the beginning of my career in medicine, I aspired to be an infectious disease physician. After a long journey through medical school, residency, and a year as a hospitalist, I started my infectious disease fellowship in Houston, Texas, in July 2019.

When COVID-19 hit Houston in March 2020 I was working at the county hospital. In a matter of days it went from consults as usual to nonstop pages from panicked health care providers seeking guidance from the infectious disease service. As infectious disease physicians we had to determine whom to test despite a limited number of tests, whom to isolate despite a diminishing supply of personal protective equipment (PPE), and whom to offer experimental therapy in the setting of so much unknown.

In a matter of weeks the hospital's usual hum of life and vibrancy went quiet, the hallways emptied of their usual traffic, and the ICUs were completely filled. By June 2020 we had our second surge of cases. I watched patients say their final goodbyes to loved ones on video chat from isolation rooms. I witnessed young people, my own age, rapidly decompensate despite all our efforts. I would drive home from the hospital in the evenings and see groups of people gathering and socializing without masks, which filled me with exasperation and hopelessness.

I never imagined that I would be in a hot spot during a pandemic or that I would be the most dangerous person for my family to be exposed to. I never imagined that I would have an actual conversation with my husband about my own code status in my 30s, just in case the worst were to happen. I never imagined how different life could be during this pandemic.

Despite all of this, I have seen amazing things. I have seen dedication to evidence-based medicine in the face of the unknown and a steadfast holding to our duty to determine what works and what doesn't, even during a pandemic. I have seen incredible strength and commitment in my infectious disease mentors and colleagues as they continue to work unbelievable hours for weeks at a time to take care of the increasing number of sick patients and to further research efforts for this new infectious disease. They have gracefully risen to meet this unprecedented occasion with strength, courage, and selflessness. I could not be more proud to be a part of this amazing field of medicine.

Being away from home has been hard, but my connection with my community of faith has sustained me in so many ways. I continue to experience God's love and promises from the outpouring of encouragement and love from family, friends, and mentors. We have been called to serve, now more than ever, and I know that together we will continue to rise to meet this calling.

Christine Akamine, LLUSM class of 2015, completed an internal medicine residency at LLUH. In June, 2021, she finished an infectious disease fellowship at Baylor College of Medicine in Houston, Texas. Houston was the nation's number one hot spot in July 2020 when she wrote this devotional. She became COVID-positive just days later. She has recovered. She is married to Zachary Taylor (LLUSM class of 2015) and in June 2021 they welcomed their firstborn, a son.

July 10

> *"He who knows no hardship will know no hardihood. He who faces no calamity will need no courage. Mysterious though it is, the characteristics in human nature which we love best grow in a soil with strong mixtures of troubles."*
> Harry Emerson Fosdick (1878–1969): American Baptist and Presbyterian pastor

My alarm is ringing for the third time this morning, and like clockwork, I press the snooze button. There are three more alarms ahead before I actually have to get up and start my day. In residency there is a peculiar oxymoron felt, where days are slow but the months and years fly by ... or so I am told.

As I write this, I am six months into my intern year, and I feel this. The days become lumped into one long stretch of day, and my only markers of time are the days off that segment this lump into more palpable pieces. I have had my share of feeling overworked, feeling unappreciated, and feeling as though maybe what I do for a patient doesn't really matter. At times my lack of reserves manifests into acting out on family, impatience with peers, and shorter interactions with my patients. And while the difficulties of my day cause me the most stress, it is because of these difficult circumstances that I get to experience blessing upon blessing with the people around me.

One afternoon I received a message on my pager telling me that a difficult patient wished to talk to the physician. At the patient's bedside I explained our plan of care, which was met with berating comments and aggressive verbal threats. This is not the first time I have had this kind of interaction with this patient, but as he was expressing his targeted comments, I started questioning my abilities as a physician and as a person. His accusations were poignant and cutting, and as I walked out of the room, I reviewed the interventions done this admission and studied each accusation brought up; I could feel the energy in my body draining with each step. Just then a nurse came to me, offered me a piece of candy, and said, "I was listening the entire time. You did a great job in there. You were very nice to him." These three sentences and this small gesture impacted my entire experience. Instead of my feeling low for the rest of the day, her affirmation liberated me from the personal weight of that interaction.

Likewise, the same hardships and pressure that have caused me stress have resulted in strong friendships with coresidents that could not have been forged otherwise. The tears and frustrations that are met with a listening ear produce a reflexive gratefulness and unconditional love to friends and family. While it is hard to serve patients, I am thankful for these difficulties that will shape me into a stronger, more confident physician. Nothing in life is ever black and white, and during those darkest times, looking at the silver lining will make all the difference; it's always there.

Esther G. Chong, LLUSM class of 2017, completed a residency in internal medicine at LLUH. In July 2021 she began a three year hematology/oncology fellowship at LLUH. Her husband, Isaac (LLUSD class of 2017), celebrates his birthday on July 10.

July 11

"For our wrestling is not against flesh and blood, but against the principalities, against the powers, against the world-rulers of this darkness, against the spiritual hosts of wickedness in the heavenly places."

Ephesians 6:12, ASV

My nurse alerts me that the family is taking my patient home.

"Absolutely not! She will die at home."

She's already getting the necessary fluids to keep her blood sugar up, but even still, the blood sugars keep dropping.

I rush into the labor unit where I've been keeping my young pregnant patient with cerebral malaria. Her aunt is actively carrying her out of the room. I intercede.

This situation has me angry. I have been fighting for this woman's life for a few days, constantly worrying, praying, checking up on her between cases in the OR. And in an instant the family wants to take her home so the village "doctor" can do his magic.

I say a prayer asking God to calm me. I arrange a family meeting and go home for a few minutes to pray for the situation.

I return to find four family members of my patient. A nurse begins translating for us from their language into French. We sit under the starry sky as I begin to hear their circumstances. They understand the woman is in a coma because she ate food bought with stolen money. She is cursed. If they could just take her to the village "doctor," she would have a chance of living. My situation is my pregnant patient has cerebral malaria. She could die here at the hospital. But she certainly would die at home. I explain cerebral malaria and hypoglycemia to the family and how she has already shown improvements. I listen. We pray. God is with us.

It is clear this battle is between God and Satan. These are Christian family members, and we speak freely about spiritual matters. Satan is happy when the family believes God does not have the power to heal this patient. He is happy when the village "doctor" is more respected than God. But my God is bigger. He is in charge of our mission hospital, and only He has the power to make the medicines, which we are giving, heal her.

I feel at peace. We each shared our case. They agree to stay at the hospital.

I continue caring for my patient. One morning I find my patient sitting up eating! The family is smiling and quickly forgives my prior impertinence. What a miracle God worked to show His power in this patient!

Soon after, she delivered a slightly premature but healthy baby—all for the glory of God! He fought this battle for me. He is teaching me patience every day as He fights the battles of which I am aware and unaware.

Danae Netteburg, LLUSM class of 2006, is an assistant professor in LLUSM's department of gynecology and obstetrics. She has practiced for the past 11 years in Chad, Africa. She is married to Olen (LLUSM class of 2007) and they have five children.

July 12

> *"The Lord directs the steps of the godly.*
> *He delights in every detail of their lives."*
> Psalm 37:23, NLT

A *patient's worst nightmare*, I thought as Dr. Senthil and the surgical oncology fellows presented a case study. It was on peritoneal metastasis of signet ring adenocarcinoma and the experimental HIPEC therapy they were incorporating into surgical resection. Few places in the United States were doing this, and Dr. Senthil was a world expert. She volunteered to lead a small group session for graduate and medical students in the translational research class that I was coordinating. I had become well acquainted with Dr. Senthil (Magi, as I had come to know her) at an AMA conference a few months before. Our respective research programs had also been featured in back-to-back articles in a recent edition of the Loma Linda University Health magazine, *Scope*. I was blessed to have a colleague that I thought of as a friend to help teach this course.

The next morning would be less fun—I was scheduled for my biannual colonoscopy. With my history of Crohn's disease I had been there and done that before. The first clue that this would be different were the words "circumferential mass" as I came out from under anesthesia. My gastroenterologist would call me the next day with biopsy results. My father had died of intestinal cancer, and my sister developed colon cancer at age 40—but she was a 15-year survivor, and I had a clean colonoscopy just 20 months before, so I was not overly concerned.

The next day, July 12, and the thirty-sixth anniversary of my father's death, I was diagnosed with colon cancer—adenocarcinoma, signet ring. That worst nightmare had become mine, and I had become that patient. I googled it—less than 1 percent survival, with median survival time of 11 months. Within a week Magi was performing a diagnostic laparoscopy—it was stage 4, and I was not a candidate for surgery.

After seven months of treatment, my tumor antigens dropped by 95 percent—something rare for this disease and stage. On Valentine's Day I got a call from Magi. She wanted to do another diagnostic laparoscopy to determine if I had become a candidate for surgical resection. On February 26 Magi and her team performed the surgery—14 hours—they got all visible tumors followed by the experimental HIPEC treatment to kill remaining tumor cells in the peritoneal cavity.

It has now been more than 11 months. I have started follow-up chemo to prevent recurrence. There is still a long road ahead, but in most places I would have been sent to hospice. My older son looks at that *Scope* magazine and sees the beginning of my article title, "Right Place, Right Time . . ." then turns the page to the photo of Magi. "Mom," he says, "it's not just about your research; it's about you and Magi. It's a miracle that would never have happened if both of you were not at the right place and the right time." He is right—God put us in the right place at just the right time.

Kimberly Payne, PhD, is associate professor in LLUSM's department of pathology and human anatomy. She directs a research lab that focuses on the development of treatments for pediatric cancer and has partnered with LLUH to form a company to bring a discovery in her lab to the market. Note: This story was submitted on June 9, 2019, and, sadly, the author passed away November 22, 2020.

July 13

> *"Whoever is generous to the poor lends to the LORD,*
> *and he will repay him for his deed."*
> Proverbs 19:17, ESV

It was a cold, misty morning, and I reluctantly emerged from under my bedcovers and tied up the mosquito net, ready to face the new day. Ryan had left an hour earlier for the hospital, just behind the clang of the mission gongs that echoed up and down the Malamulo hill. The smell of coffee brewing in the kitchen alerted my sleepy eyes to the tasks ahead, and I rummaged through my shoebox, a large wooden crate, to find my go-to misty morning Ugg boots. I had to dig awhile, and as I burrowed through the box I realized it was time for a "shoe clean-out." I selected several pairs of pumps, flip flops, sneakers, and Toms that had suddenly "burdened" my shoe collection and placed them in a large woven basket at the foot of my bed. Just as I was tossing the last pair into the "giveaway" pile one of my pajama-clad boys wandered dozily into my room. "What's that stack for?" He asked, motioning to the basket of footwear. "Shoes I don't need anymore..." I told him. "Why are you doing this now?" He inquired. I shrugged, "I don't know."

By the time breakfast was through and we began our homeschool routine, there was a familiar rattling at our chain link fence. A woman stood bravely at the gate, and above the protective barking of our dogs she motioned me outside toward her. She was an older woman, a grandmother, and she fiddled nervously with the tie on her chitenge cloth, which was wrapped tightly around her waist. I asked her if she had *njala* [hunger], and she nodded, holding her stomach. I looked down at my feet, my all-weather Uggs ruggedly keeping me warm and dry, and then I noticed her feet, standing in a pocket of water that had pooled from the night's rain, completely bare. *Sabado* [shoes]? I inquired, eyes fixed on her feet. *Palibe* [none], she replied. I took my boots off and opened the gate so we could stand side by side. Next to my now-naked foot I could see our feet were the same size. "Wait," I told her, running inside to the basket by my bed and returning moments later with several pairs of shoes and a few kilos of maize flour.

"Mommy! You made a pile of shoes for a stranger, and you didn't even know she was coming!" my son exclaimed. It's true, I didn't know she would knock on my gate that morning, but God did. He had placed in me a spirit of giving before a need arose, and the solution to both my problem and the grandmother's became evident. I needed to get rid of shoes, and she needed to receive them.

Friends sometimes ask, "Aren't you afraid that if you give to one, the next day a hundred more will appear?" I admit to thinking, *The need is so great, and there are too many people suffering for me to assist them all. If I help this one, will the bush telegraph encourage the multitudes to arrive hungry and shoeless at my door?* But there are countless times God has made provision for my limitations, and over the years He has sent me blessings, in the form of strangers, boldly rattling at my gate, "one by one."

Sharlene Hayton, BA, Human Resources and Industrial Relations from Newcastle University in Australia, is married to general surgeon Ryan Hayton (LLUSM class of 2005) and loved serving at Malamulo Adventist Hospital from 2010 to 2019. Sharlene homeschooled their three boys and enjoyed building a life in Africa to support the advancement of a new paradigm of missions focused on training Christian African doctors to become surgeons. She authored the book Kangaroo Kay: From Jungle to Teapot—An Historical Biography of Triumph and Tragedy in Central Africa *that was published in 2020.*

July 14

> *"God has wonderful plans for you—if you let Him lead and comfort."*
> Colin McCartney: contemporary Canadian author, urban youth worker, and speaker

A few days into my new career as an OB/GYN attending, I noticed an OB patient on my schedule. She was transferring her care here to be closer to her dad after her mother had suddenly died. I didn't think I was up to caring for someone with such a fresh loss for I, too, had just suffered a major loss in my life. My husband of nearly 27 years had suddenly died.

My husband had sacrificed so much for me to pursue my dream of becoming a doctor. Now that I was finished after 10 long years of schooling and residency, we were excited about our future. About a week before I was to start my new career, he suffered a massive heart attack in the middle of the night. My youngest daughter and I performed CPR on him to no avail. At age 51 he was gone.

My life was turned upside down when he died so suddenly. Missing him beyond belief, I couldn't fathom a future without him. I knew I needed to pull it together, though, to be a stabilizing force for my three daughters, 22, 22, and 19. I knew too that Steve would want me to go on and fulfill my dream of practicing medicine. To cope, I went to every grief group and read just about every book on grief I could find.

The good Lord provides for us even in our darkest hours. He brought into my life the people who could be that beacon of light to sustain me. My colleagues and support staff in the OB/GYN department were extremely caring and supportive. And the Lord directed me to read the Scriptures to comfort me and allow me to go on. Slowly over time through the Scriptures and God's angels here on earth, I was able to acclimate to a new normal and regain that sense of purpose in my life.

The Lord also knew I needed to get back into caring for others. When we care for others, we let go of a little of our own pain. Initially it was very difficult, as all the patients knew about the loss of my husband and felt compelled to reach out and comfort me. Consequently, when I met the patient who had just lost her mother, through the help of the Lord I was not only to provide care for her but to minister to her in her need.

There have been countless other patients over the years that I have been able to pray with and comfort in their times of need. Patients may come into the clinic for a specific problem but really have so much more going on in their lives. Sometimes just letting them talk is all they need, but when the Spirit leads, I offer to pray with them both, which provides that human connection that is so often lost in medicine.

I have truly been blessed not only to fulfill my dreams of becoming a physician, but also to be able to minister to patients. It is truly a privilege to care for others, a message I have shared with my three daughters, who are all RNs. Two of them work here, one in the ER and one in Labor and Delivery. Occasionally we end up caring for the same patients and hopefully make a difference in their lives.

Elaine Hart, LLUSM class of 2000, is an assistant professor in LLUSM's department of gynecology and obstetrics and assistant dean of regional campuses. In 2014 she was awarded LLUSM's Teacher of the Year. She considers it a privilege to care for her patients. She is passionate about teaching and mentoring medical students. She eventually remarried after the death of her husband and is blessed to now have five children and eight grandchildren, with more on the way!

July 15

> *"We give thanks to you, O God; we give thanks, for your name is near. We recount your wondrous deeds."*
>
> Psalm 75:1, ESV

Four miles northwest of Loma Linda University Health is a clinic in a different world. Loma Linda is a Blue Zone;* San Bernardino is a nutritional desert. Loma Linda is home to intact families; San Bernardino has more than 20 percent of its families headed by a single parent. Loma Linda is doing well; San Bernardino is broken.

In June 2016 LLUH opened the San Bernardino campus—a beautiful building housing a pharmacy, a vegetarian café, a pipeline school, and a SAC health system (SACHS) clinic, where the doctors are all from Loma Linda. Even though SACHS is an independent, federally qualified health center, patients often lump the two institutions together in their minds.

In order to care for patients suffering the health disparities of San Bernardino, SACHS clinic has a variety of services available, to include "chronic-care initiative" (CCI) teams. These are teams of four: a nurse, a psychotherapist, a care coordinator, and a community health worker. It was the pediatrics CCI team that cared for "Maria" and her "Carlosito"—the youngest of her five children, who had just turned 2 when she told their story.

Though Maria had heard of Loma Linda, she had never received care there. A few months into her pregnancy care at another clinic, she was told by her doctor that her child had congenital abnormalities, so she recommended Maria have an abortion; and to return in two weeks to finalize a plan. When she returned, Maria told the doctor, "I can hear the heartbeat—how can I end the life of my baby?" The doctor responded, "Then I cannot take care of you—you'll need to find another doctor." Maria stumbled out the door, sat down on the curb, and wept. After a few minutes a friend called and could tell she was crying and asked her what happened. When Maria told her, the friend said, "I am on my way. Now you go back in there and get a copy of your records, and I will take you to Loma Linda."

Soon she heard a very different kind of doctor say, "What do you want to do? You want to keep the baby? OK—we will be with you through everything." At each Loma Linda visit, the doctor kept saying, "There is life here. It will be OK; we will be with you." Maria was very tired during the pregnancy, but every month she saw her baby on the ultrasound and was encouraged by the staff. "I was not alone," she said. "You all gave me strength."

From birth Carlosito had many challenges; many trips to Loma Linda and the SACHS clinic. His issues were complex, so the doctors asked the CCI team to help. When the CCI nurse first met Maria, she said, "We'll help you with anything." Maria told her about the barriers she and Carlosito were facing. The CCI team began making calls and visiting their home, teaching proper asthma medication use and arranging needed home services.

What a blessing to work among people committed to serving God through medicine! At SACHS grand rounds recently, Maria recounted the care she received at LLUH and SACHS. She said that for so long she worried about him, but now Carlosito is doing so well that she is able to imagine him graduating from high school! With tears in her eyes, Maria exclaimed, "Glory to God—angels exist! You are His angels. Thank you so very much!"

*Blue Zones are regions of the world in which people live much longer than average, mainly because of their diet.

Kevin Shannon is an associate professor in LLUSM's department of preventive medicine and family medicine. He has been married to his wonderful physician wife, Karen, for 33 years. They have three children, one son-in-law, and one daughter-in-law. He loves music, medicine, and missions.

July 16

"May the God who gives endurance and encouragement give you the same attitude of mind toward each other that Christ Jesus had."

Romans 15:5, NIV

It has been said that laughter is the best medicine, but this past year has shown me that the better treatment is encouragement.

One of the early and indicative symptoms of medical school is discouragement. It may manifest itself in the recently coined term "imposter syndrome," the belief that a medical student managed to fool the admissions committee about their qualifications. Consequently, the "imposter" feels unintelligent in comparison to their peers or incapable of completing the next seven-plus years of training. As students we have been taught our whole lives that only perfection and high achievement are acceptable. Anything less than that is failure and a confirmation of our inadequacy.

But if encouragement steps in, we have a fighting chance.

I remember sitting at the top of the amphitheater studying during the middle of our second test week and questioning this whole endeavor called medical school. I sent the following text to my dad:

"Joyce can make it through and be a doctor because . . ."

A bit later I received:

"She has the gifts and calling from God to do so!"

Short, sweet, lacking any censure for doubting, filled with the kind of encouragement this world sorely lacks. A reminder to me of what I know to be true even if my emotions and circumstances screamed otherwise.

What if we were people of encouragement? As believers in Jesus, we have the greatest hope and promise of love regardless of what is happening to us or others. Why do we often bring discouragement to others?

I appreciate Paul's plea to the Romans, at the end of his famous letter, to have the same "endurance and encouragement" Jesus had when dealing with others.

The "other" could be your neighbor, patient, attending physician, department chair, dean, classmate, child, sibling, spouse, parent, stranger, friend, or anyone in between.

Encouragement means giving hope. It is the distribution of support to another person. It is reminding them of who they truly are when lies have distorted that belief. It is praying for them when they do not want it. It is "inconveniencing" yourself to have a conversation with someone who is struggling when you need to study. It is remembering a birthday and writing a card to commemorate that person's existence. It is asking someone how they are and probing beyond "fine." It is dropping a text message when that person crosses your mind because the Holy Spirit nudged you to do so. It is baking cookies and dropping them off at their house. It is being Christlike without an expectation of reciprocity. It is powerful, and it is needed. Lord, help us be encouragers in a world of despair and turmoil.

Joyce McRae, LLUSM class of 2021, is a first-year LLUH resident in the general surgery dedicated research track with current interests in pediatrics, acute care, and global surgery. She is the daughter of the Reverends Riley and Patricia McRae, two of her greatest encouragers. An early and great encourager of her pursuit of medicine was her grandmother Helen Carver.

July 17

"If anyone serves me, he must follow me; and where I am, there will my servant be also. If anyone serves me, the Father will honor him."

John 12:26, ESV

It was my first day as the one-year volunteer administrator of Malamulo Adventist Hospital and director of the LLU Global Campus site in Malawi, Africa. I had no medical background, taken no classes in health care management, and had zero experience in overseeing the workings of a hospital much less a mission hospital.

We had sold our home, pulled our kids out of a great school, and given away our business for what we felt was a clear calling. I had moved my family from Tennessee to Africa with no plan and no strategy for return. What had seemed an altruistic notion was now folly. I had made myself available to God, but had I misread His calling?

Sitting at my desk feeling sorry for myself, I began grumbling at God for "His" mistake and asking, "Why me and why here?"

And that is when it happened.

Below my office window is one of Malamulo's trademark walkways that form a spider's web of open and arched hallways connecting the wards. On that, my first day in office, I heard the most incredibly heart-wrenching chorus. It was that of an African family mourning the death of a loved one. As they walked from the hospital to the mortuary, a staff member wheeling the body covered in a tattered orange sheet, they poured out their hearts in sadness and frustration as only a distraught family could.

That which went on under my nose as I sat in my office was at a level of despair I could have never prepared for. Through the wailing and screams, the futility of my situation hit me. I could do nothing to directly affect the outcome for that family.

But then I felt God's peace in a way I can't describe. I had a clarion moment, a realization of purpose. I could indeed do nothing to directly save lives. But I could affect the care given by others. My calling was to give our clinical staff the tools by which they could positively affect outcomes.

This simple thought became my mission. My calling. God was giving me purpose through the sadness of that day. The struggles and the pain thereafter gave me strength and focus. I could remain calm in the storm because I was being carried above it.

It has now been six years since we moved to Malawi. I still have no medical ability, and am still not a trained administrator, either. The tattered orange sheets accompanied by wailing still roll below. Often the waves of futility are overwhelming. I get frustrated when I fail to meet the needs of our patients and must daily pray for strength renewed.

However, we have more of what we need, and positive clinical outcomes have risen over the years. It is my desire that in a small way, God has guided this institution through imperfection's hands. What I am sure of is that I was called for a purpose. Perhaps flawed availability is more important then skill untested.

Jason Blanchard, MBA, is currently a global administration fellow at LLUH. Born in God's country, Maine, Jason moved to Malawi when he was 4 and lived there for three and a half years. He spent six years as CEO of Malamulo Adventist Hospital and director of the LLU Global Campus in Malawi. Jason grew up with a love for nature and a desire to serve. He, his wife, Erin, and kids, Brody and Eve, live in Redlands, California.

July 18

> *"For even the Son of Man came not to be served but to serve,*
> *and to give his life as a ransom for many."*
> Mark 10:45, ESV

It hit me soon after I walked into the room to talk about his large bladder tumor revealed on the CT scan. He had pugnacious manner, surly attitude, and aggressive pessimism. He was unpleasant and negative from the first word. Every question or statement I made was met with antagonism and suspicion. Occasionally I'd look over at his wife (*did she really live with this every day?*) and wonder if she was embarrassed by this display.

We made it through the cystoscopy, which confirmed that he had a large (and almost certainly malignant) mass in the bladder. I described the surgery needed to resect it. He kept up the surly, negative attitude. I found myself struggling with the desire to return his attitude, to lash back. Choking back the cutting words I wanted to use, I finished the pre-op discussion and informed consent, and he left the office.

Later that day, after the daily deluge of patients, I wrestled with my response to this incredibly unpleasant man. Most patients in his situation are grateful for a surgeon who is ready to deal with the cancer. I was astounded by his lack of gratitude right from the start. I wondered how the people in his life put up with the poison that poured from his mouth. I asked myself (and God) how I was going to deal with the attitude after the surgery, during the inevitable post-op discussion about further cancer treatment.

Then God reminded me of Jesus' words to His disciples (when they were squabbling about who was the greatest among them): "For even the Son of Man did not come to be served, but to serve, and to give His life as a ransom for many" (Mark 10:45, AMP).

It is a foundational truth for Christ followers: Life is about serving, not about being served. When Jesus enters our hearts and institutes new management, He begins a total transformation of everything that we are. He takes a wrecking ball to the natural, human desire of being served, of receiving, of being admired and thanked and praised. Because when we could give nothing at all to God, He met our deepest need. "God demonstrates His own love toward us, in that while we were still sinners, Christ died for us" (Romans 5:8, NKJV). When I remember God's gift of forgiveness in Christ, gratitude fills my heart and displaces the quid pro quo mindset that wants to pay back evil for evil. His love enables me to serve even ungrateful, unpleasant people.

This reminder completely changed the paradigm with my difficult patient. God loved me and served me and met my needs—and continues to do so every day! I am free to give back His love to the people around me—patients, friends, coworkers, employees, acquaintances, even enemies—as He strengthens me through His Spirit.

David Elkins, LLUSM class of 1997, practices general urology in Salem, Oregon, and is married to Gina. They have four children, including Daniel (LLUSM class of 2022) and Joseph (LLUSM class of 2024). David and Gina enjoy reading, hiking, fitness, and exploring God's world.

July 19

> *"The LORD is near to those who are discouraged;*
> *he saves those who have lost all hope."*
> Psalm 34:18, GNT

Dani was a 2-year-old girl in an impossible situation in the cardiac ICU. She had multiple surgeries on her heart that left her critically ill. Her chest was open, covered only by a sterile sheet of plastic. She was successfully taken off the heart lung bypass machine (ECMO circuit) the day before, but today she was in trouble. A bronchoscopy to clean her lungs turned deadly when thick, cement-like secretions combined with old blood completely plugged the bronchoscope and lodged securely into her airway.

Her oxygen saturations plummeted from 100 percent to an alarming 70, then to unreadable as we vainly tried to clear the secretions with tiny forceps. As we frantically called ENT surgeons to come, her heart stopped and Dr. Martens (pediatric cardiac surgeon) began compressing her tiny heart with his thumb through the thin plastic that covered her open chest. We briefly got her heart to beat again with normal oxygen levels, but we knew that if we couldn't clear her airway, she would die. The room filled with nurses, respiratory therapists, doctors trying to keep her alive. As I took my turn to compress her heart, I remember praying silently for Dani and the team. We brought her parents to the bedside along with our chaplain Saul Barcelo. They asked for music to be played so that she could hear something positive.

When Dr. Park (ENT) arrived, the only way to remove those cement-like secretions was to remove her lifeline, her breathing tube. In a choreographed effort we removed the tube and the surgeons went in with their rigid scope and forceps. As her oxygen levels dropped and her heart gradually stopped, we replaced her tube and restarted chest compressions. This dangerous dance went on four more times. Finally, most of the "chunks" were removed, but the only way her oxygen stayed up and her heart kept beating were impossibly high ventilator settings. In a span of four hours she received almost 30 doses of epinephrine and multiple rounds of CPR.

As our chaplain prayed with the family at the bedside, we settled her on the ventilator, and watched as her oxygen levels remained stable. Would her heart remain stable? Would her brain be OK? For the first time in hours her heart beat on its own, and as I silently thanked God, I heard the music now playing—Danny Gokey, and the last line of his song "tell your heart to beat again." Unbelievable!

Her heart never stopped again after that, and she was discharged home sometime later, completely intact neurologically and playing like a 2-year-old should. She should not have survived that impossible ordeal, but I know God was there guiding the team to help fix her broken heart.

Whether in your personal life or with your patients, you may have a day when things really seem hopeless, and it is in those times that God can take over, put His hand on your heart, and help it to beat again.

Merrick Lopez, LLUSM class of 2005, is an assistant professor in LLUSM's department of pediatrics. He works in pediatric critical care at LLUCH and is the medical director of the PICU. He is married to Lynne Yulip-Lopez (LLUSN class of 1999). They have three children: Mia, Lucy, and Kyle.

July 20

"I don't know what your destiny will be, but one thing I know: the only ones among you who will be really happy are those who have sought and found how to serve."
Albert Schweitzer (1875–1965): German Lutheran theologian,
physician, humanitarian, and Nobel Peace Prize Laureate

I do know, without a doubt, that God designed me to be a missionary and a surgeon. This knowledge has made my job so much easier.

Five months after I arrived in Liberia, Thomas Scotland was assigned to me for his intern surgical rotation. He impressed me as dedicated, compassionate, and eager to learn. He was with us less than a month before Monrovia was swept under a wave of Ebola, killing thousands, including hospital staff. Ninety percent of Monrovia hospitals were closed. And then during a Ministry of Health meeting, a cry went out for volunteers to work in a newly established Ebola treatment unit (ETU) run by a team from Uganda.

Thomas called me after that meeting to explain that he wouldn't be coming back to work, as he was one of the four who volunteered to work in this psychologically and physically difficult ETU setting. Let me put this into perspective for you. At the time there were only 120 treatment beds for Ebola patients in the city. There were probably hundreds, maybe even thousands, of cases in the city, and the few beds were already overwhelmed. They were lined up on the streets, some alive, some dead, many in far advanced stages of Ebola. Our ETU was not yet opened; nobody was quite ready or prepared to handle this epidemical surge.

Thomas would come check on me on his days off, explaining the safety and treatment protocols to reassure me that he was doing everything possible for his personal safety. He would also tell me what Ebola patients looked like, what the most common symptoms were, and the disease's progression. We didn't have adequate laboratories; no imaging was available. All we knew was that the Ebola patients looked desperately ill.

I spoke to Thomas again a few weeks later. He sounded committed and cheerful. But the emotional strain of watching people die horrible deaths, witnessing 80 to 90 percent of a family wiped out, and seeing the pain of the single survivor took its toll. Even so, Thomas persevered in doing what he decided to do, because it needed to be done. Thomas died two weeks later.

I want you to see Thomas Scotland, and many others who experienced the Ebola crisis, as the heroes they were, as they refused to leave others in misery, pain, and death. He saw a job that needed to be done, and he saw an environment needing the skills he possessed. He couldn't turn his back. His story is the inspiration for each of us when we face our own times of trouble. You won't need to go looking for it—it will find you. Whatever the crisis, I want you to remember three things. First, you're human. Despite what we ask you to do, you are not God. You will make mistakes no matter how hard you try. Understand your limitations. Forgive yourself. Learn from it, and move on.

Second, you are not alone; you have friends, colleagues, and family. You can ask them for advice and assistance. It is not a humiliation to ask for help. It is inviting someone to work with you to achieve a better goal. It is humbling and exhilarating to watch the forces come to your aid. There is no burden that doesn't become lighter when you call for help.

Finally, be brave. Be brave like Thomas Scotland when you decide to risk everything because someone needs you. Be brave in times of trouble. Be brave.

Gillian Seton, LLUSM class of 2008, is an assistant professor in LLUSM's department of surgery, division of general surgery. She completed her general surgery residency training at the University of Utah. In February 2014 she went to Liberia for her deferred mission appointment placement, arriving just before the Ebola outbreak. Currently she is working at Malamulo Hospital in Malawi, Africa. Note: This story is an excerpt from her LLUSM commencement address to the class of 2016.

July 21

"See what great love the Father has lavished on us, that we should be called children of God! And that is what we are!"
1 John 3:1, NIV

When I was in pediatric residency at LLUCH, we were required to do overnight call on the pediatric hematology/oncology unit. On one particular night I received a call from a nurse who said that her patient, a teenager well known to the unit, was complaining of pain. I had taken care of him previously, and he was what one might consider a typical teen. He was stoic and independent, wore trendy clothes and studded earrings, and usually donned a snap-back baseball cap to hide the bald head that resulted from multiple rounds of chemotherapy. He was always so calm and collected, and was the last person I thought would be in pain. In my tired and burned-out state, I reasoned that he was probably just being overdramatic and wanted some attention.

It was late in the night, and I was not in the mood to be bothered, especially since I was in the middle of a nearly 28-hour call. The nurse specifically asked if I would come to this patient's bedside because she was concerned about his pain. Frustrated and losing my patience by the second, I begrudgingly got out of bed and went to see him. When I entered the room, I was not prepared for the scene before me. I saw a frail and skinny kid hunched over at the side of his bed, wincing in pain, with a few nurses there comforting him. As I got closer, I heard the faint sound of sniffling: He was crying. In an instant my heart dropped, and I was overcome with guilt. A person was in pain, and it had made me upset that I was being called to help. It made me realize that I had become so jaded and burned-out with residency responsibilities that I forgot the reason I went into medicine in the first place. My profession called me to be selfless, but I was being selfish. Because of that humbling experience, I renewed my vow to be a stronger advocate for my patients. I am still a work in progress, and I still feel the burnout at times, but I want to be a better doctor and a better Christian to those around me.

As physicians we are called to be co-workers with Christ and to further His healing ministry. It is easy to get bogged down with the stresses and difficulties that come with a career in medicine, but it is in times like these that we must look to Jesus and remember our calling. We have a responsibility to show others the love and character of God, and we must not lose sight of that. The trials and tribulations of this world will try to bring us down, but with God's help and with the support of each other, we can bring forth His kingdom and His healing love to those who need us the most.

Bradley Cacho, LLUSM class of 2014, is an assistant professor in LLUSM's department of pediatrics, division of neonatology. He and his wife, Erica, share two crazy but lovable dogs.

July 22

> *"For by grace you have been saved through faith. And this is not your own doing; it is the gift of God, not a result of works, so that no one may boast."*
> Ephesians 2:8-9, ESV

Grace. Daberechi. A book—*Morning Rounds*. Me, a Nigerian man who grew up in urban slums. Eleven years in America. College. Studying medicine in Greenville at the University of South Carolina. These things came together and bent the trajectory of my life journey. Five months ago after Zoom graduation, I sold almost everything I owned and began the four-day drive from Greenville to Loma Linda for internal medicine residency training.

Daberechi is a Nigerian Igbo name meaning "lean on God." I have known Daberechi since college. She gave me weekly rides to Sunday church services. With a charming smile and a melodious laugh that often ended with a snort, she lifted my spirits. Her presence warmed and cheered every room she walked into. Yet she also had a gift of listening and caring. When I struggled with studies, I confided in her. When my faith cooled, I spoke with her. She always reminded me that God's grace had been sufficient. Perhaps sensing my struggle, she one day told me, "I've found a gift for you. I've found a book. You're not alone. I hope it brings you inspiration, insight, and context." She gave me the book *Morning Rounds*.

Just inside the front cover was a note from editor Donna Hadley (LLUSN class of 1975). The book contained "stories that gave pause to think of spiritual implications. Stories that inspired. Stories that provided insight into life's lessons." Most authors, like me, were somewhere on a journey of service in the medical professions. All had connections to a place I had not heard of before called Loma Linda University School of Medicine.

From Wil Alexander's* January 1 "Life Lessons" to Marino De Leon's December 31 story of baseball Hall of Famer Roberto Clemente's humanitarian service, I looked forward to each story and reflection. De Leon summed, "We can commit daily acts of service and excel in our career of choice." As days passed, I read and sometimes reread vignettes from the book. The real experiences in these personal life stories resonated with me. I felt increasingly connected in spirit to the students, faculty, and alumni of the Loma Linda University School of Medicine. I struggled, learned, and grew together with the book's authors.

I soon did a web search. I saw an institution that made its motto "To make man whole" and its mission "to continue the teaching and healing ministry of Jesus Christ." I imagined a health care environment in which faith might connect me to patients and colleagues. I applied to the Loma Linda University Medical Center internal medicine residency program. On the day of my interview, December 17, 2019, the serene snowcapped mountains seen during my drive from Los Angeles to Loma Linda presaged my imminent interviews. During the interview and meetings I sensed the spirit that birthed the book that inspired my journey to Loma Linda this past July.

He worked through my friend Daberechi to provide me with *Morning Rounds*, setting me on the course that has led to this very moment of reflection. Now as a resident, I reflect on Lecrae's lyrics in "Lucky Ones": "I don't believe in luck; I believe in Grace." It is only by God's grace that I am here today.

*For Wil Alexander's bio, refer to the devotional on January 18.

Chibueze Ubah is a first-year internal medicine resident at LLUH. He was born in the small city of Aba in Abia State, Nigeria. He moved to the United States in 2009 after being blessed with an academic scholarship to attend South Carolina State University, where he received a BSc in nursing. He worked as a critical care nurse for three years in Columbia, South Carolina. Eventually he was accepted to medical school at the University of South Carolina School of Medicine Greenville.

July 23

> *"And who knows whether you have not come to the kingdom for such a time as this?"*
> Esther 4:14, ESV

I've always held medical missionaries in awe. Like many of us, I grew up on the stories of the brave doctors and nurses who committed their lives to serving the needy in the far corners of the world. During my time at LLUSM, there was always something in the back of my mind that entertained the hope of at least short-term medical missions. I sincerely prayed for God to open doors for me, and He did, allowing me to match into the competitive specialty of otolaryngology (ear, nose, and throat). *Well*, I thought, *I suppose they need head and neck cancer surgeons in the mission field*. But unexpected doors kept opening: almost before I knew it, I found myself in a rhinology (nose and sinus surgery) fellowship. How could that ever be of use in the mission field?

Time went by, and I was eventually entrusted with directing Loma Linda's otolaryngology residency program. "If I can't use my skills in the mission field, I'll get my residents excited about using theirs," I reasoned. Our department searched for a mission hospital to visit, and connected with LLUSM alumni Joel Mundall and Jason and Belen Lohr at Hospital Adventista Valle de Ángeles (HAVA) in Honduras. Before we knew it, our little ENT team had spent a week at HAVA, experiencing the joy of using our talents to serve the lovely Honduran people.

On Sabbath morning my resident, Dr. Darron Ransbarger (LLUSM class of 2007), and I were rounding on our postoperative patients when a woman appeared at the back door of the hospital. With her were her two young daughters, who looked to be around ages 4 and 7. The nurse tried to explain to the woman that the hospital was closed for Sabbath. I watched from the nurses' station as the woman began to explain why she was there. Her family lived in another city, several hours away. During the past few months her younger daughter had developed blockage and foul drainage from one side of her nose. There were no ENT doctors in her town, and the local physician had suggested she travel to the capital city, Tegucigalpa, to seek help. After a long bus ride to the city, she was distraught to find that she could not afford to see the doctors she'd come for! Just when she didn't know what to do, she heard an advertisement on the radio: a team of ear, nose, and throat doctors from America were visiting HAVA! She and her daughters caught the bus up into the hills where our hospital is located and arrived on Sabbath morning.

The nurse apologized to the woman that the ENT doctors were no longer seeing patients. She burst into tears, and I asked the nurse what was going on. As she explained, I listened in growing amazement. This child needed a nose specialist! God had planned this all along. I supervised as Dr. Ransbarger looked into the child's nose with his otoscope. It was a foreign body—green, a bead or something (kids everywhere love putting things up their noses). We broke open our instruments, which were already packed for the trip home, and carefully reached into her nose and plucked out—a sprout. I thought I'd fallen into an Eric B. Hare* mission story. Clearly, this was the tip of an iceberg. We set to work again, and a few minutes later, with both patient and doctors sweaty and a little tearful, it was out—the whole huge, sprouted bean. I still have the picture of the little girl and her sister standing in front of HAVA. It reminds me that no matter where God leads us in life, if we are willing, He will use us.

*Eric B. Hare was a missionary in Burma (now Myanmar). He is best known for his mission stories, which thrilled children at summer camps and camp meetings for years.

Christopher Church, LLUSM class of 1996, is a professor and residency program director in LLUSM's department of otolaryngology, head and neck surgery.

July 24

> *"Jesus said to her, 'I am the resurrection and the life. The one who believes in me will live, even though they die; and whoever lives by believing in me will never die.'"*
>
> John 11:25-26, NIV

Newly married to a medical school classmate and just beginning the season of residency interviews, I felt as though we were invincible. One evening my husband (it still felt strange to say "my husband") came home from his inpatient internal medicine rotation with a somber expression on his face. Careful not to violate HIPAA, he told me only that he was caring for an elderly retired physician whose prognosis was poor and that her husband, also a retired physician, had been a constant presence at her bedside. The husband had shared with him that they, too, had met in medical school at Loma Linda.

That night I lay awake, imagining what must be going on in the LLU Medical Center up the street and drawing parallels between that physician couple and ourselves. Tears ran down my cheeks quietly as I pictured the scene.

She lay in the hospital bed, her chest gently rising and falling. She seemed peaceful, and her husband at the bedside was relieved. She had been admitted several days ago, and her condition had not improved. The conversation with the team to discuss her goals for end-of-life care had been necessary, but now he was sitting with the weight of the words on his mind. He was a physician and had spoken those words many times during his long and successful career, but always to other families. It was so much harder to hear the words spoken in regard to his beloved, also a physician who had had a long and successful career of her own.

He thought back to how driven she was in medical school, laser-focused in class and studying for hours at a time with barely a break. It took considerable effort to convince her to spend any time with him at all, let alone go out on a date! She agreed to a walk with him after supper as a sensible study break and exercise at the same time. Their evening walks continued, and she came to know him as a kind and thoughtful man, certain he could make the world a better place through the practice of medicine. She began to look forward to those walks and they continued through their courtship and marriage, wherever they lived, later pushing a stroller or watching children ride bicycles ahead of them, whenever they were able (meaning both not on call).

He grieved the loss of that time together, sharing the joys and heartbreaks of the day with her. She understood more than anyone else because she was a physician too and had taken the same oath as he.

There was one other detail my husband told me. Her husband had said to mine, "I know I will see her again in heaven."

Though our respective stories were separated by 70 years of history, I found comfort in our risen Savior, who has promised to make us whole again.

Kyra Brusett Eddy Piñango, LLUSM class of 2012, practices full-spectrum family medicine with OB in her hometown of Livingston, Montana. Her husband, Henry Piñango (LLUSM class of 2012), practices internal medicine and is the hospice director at Livingston HealthCare. July 24 is their wedding anniversary. They have two children, Tiago and Vivian.

July 25

"He will not let your foot be moved; he who keeps you will not slumber."
Psalm 121:3, ESV

I believe our God is a personal God. He's there when we need him, especially in our most difficult times, and even if we might not realize it. I like to call the moments God reveals himself to us—often in surprising or unexpected ways—divine appointments. Perhaps you've experienced them too.

During my son Greg's nearly two-year battle with a brain tumor (a glioblastoma multiforme), I learned to be more aware of God's presence in our everyday lives. Greg assured me that God is omnipresent; we need only to pay attention. I am confident that each one of you has had events happen in your life in which, unexpectedly, things come together to illustrate God's perfect timing and His presence in your lives. A divine appointment!

May I share a few personal ones?

Soon after Greg's diagnosis a hummingbird decided to build her nest in a bush outside a window at eye level just behind Greg's desk at home. She proceeded to lay her eggs and sit on them. Soon the baby hummingbirds hatched, and eventually fledged. Thus, Greg witnessed God's creation and felt his caring and loving presence every day—a heavenly appointment with a tiny bird.

On another occasion Greg was having a rough day and decided to go to one of his favorite places: The Guitar Center. As he walked up to the store, a homeless man accosted him and asked for money. Greg stopped, gave him some money, and asked the man why he was there, which started a conversation. The homeless man told Greg he detected a sadness. Greg shared about his brain tumor, and the man wanted to know his name; he would pray for him. He then gave Greg a hug! Greg walked away feeling as though he had encountered an angel. A divine appointment?

A few weeks later I had gone with Greg for a proton treatment. We were sitting in the waiting room feeling anxious when a beautiful woman dressed in turquoise and wearing a stunning turquoise butterfly necklace came over to us. She took Greg's hands, looked into his eyes, and said she felt God wanted her to comfort Greg. She spoke words of encouragement and love and assurance of God's presence in his life. Then she was gone. We were never to see her again. I inquired at the receptionist's desk who the woman might be, but the receptionist had never seen her before. Again, we felt she must have been an angel. A divine appointment?

I tell you these stories because I want each of you to experience divine appointments in your lives. I am sure they are happening; simply open your hearts and eyes.

We will never know all the divine appointments that happen at any given time in our various Loma Linda hospitals, but I do know they are staffed with caregivers who serve as someone's angel countless times every day.

God bless you; I wish for you many divine appointments.

Dixie Marcotte Watkins is a graduate of LLUSAHP clinical laboratory sciences class of 1962. She is married to Hubert C. Watkins (LLUSM class of 1962), and is the mother of four, including Greg Watkins (LLUSM class of 1987) and Barry Watkins (LLUSM class of 1993). Dixie and Hubert live in Redlands, California.

July 26

> *"For this world is not our permanent home;*
> *we are looking forward to a home yet to come."*
> **Hebrews 13:14, NLT**

The Ice Bucket Challenge promoting amyotrophic lateral sclerosis (ALS) awareness was a popular new fad during my third-year internal medicine rotation. At that time I just so happened to be consulted for an admission on a patient who had ALS, a relentless neurodegenerative disease resulting in progressively worsening muscle weakness, affecting the arms, legs, and eventually the respiratory muscles. John was 56 years old, married with one son, and presented with respiratory distress because of his inability to clear his secretions. His diaphragm was so weak that he could not speak and had to communicate with me using his phone. Every breath took significant effort.

After building more rapport with John, I asked him what gave him the strength to persevere during this illness. His answer was "family," a common answer I receive from patients. As I dug deeper, he told me they used to attend church regularly prior to the beginning of his illness one year before. Since then he had lost his faith in God. "Why does God want me to suffer?" he asked. "My dad died from a heart attack. Why couldn't I be so lucky?"

Thinking about his dreadful and debilitating disease in that moment, I couldn't help wondering, *Why does such a terrible disease exist? What did he do to deserve this?* Everything I knew about anatomy, physiology, embryology, and cell structure and function made it difficult to deny that there is a God. His handiwork in the way our bodies were formed, how all the organs work together perfectly down to the molecular level with mechanisms that are so sophisticated, are undoubtedly the greatest creation He has ever made. Yet it also sheds light on how far sin and corruption, leading to disease and brokenness, have led us astray from God's original, beautiful design. My thoughts were racing, and my brain was overheating as I searched for an answer. All I could say was that God did not want him to suffer, that God was actually heartbroken in his suffering, but also that our wisdom was so limited compared to God's infinite wisdom. I asked him if he would like me to pray with him, but he declined.

A week later, the day before his discharge and my last day on rotation, I came in early to spend more time with him and his wife. We addressed his physical concerns and got everything squared away for his discharge. As I was about to leave, I felt an urge just to ask again if he would like to pray together. He said yes. I prayed over him and his family and thanked God for giving him a meaningful life and precious time. I prayed that He would strengthen our faith in the hope that we have a far more wonderful home waiting for us. For this time on earth is so short in light of eternity, and this world truly isn't our home, we are just passing through.

William Angkadjaja, LLUSM class of 2017, completed his family medicine residency at LLUH in 2020 and is currently working in private practice. This patient encounter took place at Kettering Hospital, Ohio, when he was a third-year medical student. He was lucky to have met and married his classmate Julia, who is an ophthalmologist in Redlands, California. They were engaged July 26, 2016.

July 27

> *"He is the one you praise; he is your God, who performed for you those great and awesome wonders you saw with your own eyes."*
> **Deuteronomy 10:21, NIV**

Our first father/daughter mission trip took place many months ago in Holguin, Cuba. I just knew we would witness God's guidance and see, firsthand, numerous miracles that would help strengthen our faith.

One of the first miracles took place even before we took off for Cuba. We had more than 280 pounds of food, medication, medical supplies, 600 pairs of glasses for the eye clinics, and plenty of clothes for all ages. Once at the airport we learned that there was a limit to the number of bags we could check and carry on, and there was a weight restriction for each of the bags. We were allowed two checked bags per passenger, with a maximum of 70 pounds per bag, plus we could take a carry-on for each of us, with a weight allotment of 22 pounds per person. We each maxed out our carry-on weight, and my daughter's two bags that were to be checked had slightly less than 70 pounds apiece, so they were good to go. My two bags weighed 78.5 pounds and 64.5 pounds, so unfortunately together they weighed 143 pounds We had spent so much time carefully picking out and sorting all the supplies we would need for the trip, so it would have been a huge letdown to leave anything behind.

As I was silently hoping for something miraculous to happen, I was impressed to try to repack and move the items from one of my bags to the other. Hoping for a tangible miracle, I placed each bag back on the scales. The weight on the digital scale showed 68.5 pounds for the first bag, and 69.5 pounds for the second bag—a total of five pounds had disappeared from my bags right in front of our eyes!

I turned to my daughter and said, "Sarah, this is our first divine intervention on this trip."

The airline agent gave us a nod and smiled. We couldn't believe what we had just witnessed! We miraculously had lost five pounds from our luggage, and Sarah and I were beaming with thankfulness at what the Lord had just done. As we boarded the plane, I couldn't help thinking, *If God can help our luggage lose five pounds, I wonder what else He has in store for us on this trip!*

Josif Borovic, LLUSM class of 1997, lives in the Los Angeles area and works at White Memorial Medical Center as a pain management specialist. He loves to take mission trips with his daughter Sarah, who recently completed her freshman year at Southern Adventist University in Tennessee, majoring in biology. She plans to follow in her dad's footsteps when it comes to mission work and her choice of profession.

July 28

"Jesus wept."
John 11:35, NIV

Each of us has faced death—spouse, children, parents, friends, or coworkers. An understandable reaction is to ask why. We all know that we are mortal and that one day we will die. When the day comes, however, it may be perceived as premature and unfair, especially when accompanied by tragic accidents or homicide.

During my first week as a missionary physician at Bella Vista Hospital in Puerto Rico, I had to convey news of a mother's death. The numerous family members began to scream and fall down on the floor, wailing with tears—not an atypical cultural response. In Puerto Rico a common response to petitionary prayer for divine intervention was *Si Dios quiere* [If God wills].

A common reaction to death is to rail against God and ask why. Although He never gives us an audible answer, many of our well-meaning clergy, family, and friends are often far too eager to give us one. In their desire to console, they commonly say that it is God's will or that He moves in mysterious ways. Although some may find solace in that premise, I find it theologically unsound and morally preposterous. What kind of loving God would will the death of an innocent child? In a larger sense, of course, death is within God's will as a deeper, albeit unwelcome, consequence to giving humanity free will. But to ascribe the death of an innocent child to some secret or unfathomable reason known only in the mind of God forces us to seek some personal purpose that is not there. Certainly good can come from death, but that would not be its purpose.

When Jesus' good friend Lazarus fell gravely ill, Jesus was sought out to come quickly to heal him. Curiously, Jesus took His time, saying that Lazarus was sleeping, which meant that he was dead. When Jesus arrived, Lazarus had been dead for four days, and his body was beginning to smell. Many of those present said that if only Jesus had come earlier, He could have kept Lazarus from dying. As Jesus was taken to where he was laid, Jesus wept. The Son of God cried. After the stone was removed, Jesus said, "Lazarus, come forth!"

We may never know why Jesus cried. Some think that He was moved in sadness or was simply grieving with those around Him. I think He cried because, after all the miracles He had performed, He was dismayed that so few had faith to believe that He could raise Lazarus up.

But Lazarus died a second time, and Jesus was not there—just as He is not here now to raise up our loved ones. But in the resurrection we will see them again. Thus, we should not grieve as others without hope, because He is the resurrection and the life.

Gregory Wise, LLUSM class of 1973-B, spent six years in mission service in Puerto Rico. He then became head of general internal medicine and geriatrics at LLUSM, and later served as chief medical officer at Kettering Health Network in Ohio. Today he is editor-in-chief of primary care reports.

July 29

"And she [Hagar] called the name of the Lord that spake unto her, Thou God seest me: for she said, Have I also here looked after him that seeth me?"
Genesis 16:13, KJV

That the same God who is occupied with the affairs of an ever-expanding universe with billions of galaxies notices a runaway servant girl is a story that should greatly comfort you and me in the daily struggles of our lives. Hagar, whom Abram had honored to become his second wife (a decision not endorsed by God), finds herself in the desert in an attempt to flee from her mistress, Sarai. There in the moment of her desperation, the angel of God reveals to her that she was pregnant, delivers the name of the child, and reassures her of the great blessings in store for Ishmael.

I was awakened by my pager at 2:00 a.m. one morning to come see a patient in the emergency department with abdominal pain. I got up, rubbed my eyes, walked down a flight of stairs, down the hallway, and into a section of the emergency room where this patient was. I listened to her complaints, examined her, reviewed the CT scans and labs with the students and residents, and came back to discuss the plans with the patient. This is a routine that I have repeated by now hundreds, if not thousands, of times. Just before walking away, the patient said to me in a soft voice, "Sir, may I talk to you for a minute? I have been lying in this bed for more than eight hours, with my pain getting worse. I have not prayed in a long time, but I felt compelled to do so because of the worsening pain. I asked God to please send me someone who could help me. As soon as I opened my eyes, I saw you walking in the hallway. Before I even knew you were coming to see me, a voice said to me, *This is My servant that I have prepared to attend to you.* In that instant I felt a sudden calm and peace. Right after that, you came over to talk to me." She thanked me, and I left, barely able to hide my emotions from the surgical residents. To know that this time I was used by heaven in direct answer to this woman's prayer is both profound and humbling. Only eternity will reveal the true impact of this interaction on both of our lives.

In a world that is becoming increasingly impersonal, it is not always easy to conceive of a personal God who is actively "roaming" the hallways of our institution, seeking to place us in contact with patients/people. Yes, sometimes as a direct answer to a prayer for help. He sent an angel to comfort and minister to an upset runaway maid in the desert. Sometimes He sends angels with wings, and sometimes He sends angels in scrubs. "God never leads His children otherwise than they would choose to be led, if they could see the end from the beginning, and discern the glory of the purpose which they are fulfilling as co-workers with Him" (Ellen G. White, *The Desire of Ages*, p. 224-225). Dear friend, may you and I be available today to be used by God for the accomplishment of His purpose, for herein lies the true meaning of our profession.

David Turay completed his surgery residency at LLUH in 2010 and is an associate professor in LLUSM's department of surgery, division of trauma. He was the 2019 LLUSM commencement speaker. His passion is to encourage colleagues and medical students never to forget the treatment of the "whole person," especially in an increasingly busy and impersonal world. He is a sincere believer in the impact our spirituality has on our health and recovery from disease.

July 30

"God is light and in Him is no darkness at all."
1 John 1:5, NKJV

We had earned our keep aboard the *Palikir* this week. The medical and dental teams worked hard on every atoll, but this was nearly impossible when we got to the equatorial heat on Kapingamarangi. The medical team was exhausted from removing at least one mole from almost every island villager. They had just lost one of their own to melanoma. The dental team always worked hard on every island.

The heat and humidity had sapped our energy. Our mentor, Dr. Ron Thomas, was in charge of the galley on board the *Palikir*, and he was running low on food to feed our hungry team members. Nevertheless, we planned a final-night vespers for the villagers.

We had sensed a darkness on this island drifting down from an unbelieving, ungrateful chief. This was countered by the resident Adventist schoolteacher, Kyoce, our friend from previous trips to another atoll.

There were four of us with enough energy left to come ashore for the scheduled meeting. We planned to share music with Kyoce, who played guitar and sang beautiful spiritual songs. After that we gave a health talk and a homily from the Bible.

We sat on the beach surrounded by palms and fading colors of a sunset beyond imagination.

There was one minor glitch—no one came. Our pastor, Eddie Dopp, thought he had achieved buy-in from the chief.

But there we sat in the ever-thickening equatorial darkness. For an hour. Alone and feeling rejected.

Then God moved. He put it into our heads to sing. Why not? We had two guitars and four voices. We started timidly with "This Little Light of Mine."

By the end of the first verse we felt a bit better. By the time we got to the "neighborhood" verse, we had caught a glimpse of something.

A light from one swaying lantern in the distant darkness. It was Kyoce, followed by villagers and their reluctant chief.

We sang together. We talked about health and wholeness. We talked about the way in which Jesus had shown up on this obscure island on the equator.

At the program's end the villagers filtered back to their huts while Eddie and I sought out Kyoce.

Kyoce's guitar was almost unplayable, and we had two new Taylor guitars. We prayed with him and talked about how he was God's man on this island. Hugs and tears, and then we handed him one of the new guitars.

An appreciative look, and then our goodbyes.

Let it shine, Kyoce. Let it shine.

Philip Broeckel, LLUSM class of 1976-B, has been in the department of emergency medicine for Scripps in San Diego since 1984. He has a particular interest in planning mission trips with Eddie Dopp, the pastor at Oceanside SDA Church. He and his wife enjoy their three kids and four grandchildren.

July 31

> *"Teach us to number our days, that we may gain a heart of wisdom."*
> Psalm 90:12, NIV

The pager vibrated against my hip. I had turned off the noisy beep months ago, as a Pavlovian-induced chest pain was triggered when I heard other electronic tones, such as those from the microwave. As a urology resident, I was on loan to the general surgery department for my first year of training.

As is not uncommon in a surgery residency, I was trying to do too many things with 15 minutes. This page came at an unfortunate point. I had promised my chief resident that I could cover a colon surgery, and separately told a urology attending I would stop by to review my work on a manuscript. I looked at the phone extension on the page, did some mental time calculations, and headed toward the emergency department to see a consult. Twelve minutes later I was running, or at least moving quickly while wearing clogs, toward the urology department.

Even though it was not particularly logical, I felt as if I could discuss my research in three minutes. But as any researcher will tell you: lab meetings are never a hurried affair. Thus, I arrived at the operating room late. For the reader not accustomed to operating room culture, this is about as optimal as eating a rock.

What follows is a transcript of the conversation. Please note the full effect is better in this particular attending's Italian accent.

Attending: "Wayne, you need more fiber in your diet!"

Wayne: "I am not sure I understand, Sir."

Attending: "There are only two reasons you would be late to my OR: (1) you are dead—which you are clearly not—or (2) you are constipated. Given the options, I will now refer to you as 'Slow Transit' Brisbane."

Let me assure you, this new name form became popular among the other interns as well! The tasks we would like to accomplish invariably outlast the number of minutes available to allocate appropriately. Thus, how we distribute our time is an ultimate determinant of our values. It has been seven years since my intern year, and I have triaged multiple demands for time. Yet nothing provides more clarity and focus than thinking about what I would like to accomplish before my time eventually runs out. I ultimately chose to become a urologic oncologist because I love being part of how people decide to spend time once they have a cancer diagnosis. No matter what obligations you have today, take five minutes to reflect on what is truly important, and spend your minutes on that. It is undoubtedly time not wasted.

Wayne Brisbane, LLUSM class of 2013, recently completed a fellowship in urologic oncology at UCLA in June, 2021. By the publication of this book, he will have finished the 12 years of training prerequisite for finding a "real job." Besides an education, this time has yielded two boys (Charles, born 2016, and Benjamin, born 2019) and strengthened the love between Katie and him (married 2010). Aside from the aforementioned dates, the time at Loma Linda was among the "happiest and most fulfilling of the past decade."

AUGUST

☙ TEAMWORK ☙

"Alone we can do so little; together we can do so much."

HELEN KELLER (1880–1968)
American political activist and first deaf-blind
person to earn a Bachelor of Arts degree

August 1

> *"Go to the ant . . . ; consider her ways, and be wise."*
> Proverbs 6:6, KJV

Children hospitalized for a lengthy period can attend special school classes held by child life education that provide a much-needed service within the children's hospital.

During a natural science class the subject was ants. Students in the class listened intently as the teacher described some of the rules that ants live by. She added, "Queen ants are the founder and leader of the colony, and some can live up to 30 years in an underground chamber sometimes 25 feet deep. Drones become the fathers to the eggs the queen ant lays, and worker ants that are female forage and protect the colony." The teacher added, "Did you know that a worker ant can carry up to five times her weight in food, and some ants can move more than 50 times their weight? Why do you think this is so?"

Seven-year-old Jimmy with a precocious reputation responded, "Because she is not unionized."

The teacher, caught off guard and wanting to instill in Jimmy and her students the importance of teamwork, replied, "That's true, Jimmy. As part of a team, they are able to provide for the needs of the ant colony while living up to their various abilities. In this case, participating in ways that provide for the colony may be similar to how we can help and support each other."

Jimmy was silent for a moment and then replied, "I wish I could be like a worker ant."

The teacher asked why.

"I want to be useful," Jimmy said.

Sensing an opening, the teacher gently reminded her class that ants make use of every moment that they have. In all their endeavors they utilize drive and illustrate resourcefulness—two laws necessary for teamwork and success.

Many of us carry a load that is made lighter by the vision that we too are part of a huge team participating in His service. As we reflect on Jimmy's answer, his casual response gels. Sharing in the healing ministry of Jesus contributes to the benefit of others and, on a personal level, generates a sense of optimism, peace, and well-being. Jimmy's off-the-cuff remark reminds us of the depth of His creation in nature, which carries over to our own sense of purpose and well-being. There is so much we can learn from God's creation in nature.

Leigh Aveling graduated from LLUSR with an MA in ethics and church ministry, earned a DMin from the Claremont School of Theology in California, and is an LMFT. He currently works as a chaplain at LLUMC and is associated with the School of Religion, with a focus on relational studies and ethics. He is the father of four boys.

August 2

"God gave Solomon wisdom and very great insight, and a breadth of understanding as measureless as the sand on the seashore."
1 Kings 4:29, NIV

Retirement allows time for reflection, bringing focus on what is really important in life. In my case these reflections take me back to Loma Linda, where I spent 45 years, my entire nursing career, and where I was particularly blessed by the influence of three wise men.

My early days in Loma Linda were spent in the School of Nursing, from which I graduated in 1971. I was naturally attracted to cardiothoracic surgery and thrived in this setting for many years under the direction of the chief of the department, Ellsworth Wareham (CME class of 1942). This wise man opened new horizons for this young nurse, taking me to the ends of the earth with the overseas heart surgery team and challenging me to be the best patient advocate I could be, wherever I served. Dr. Wareham's presence was always larger than life, and his quiet confidence created a peaceful and healing environment for both patients and staff.

My travels overseas with the heart surgery team introduced me to a second wise man, Roy Jutzy (CME class of 1952), chief of cardiology, who tirelessly traveled near and far as Loma Linda's ambassador, identifying patients who were in need of cardiac surgery. In Roy Jutzy I saw absolute kindness, authenticity, and cheerfulness of spirit. I wanted to be just like him in my interactions with others. In 1985 I began working exclusively with Loma Linda's fledgling heart transplant program, giving second chances to babies and adults with incurable heart disease. Here I flourished under the influence of a third wise man, Leonard Bailey (LLUSM class of 1969). From him I witnessed compassion, tenderness, and creativity on a daily basis. I learned the importance of sharing our expertise with others in a spirit of genuine generosity without thought of any gain. I was witness to true humility.

I am blessed beyond measure to have spent my working life in the presence of these great Christian role models. For me, they exemplified Loma Linda University Health's motto, "To make man whole," in their day-to-day lives. Time spent in their presence has helped to make me become "whole" as well. And I believe that the world would be a kinder place if more people could be exposed to these core qualities that reflect the teaching and healing ministry of Jesus Christ.

Joyce Johnston Rusch, LLUSN class of 1971, is a retired nurse now living in Oregon. Both she and her husband, Roy (LLUSM class of 1965), cherish their ties to LLUH.

August 3

"Listening is one of the loudest forms of kindness."
Anonymous

It was the first week of my third year of medical school, and I was on call at the Jerry L. Pettis Memorial Veterans Medical Center for my internal medicine rotation. A new admit was waiting in the ED. I located my patient in the corner of the room. As I approached the curtain, my mind went blank, but my heart raced, as it often did when I'm nervous. As I turned the corner, my eyes met a man shaking uncontrollably. Moving quickly to the bedside, I asked, "Sir, are you OK?" No answer. I assumed quickly that the man wasn't having a seizure, and didn't see any visible signs of injury. Breathing a sigh of relief, I addressed the patient again. The first words out of his mouth still ring in my ears as I write this: He shouted, "I just want to die!"

Now, I'm not usually the toughest person, but I also don't consider myself an emotional person. However, when I heard this fully grown man shout those words and start sobbing hysterically, tears filled my eyes. What could I say to that? I froze. "Sir," I said with a trembling voice, "Tell me what's going on." After a moment he caught his breath and began to explain his story. A disastrous family situation, broken relationships, poor health care, and much more filled the air as this man poured out his bleak life story. I tried to calm him down with such classic phrases as "It'll be OK, Sir" or "We are going to get you through this" or (my personal favorite) "That's really tough." Very naive comments from such a young and inexperienced "practicing physician." All the while, the man was pulling at his hair and repeating, "I want to die, and no one cares." Minutes running by, I resorted to grabbing his hand. The physical contact significantly calmed us both down. Who knew the last time he actually had someone show him love in any capacity, much less physical contact? I sat down in a nearby chair to hear his story.

Time passed, and he was admitted to the floor, so I returned to the workroom. Taking a seat, the resident leaned over and said to me, "It's not easy being a doctor," and I thought to myself, *How am I going to become a doctor and not get emotionally attached to my patients?* Completely engrossed in the patient's circumstances, I learned that day that I have a long way to go in understanding how to work through these kinds of situations. I honestly think I did do some things right that day, such as holding the man's hand and sitting by the patient's bed. However, I know I have much to learn in practicing wholistic medicine. All I do know is that when I entered my patient's room the next morning, my eyes were met by a man with a smile on his face and a fresh perspective on life, greeting me with a "Good morning, Doc!" I guess I chose medicine for times like these.

Paul Miller, LLUSM class of 2020, is the son of two MDs, and proud to be carrying on the family's name in medicine. His family showed and taught him to take the time to listen to others and display Christ's love and kindness at every opportunity.

August 4

Proposed LLUSM White Coat Ceremony, 2022

Reflections as my firstborn matriculates to LLUSM …

Loma Linda University School of Medicine now has a white coat ceremony at the beginning of the school year, which they didn't have when I attended. As they read the names of the first-year students and coated them, the church, which was packed, erupted in whoops, hoots, hollers, and cheers. I, in contrast to the celebratory air around me, felt sobered.

Oh, LLUSM, I silently entreated, we are offering you our firstborn, not by our choice, but by her choice. Because she made this decision, we are also aware of the incredible privilege she has to be in this class. You will transform these bright, innocent, naive young people through an inundation, a virtual deluge of facts that will rapidly change in our high-tech, high-speed, information-laden world. You will bring them into contact with indescribable suffering and miraculous healing. They will witness professional health care workers in all their humanity, including heroism, gentleness, and grace, along with those who will be cynical, burned-out, or harsh with them and make them question if this journey is all worth it.

Regardless, these children will emerge changed. They will have lost their innocence, and they may lose permanently the capacity for joyous spontaneity. They will emerge as professionals. They will grow closer to these classmates in a special bond that outsiders cannot fathom. Marriages and relationships may disintegrate, but new ones will be formed. They will be bruised and at times broken by what they see and hear, but my hope is that they will continue retaining their core humanity, some human decency, and a capacity to find hope and beauty in their future lives.

Class of 2020, future colleagues, my beloved child, it is holy work in which you now embark. May you be reminded, whenever necessary, that it is His work in which you are now engaged, and may you always feel His steps alongside yours.

Waylene Wang Swensen, LLUSM class of 1986, is a radiation oncologist at University of Washington. She is married to Ron Swenson (LLUSM class of 1984). The above was written in 2016 for her daughter, Sasha (LLUSM class of 2020), at the white coat ceremony on Sasha's first day of medical school.

August 5

"We are His hands to touch a world that's broken. We are His voice to cheer the wounded soul. Shining the light of love that lives in Jesus, we are His comfort, His healing love."

"Healing Love," Wintley Phipps (1955–) and John Stoddart (c. 1972–): American singers and songwriters commissioned for the LLUH school song

Though I had gone on several mission trips as a medical student and resident, this was my first experience as an independent practitioner. This trip was also unlike the others because I was responsible for leading our group. I was nervous because I had never been to the Philippines before, and was not familiar with their culture.

Despite my anxiety, I had lofty ideas for our project: I envisioned a spacious auditorium with multiple booths offering medical services, dental care, physical therapy, pain management, spiritual counseling, and even sessions in hygiene, nutrition, exercise, and massage. When we arrived on site, space was limited, with only a handful of staff; I was immediately discouraged by our limited resources.

Initially the villagers trickled in slowly, but within hours dozens of families were waiting in the parking lot. The staff was organized, efficient, and helped streamline the entire program. Most patients had common complaints: coughs, colds, urinary infections, and diabetes.

After several days we had barely made a dent in our inventory and still had plenty of supplies. I was again disheartened, and regretted purchasing so many advanced medications, some of which were never used, especially the ones for congestive heart failure and stroke.

On the penultimate day of our trip, we decided to make a house visit to the village elder. She was too sick to commute to our clinic and refused to leave her home. When we entered the doorway, a dozen family members surrounded us. I was shocked by what I saw: an elderly woman whose entire body was swollen with water. Her lungs were wet with congestion, her legs were mottled from poor circulation, and her skin was ulcerated with wounds as a result of immobility from a recent stroke. After finishing my history and exam, I prescribed her medications that would help offload the excess fluid, treat her skin infection, and prevent a second stroke. Miraculously, all the medications that I thought would be wasted were ultimately used for her multiple advanced medical diseases!

As we drove away, I was awestruck and humbled: awestruck because I genuinely believed that God brought us to one another, and humbled because despite my lack of faith and constant doubt, God showed me that He was in control. His plan is always bigger and better than my own. How else could He have coordinated for an internist to treat a village elder with congestive heart failure? How else could our partnership with the local church have led dozens of souls to accept Bible studies, personal prayer, and spiritual counseling? He cares so much for each individual soul that He would equip an entire health care team with personalized medications, even to deliver it within a remote village. God's love for us has no limitation in space or time!

After finishing up with our final patient, the pitter-patter sound on the tin roof turned my gaze outside, where I beheld the most beautiful rainbow. I spoke a prayer of thanksgiving and for His promise of "Immanuel," God with us.

Denny Hong, LLUSM class of 2015, is an internist in the deferred mission appointee program. He and his family are currently working with Adventist Health International in Kenya. They all desire to lead others to Jesus, the true source of healing.

August 6

"I will give you a new heart and put a new spirit within you; I will take the heart of stone out of your flesh and give you a heart of flesh."
Ezekiel 36:26, NKJV

A young, recently married woman with a heart problem since birth met a world-renowned cardiologist around 1946. After fluoroscopy of her chest, he told her she had an atrial septal defect (ASD) the size of a quarter. He informed her she should not have children, would become a cardiac cripple, and would die before she was 40. Heart surgery was not an option at that time.

She went home and lived life, forgetting his prediction. She had three children, raised them, and went about all the family activities, maybe not as fast as the kids, but they didn't mind.

She had excelled in school, regularly bested the "preprofessional students," and trained to be a teacher. She chose to teach special-needs students, patiently helped them learn their phone numbers and addresses, knowing they would need to relearn them next school year. She loved children.

By her working, she and her PhD husband, also a teacher on denominational wage, through sacrifice and commitment to education, were able to put all three children through academy, college, graduate school, and medical school without debt.

When her son was in medical school, he tried out his stethoscope, listening to her 55-year-old heart, hearing a very loud murmur.

When she was in her early 70s, she needed presurgical clearance for a cholecystectomy. Her radiologist son read her most abnormal chest X-ray: heart size was three times normal, filling most of the chest, and pulmonary arteries, typically finger size, the size of the wrist. His first thought was this has to be the wrong X-ray for this normal-appearing woman, who took only blood pressure medicine.

The cardiologist balked when she said she had an "ASD the size of a quarter," thinking rheumatic heart and valve disease, "since ASDs don't live this long," and ordered the full workup. The echo techs all swarmed around as they scanned her heart with color-flow, never having seen such abnormal dynamics. When she returned for the follow-up appointment, the cardiologist diagnosed an "ASD the size of a quarter!" They figured her blood recirculated three times through her lungs before it went to her body. The cholecystectomy went off without a hitch.

She lived a full life, active in church, school, home, and family. She always had something uniquely special for each grandchild.

She succumbed to a stroke from a paradoxical embolism at the age of 78. She had doubled the original prediction. Her gravestone is engraved: "Great Heart."

A living miracle, my mother.

She lived a full life, not a cardiac cripple; she had a brilliant mind, and chose to patiently teach disabled children. She depended on the Lord for daily health and strength. In her humble way, she touched all those around her who had no idea what was happening inside with each heartbeat. We witnessed a lifelong miracle.

Robert Hewes, LLUSM class of 1976-B, is an interventional radiologist at AdventHealth in Daytona Beach, Florida.

August 7

> "The LORD will keep you from all evil; he will keep your life. The LORD will keep your going out and your coming in from this time forth and forevermore."
>
> Psalm 121:7-8, ESV

August 1967 a group of junior and senior dental students were privileged to go on one of the first Loma Linda University School of Dentistry service learning mission trips. Faculty advisor Don Peters (LLUSD 1961, 1969, 1974); Gary Cornforth (LLUSD 1968, 1975); Virgil Erlandson (LLUSD 1968); Fred Mantz (LLUSD 1969, 1973); Quint Nicola (LLUSD 1969); Richard Parker (LLUSD 1968) and his wife, Bonnie; and Hank van den Hoven (LLUSD 1968) were excited to go to the beautiful country of Guatemala, Central America. We used a mobile clinic donated by the Student Association of Thunderbird Adventist Academy in Arizona. Sometimes the team had a panoramic view as they traveled through a village riding on top of the mobile clinic. Immersed in the culture of rural Guatemala, we stayed in local churches or simple motels. The people were very appreciative of the dental clinics held on church porches, schools, or village centers.

In one village many of the locals had decayed or missing front teeth from sucking sugar cane. One 16-year-old girl with a beautiful smile wanted her two perfectly good upper front teeth removed. We soon discovered the reason—she wanted her front teeth removed to be like her peers. Needless to say, we didn't remove her front teeth but reassured her of the importance of keeping her own teeth!

After the main group of students returned home, the Parkers stayed another week, visiting with Richard's cousin, Lynn Baerg, Guatemala Mission president; his wife, Sharlet; and two children, Deborah, 7, and Michael, 8. We took a special weekend to enjoy the country's picturesque beauty. Sharlet noticed a field of wildflowers and asked to stop the van to take a closer look. Michael and his mom got out and crossed over to the other side of the road. Deborah decided that she too wanted to see the flowers up close and slipped unnoticed out the open van door. There was a thud and screech of brakes as a passing car hit Deborah, sending her flying through the air and landing on her head some distance in front of the van.

No emergency medical care was available in this remote area. The best we could do was to put semiconscious Deborah, bleeding from the ear, with no apparent broken bones, in the van with her dad frantically driving while all of us prayed that God would intervene. We were about an hour to Quetzaltenango, where we knew medical care would be limited. By the time we arrived at the hospital, Deborah was waking up. Providentially there was a visiting neurosurgeon, seeing patients there only for that day, which was a miracle! After looking at the X-rays and observing the patient, the doctor reassured us that even though she had had a concussion, with several days of rest she should be fine.

We think back to that traumatic and eventful trip with gratitude for God's miracles of healing and protection.

Bonnie R. Parker, La Sierra College (now La Sierra University) BS 1966, resides in Yucaipa, California, with husband, Richard (LLUSD class of 1968). They have enjoyed mission service in Micronesia, mentored many dental students at LLUSD, and are active on many service learning trips. They have three sons and eight grandchildren. August 7 is their wedding anniversary.

August 8

Grand Opening of LLUMC and LLUCH, 2021

> *"I alone know the plans I have for you, plans to bring you prosperity and not disaster, plans to bring about the future you hope for."* Jeremiah 29:11, GNT

The seismic mandate from the California legislature to the Loma Linda hospitals was clear: Replace the iconic cloverleaf towers or close. The deadline for compliance was December 31, 2019. But how do you raise $1.5 billion to build an entirely new adult hospital and a large addition to the children's hospital with extremely limited cash, weak financial performance year after year, and a marginal credit rating? With much soul searching and prayer, campus leadership went to work and formulated a $1.5 billion plan. The plan was audacious. It had three essential components:

First: The hospitals would have to be successful in qualifying for $165 million under two state grants designed to fund only children's services. The experts said it couldn't be done. They said: (1) state officials would never accept a building design with a common pedestal supporting a separate adult tower and a separate children's tower even though the design was cost-effective and efficient (the design would mix the adult and children's hospital space, disqualifying the design for grant funding); and (2) state officials would never approve the distribution of taxpayer-funded grant dollars to our not-for-profit religious (Christian) hospitals—separation of church and state would preclude such!

Second: The hospitals would have to raise more than $230 million in philanthropy. The experts said it couldn't be done. They said: (1) the hospitals had no proven track record for raising large sums of money; (2) the alumni pool was small; and (3) the hospitals did not have large philanthropic foundations.

Third: The hospitals would have to raise more than $1 billion from the commercial bond market. The experts said it couldn't be done. They said: (1) the hospitals had a poor insurance payer mix with too many patients relying on the state Medicaid program; (2) the hospitals had years of weak financial performance; (3) the credit rating for the hospitals was at a low level, and the New York bond market would reject any bond offering.

Today, after years of planning, perseverance, and prayer, we see that which was once thought undoable—done.

The building: The building design consists of a common pedestal with a separate adult tower and children's tower that is a model for cost-effectiveness and efficiency.

The grants: The state has fully funded the $165 million in grants for the children's hospital.

The philanthropy: The Vision 2020 philanthropy campaign began with a $100 million lead gift; it then grew to yield more than $230 million in gifts for the hospitals and more than $210 million for the university. Vision 2020 opened the giving hearts of alumni, patients, and friends of the hospitals and the university in unimaginable ways.

The bonds: Under three separate bond offerings, more than 50 bond investment firms from New York to Los Angeles purchased more than $1 billion of the hospitals' bonds.

What about the experts? Well—the experts were wrong. Today is not a day for boasting, but a day for humility—humility in the realization that doors were opened in mysterious and inexplicable ways in order to allow for the construction of the new hospitals. In the beautiful words of Jeremiah, God has given the hospitals: a future and a hope.

Kerry Heinrich, JD, has served as the chief executive officer of the six hospitals within the LLUH system since 2014. He is married to Judy (LLUSD class of 1988). His son, Christopher (LLUSM class of 2020), is a resident at Mayo Clinic in Minnesota. His daughter, Katherine, is a graduate (2019) of the LLUH Business Management Residency program.

August 9

"Commitment is an act, not a word."
Jean-Paul Sartre (1905–1980): French philosopher and Nobel Prize Laureate in Literature

It was the first day of medical school. Excitingly that meant two weeks of being assigned to a clinical setting, a sort of orientation into our futures as physicians prior to digging into the books. My assignment was geriatric psychiatry. Having spent a semester of my undergraduate studies visiting a psychiatry ward, I was looking forward to having similar interesting conversations with patients. A specific gentleman really stood out to me. "I always liked math and computers, so I finally wrote a book about the robots I invented. These creatures, as I call them, are able to find their own food and they are emotionally intelligent. Here, read all my calculations and blueprints. You can buy the book online too. Did you know you can be your own publisher?" I held his book in my hands, and leafed through the pages, filled with ambitious claims that held no cohesive ideas. He also went on to describe two other books he had published, one on psychiatry and the other on agriculture.

When I asked him why he came to the psychiatric hospital, he said, "My wife told me I was getting crazy again. Sometimes I do that, so I came here before I did anything dumb." As we continued to talk, I learned that he had issues since his early 20s, and now being in his 60s, he explained how he had finally learned to deal with his "untrustworthy brain." "You see, living with my brain is as if I am always carrying two buckets with a yoke. Sometimes one bucket gets too full. It can be repetitive thoughts, sounds, or sadness. Most of the time I am good at ignoring it, but now it got too heavy," he explained. He was a pleasant gentleman, socially aware, asking me questions and interacting appropriately.

Impressed with his coping abilities and wanting to learn more from this well-adapted patient, I asked about his support system. "Well, my wife doesn't care about me." This seemed more likely a response stemming from his pathology, since he went on to explain how he had been married for 40 years to the same woman. When the treatment team called her to ask about his medications, she had everything organized and asked how he had been doing.

It was surprising to see a couple who had lived through so much heartache together, especially such an alienating situation of psychiatric problems. As I continue to meet patients who have so easily lost their mental capacities, the very thing that gives us our human power, it is difficult not to feel weary of our fragile minds. I will dare to take a lesson from others' suffering, though I could never claim to understand their difficulties. I will claim the importance of community. His weak mind was made stronger when supported by another's, someone who stood by his side and has thus helped him navigate through life. I thus pray for the strength to help and the humility to be helped.

Giovanna Sobrinho, LLUSM class of 2016, is from Mato Grosso, Brazil. She completed her residency in psychiatry at USC Keck School of Medicine and now practices at the West Los Angeles Veterans Affairs Medical Center. She met her husband, Michael J. S. Lee (LLUSM class of 2016), in medical school. He sees the brain from a different perspective as a neuroradiology fellow at UCLA.

August 10

"For this reason I bow my knees before the Father, from whom every family in heaven and on earth is named."
Ephesians 3:14-15, ESV

My neck itches. I think it's the tag still attached to my white coat's collar: *Is it because it's new, or because I might need to return it?* That's why they don't embroider our names as first-year medical students, giving us only removable badges along with a gold Humanism in Medicine pin. Well, here I am. And here's the elevator to the sixth floor, and my first patient.

Adjusting my stethoscope around my neck, I hear my physician-professor's voice. These two weeks before classes begin are the closest you'll ever be to the patient's experience. From now on, you'll move further and further away from knowing what it is like to know nothing at all about medicine. Remember this feeling. A third-year leans over to her classmate, laughing. A first-year just asked what hypertension was. I said high blood pressure, and he wrote it down! They try to stifle their chuckling. I try to cover my book. "Hypertension = High Blood Pressure" written only minutes before.

Doors opening; my third-year mentor turns. "Let's go see your first patient. She has a classic murmur." Classic. More than your usual lub-dub. You gotta hear it: It will help you this year. You'll never forget it. So we walk toward the patient's room, this patient whose heart will be our textbook.

I look down at our list as we walk past bed 2, 55-year-old male, pancreatitis; bed 7, 31-year-old female, sarcoidosis. Here was our patient: bed 11, 89-year-old female, failure to thrive. Her weight: 76 pounds. My mentor was already listening to her heart: hand upon stethoscope upon intercostal spaces, tracking the murmured conversation of her heart under the withered expanse of her breast, each space grooved in striking topographic clarity. I was next. I remembered an instruction from days before: As you listen, place your other hand on your patient. The touch may be comforting. I rested my hand on her shoulder and placed the stethoscope. I heard the slow, clear plod, but no murmur. I looked at her face: knowledgeable skin stretched, taut, thin as my knowledge, between its bony eminences. Her eyes were mostly closed. Did she see me? The room was dim.

As I looked at her closed eyes, panic turned first-year ignorance into beads of hot shame. Still no murmur. Maybe I should close my eyes, I'll hear better. Still nothing. But what was that rub, that sensation? My eyes opened to see her hand, resurrected from the hospital blanket, over mine, her thin left thumb lightly grazing, reassuring my stethoscope-bearing own. Murmur forgotten, I began to rub her shoulder softly, still holding the stethoscope, my only excuse to stay. Her eyes still closed, our hands holding each other, as she taught me something I would never forget: "Failure to thrive" is not my name.

Karl Wallenkampf, LLUSM class of 2021, graduated from LLUSR with an MA in bioethics in 2020. He and his wife enjoy hiking, reading, writing, and exploring around their new home in St. Louis, Missouri, as Karl begins residency in the Washington University Barnes-Jewish Hospital internal medicine program.

August 11

> *"Each day is precious when we consider what we can do to serve God and His Kingdom."*
> Elizabeth George (1944–): American author and Christian Speaker in
> Moments of Grace for a Woman's Heart

He was a lovely healthy baby. His mom's pregnancy and labor had been uneventful. There were no baby monitors yet, but as the head emerged a tight cord was wrapped around the neck. I was able to quickly clamp, cut, and proceed with a rapid safe delivery in the little mission hospital extension. After some stimulation and quick prayer, his little body pinked up and developed more tone, and finally there was a good cry that brought joy to all of us in the room. There was no more evidence of anoxia. We watched him grow and develop normally.

Several months later we had gone to town (40 winding miles with people, bicycles, goats, etc., to dodge) to buy groceries and supplies. On our town trips we often had lunch with the baby's mission family. They would take care of our little girl while we quickly did our shopping and business. On this day they were concerned about their small son. He had a high fever and was lethargic. His little body would jerk with noise. A quick call to the missionary neighbor to come and care for the other children, while his mom drove, and we "raced" out to the mission hospital. I held him the whole way there in case he needed CPR. Each breath was a prayer as the malaria test was negative, but the WBC was very high. The spinal fluid was white like milk. Fluids and IV antibiotics were begun. The staff all held hands and knelt around his crib and earnestly prayed that if God would heal him, help it to be complete so that he could work for the Lord, but that if He was not to be completely healed, to allow him to go to sleep in Jesus. Convulsions continued the rest of the day and night. Early in the morning his little body ceased convulsing. We continued to pray, and he recovered, seemingly fully.

Fast-forward two years. The mission family had gone on a retreat to a lake area and everyone was enjoying a picnic, water time, and periods of fellowship and worship. While they were talking in a group at the shore, someone looked for our miracle boy; he had run out into the lake, and fortunately *his feet were above the water*. Rescue was quickly done! He was not injured, but we all solemnly thanked God for his life *again*.

Another two years or so passed, and a group were playing in the yard. We glanced out to see what the children were doing, and alas, our little soldier had climbed up on the tongue of a utility trailer, and the owner, not knowing he was there, was getting ready to drive out of the yard. A quick yell, and we were able to stop them before anything happened to "our" little missionary boy.

Forward another 45 years, and a brain tumor now threatens "our" boy turned man and his teaching career. We pray that once again he will be delivered so he can continue serving His Lord.

Rheeta Stecker, LLUSM class of 1963, graduated in the same class as her husband, Elton. They served in Africa for 13 years and in Hot Springs, Arkansas, as family physicians for 40 years. Both retired at age 80. Teaching health principles in community and church venues has been their passion.

August 12

"Perseverance is not a long race; it is many short races one after the other."
Walter Elliot (1888–1958): British politician

Being in the dark was nothing new to me. As a radiology resident, I was comfortable in darkened reading rooms, bantering with my fellow residents while interpreting and dictating imaging studies. But this was different.

Instead of my usual shirt, slacks, and shoes, I was swaddled in a cocoon of white sheets and white bandages. The faint rhythmic beeping of a cardiac monitor suggested I was in a hospital, but the soft, subdued words floating over and around me made no sense.

And then I looked down. *They were gone.* My legs and my right arm were gone. The dark room was the ICU in the Unfallkrankenhaus, the trauma hospital in Salzburg, Austria, and the nurses were speaking German. My life had turned upside down. Things would never be the same again. With the love and help of my husband, Dave Hodgens, I started to reinvent myself.

As the months of rehabilitation went on, I was overwhelmed with gratitude for my upbringing and medical education. The ties to medicine were strong. My father, Albert Olson (CME class of 1949), was a member of CME's pathology department in the fifties, sixties, and early seventies. It was a very small, close-knit group consisting of Drs. Small, Dybdahl, Wat, Judefind, Olson, Thrasher, and Stilson (all CME graduates).* Sifting through memories for role models with disabilities, I was pleasantly surprised to remember two successful pathologists—Alan Loeffler (CME class of 1954), who was deaf; and Tim Greeves (faculty at White Memorial Medical Center, now Adventist Health White Memorial in Los Angeles), who was quadriplegic. *If they can do it, I can do it.*

And then one day my mentor, Ike Sanders (CME class of 1955-AFF), reminded me of Walter Stilson (CME class of 1934). Why hadn't I thought of him before? Of course! He was a radiologist who'd lost his arm at the shoulder as a young person. Even though I'd known him most of my life, I hadn't remembered him as a disabled person. Surely *if he can do it, I can do it.*

During the next 30 years my disability became an asset. As the director of breast imaging at the University of California, San Diego, I was privileged to interact with thousands of women, many of whom were scared and facing the unknown. When I entered the exam room with my cane and bilateral prosthetic leg toy-soldier gait, there was immediate empathy. My optimism was obvious and reassuring as I explained what needed to be done. I left them with the courage to seek the medical and spiritual help that would guide them through the journey ahead: *If she can do it, I can do it.*

*Carrol Small, class of 1934; Gerhardt Dybdahl, class of 1941; Bo Ying Wat, class of 1949; Thomas Judefind, class of 1935; Thais Thrasher, class of 1957; Donald Stilson, class of 1946.

Linda Olson, LLUSM class of 1976-A, is emeritus professor of radiology, University of California, San Diego, and is married to David W. Hodgens (LLUSM class of 1976-A). She was LLUSMAA's honored alumnus in 1994, and a recipient of LLUSM's Women in Medicine Courage Award, 2012.
Note: The accident occurred in 1979. The author writes about it in Gone: A Memoir of Love, Body, and Taking Back My Life, by Linda K. Olson, published in 2020 by She Writes Press.

August 13

> *"Bless the LORD, O my soul: and all that is within me, bless his holy name. Bless the LORD, O my soul, and forget not all his benefits: Who forgiveth all thine iniquities; who healeth all thy diseases; Who redeemeth thy life from destruction; who crowneth thee with lovingkindness and tender mercies; Who satisfieth thy mouth with good things; so that thy youth is renewed like the eagle's."*
>
> Psalm 103:1-5, KJV

It was early in the morning when a young Malawian woman came to Blantyre Adventist Hospital. Abdominal pain and nausea prompted pancreatic testing, and although these results were mildly elevated, her physical examination and abdominal X-rays suggested bowel obstruction. In the early-morning hours of the following day her blood pressure was unrecordable. I was called, and upon arrival found her peripheral intravenous line not functioning well. I looked for a central line, but could not find one. The anesthetist made multiple attempts to place an alternate peripheral line, but this was unsuccessful. I thought she would not survive and was surprised when she was alive for morning rounds.

The surgeon had found and placed a central line. Nursing staff made a difficult transfer to the ICU. Her blood pressure remained unrecordable despite infusion of fluids. Vasopressor infusion and antibiotics were administered shortly thereafter. I was surprised when her blood pressure suddenly improved, and within minutes the vasopressor was weaned down, and then stopped. To me she appeared "drowsy, answers questions, moderate respiratory distress" and her abdominal examination showed "absent [bowel sounds], markedly distended." Abdominal ultrasound showed moderate free fluid. I notified the surgeon that she was stable for surgery.

More than 29 hours after her arrival, she was taken to the OR. On exploratory laparotomy, more than two liters of dark-brown fluid were seen in the abdominal cavity, with moderate necrotic tissue in the peripancreatic area. The spleen was seen floating in the cavity, with only the connecting blood supply. The entire stomach was gangrenous and perforated. The operative procedure included a splenectomy, debridement of necrotic tissue in the peripancreatic area, total gastrectomy, closure of duodenum, and esophageal anastomosis to the jejunum. She returned to the ICU, intubated. Her blood pressure was low, but then improved with continued infusion of fluids. Although her postoperative course was complicated by pneumothorax, pleural effusions, and reintubation, she was following commands and writing to nursing staff four and five days after surgery, respectively. Recurrent mucus plugs, requiring reintubation two additional times, made weaning off the ventilator difficult.

Fourteen days after surgery she was extubated. The next day she was able to move from her bed to a wheelchair and speak. A visiting nurse from LLUH was astonished at her "unheard-of" recovery—and without any bed sores! We recognized the healing power of God and planned to bring her to morning worship the next day as a living example. As I walked toward the ICU, I heard nursing staff singing "The Great Physician" in Chichewa—my most cherished memory of Malawi so far.

David A. Saunders, LLUSM class of 2006, is an adjunct assistant professor in LLUSM's department of medicine. He visited Malawi in January 2011, started working at Blantyre Adventist Hospital in February 2012, and returned to the United States in April 2019.

August 14

"Do not be conformed to this world, but be transformed by the renewal of your mind, that by testing you may discern what is the will of God, what is good and acceptable and perfect."
Romans 12:2, ESV

My pager beeped, again. My night was only beginning, and the second family was questioning the day shift medical team's plan. Both were patients with extended stays and complicated histories; the first had a metabolic disorder needing a sophisticated baby formula, and the second had chronic respiratory failure requiring a detailed discharge plan. I quickly scanned their notes, soaking in the details. The day team had talked to many consulting specialties and would be better suited to answer the questions, but they were gone. I paused, sighed, and walked into the first room.

The room was dim, with the sunset peeping through the tall windows. The hospital crib had a bright patchwork bear in one corner, and a pink "Get Well" banner hung on the wall. The young family was huddled together on the hospital pullout, and dark circles with weary lines framed the parents' eyes as their questions began. "Why did we pick this formula?" "Why did we change the flow rate?" Their thoughts were tinged with exasperation, and the unspoken "What if this doesn't work either?" These answers were tough; I was only a small part of the team. We talked through several scenarios before the dad put his head in his hands. "Work kept me from being a part of the family rounds today, and my wife feels overwhelmed by the big team." Their frustration covered a future of unknowns as they grasped to understand what being in the hospital meant for their family.

I entered the next room wearing a mask and bright yellow gown required by safety precautions. As I stepped into the room, the mother's words tumbled out. "Why do we need home health nursing? Do you not trust me?" She described caring for her child at home, and mistrust of the medical community seeped through her words. Home health nursing felt like a slight. I listened until she slowed; circumstances left no easy solutions. Her shoulders slumped, and she sighed, "I understand." More than anything, she wanted her son to have a full life, preferably away from the hospital.

Sometimes we take the brunt, entering a story when frustrations build and tempers flare. Our broken world takes its toll on our patients, and we are tempted to personalize the attacks. When we do, we feel resentment. We want to stop the feeling, but don't know how. No easy answer exists, but God has left us a promise. God can change the way we approach these situations, keeping us from buckling under the weight of sin or its consequences. Instead of the frustration or anger, we see the loss of a dream, a miscommunicated thought, or a failed attempt. May our devotional time today be renewing, encouraging us to claim God's promise to be unchanged by what we encounter in this world.

Shelby Tanguay Weber, LLUSM class of 2017, is in residency training for general pediatrics, general psychiatry, and child and adolescent psychiatry in Cincinnati, Ohio. She and her husband, David (LLUSD class of 2018), enjoy scuba diving, snowboarding, camping, and spending time with family.

August 15

> *"My command is this: Love each other as I have loved you."*
> John 15:12, NIV

It was a busy morning as I tried to closely follow my assigned third-year medical student through the LLUMC Labor and Delivery unit. We had already seen two births and were trying to finish up morning rounds with our attending before another mom was ready to deliver. Oddly enough, I felt a sort of kinship with the two babies I had seen enter the world earlier that morning. They were so new, full of potential, and totally unaware of what life would soon be like. That was kind of like me, a first-year medical student who had just been born into the world of medicine only a week before. As the day progressed, things started to slow down and my third year suggested it was a good time for me to do my patient interview assignment. Since we were in the Labor and Delivery unit, I would be interviewing one of the postpartum mothers. The guidelines were simple: First-year medical students (me) were supposed to interview a patient so we could practice active listening while they told aspects of their medical journey.

Walking up to my patient's room, I felt a tinge of nervousness and a blizzard of questions started to whiz through my mind. Should I shake the patient's hand? Where should I stand? How should I start the conversation? Do you think she'll be able to tell that I have absolutely no idea what I'm doing? I almost forgot why I was going into the patient's room in the first place.

As I entered the room, I politely introduced myself as a "student doctor" and explained the purpose of the interview. Within seconds of the introduction the patient asked if I wanted to hold her newborn baby as she organized her hospital bag. I was caught off guard. *Wait, did I hear that right?* I thought. But... I couldn't say no; who could resist holding a baby?

I gingerly picked him up from the bed and slowly placed him in the crux of my forearm. As his mom packed her things, I realized that I had never held a baby that new or small. At only 5 pounds 12 ounces and less than 24 hours old, he felt weightless and so fragile as I cradled his tiny body. I studied his face, gazed into his deep brown eyes, and felt so honored and privileged to hold his new life in my hands. This newborn was a one of a kind masterpiece, carefully fashioned inside his mother's womb by our brilliant Creator. He was and is a reflection of God's perfect image, and someone who is treasured by our Lord. But as I stood there in awe, I realized that every human ever born into this earth was created in the same manner. From the person who had cut me off on the way to the hospital, to the rude woman at the coffee shop, all are claimed by God as one of His own.

My first patient experience taught me that every patient I will interact with is a privilege and honor, even though some may not feel like it in the moment. Each life that I will care for is just as precious, valuable, and wonderfully made as the tiny life I first held in my arms. Regardless of how I perceive someone to be, I am called to recognize each person's inherent worth in Christ, and to love them unconditionally without reservation. Just as Christ first loved me.

Lindsey N. Kim, LLUSM class of 2023, was born in Southern California but raised in the Pacific Northwest and looks forward to seeing her family with each trip home. Ever since she was 4 years old, she knew she wanted to become a doctor. She feels incredibly blessed to be able to study medicine and work toward realizing that dream. In her free time she enjoys exploring new restaurants, traveling near and far, and being in the company of her friends.

August 16

"And he sent them to preach the kingdom of God, and to heal the sick."
Luke 9:2, KJV

It was supposed to be a routine flight to Baramita, a remote village in northwest Guyana, South America. Mission pilot/RN Laura LaBore was to transport three engineers to check on the status of a new health hut construction project. Suddenly, after landing and deplaning, two women rushed to her: "Please, there is a man who was attacked by another man with a machete last night and is bleeding badly. Would you be able to fly him to the hospital?"

Laura needed to triage the situation. She was hoping that she could just take the patient back to the hospital in her home village, Mabaruma, to save fuel and time. While the Mabaruma hospital wasn't equipped to handle difficult cases, such as surgeries, they did have basic supplies for suturing wounds, and she hoped that that would suffice. Unfortunately, this was not the case. While climbing a bank of slippery mud to reach the house, several men carrying the patient in a hammock met Laura on the trail. They laid him down on the grass so Laura could take a look at him. She noticed several deep slash marks from a machete on his arms, chest, and face. Upon removing his sweatshirt, she could see he had a compound fracture with his elbow bone exposed. He needed a medevac to get him to the city hospital.

He had bled all night; the local clinic worker was too intoxicated to care for him. It was now 10:00 a.m. Laura ran to the health hut, searched, and found an IV kit and some saline solution. She prayed to God for guidance. It had been awhile since she had started an IV and, in his dehydrated condition, it could be difficult. However, she inserted the IV on the first try! She breathed a word of thanks to the Great Physician. With an audience of villagers, she worked on the man. Once stable, they helped her load the patient into the plane. During the flight she had to fly and change the IV bag because no one else was on board. The ambulance met her at the city airport and whisked him to the hospital. Mission accomplished!

A Cessna 182 has four seats. As a result of the medevac, she left the three engineers from her planned flight at Baramita. She needed to return to Baramita to get them. Upon landing, a new group of people met her with another man, this one with a cloth diaper around his head and other bandages on his neck. They said that the man she just flew out had attacked him, but others said that this one was the attacker. Regardless, he didn't need a medevac, but suturing was required. Laura contemplated just doing it herself, but it was getting late, and she learned there was a doctor in the next village. So she loaded her stranded passengers and flew him there, then, gratefully, home. In thinking back on the day, she was amazed at how God had blessed, and used her to share God's love in this remote community.

Bill LaBore and his wife, Laura, spent 10 years in Guyana, South America, and three and a half years on the island of Palawan in the Philippines. They served with Adventist World Aviation, whose mission is to serve isolated missionaries in need of air support. This story occurred in 2009. The LaBores now reside in Calimesa, California. Today, Bill is a development officer with the Office of Philanthropy at LLUH and Laura is a home health nurse.

August 17

*"Fear not, for I am with you; be not dismayed, for I am your God.
I will strengthen you, Yes, I will help you, I will uphold you with
My righteous right hand."*

Isaiah 41:10, NKJV

Ever since my first mission trip to Venezuela during my junior year of academy, I dreamed of doing long-term mission work. Going into radiology was a tough decision for me because I was afraid I'd have to give up my dream. I didn't give up all hope, however, and in my last year of residency I contacted Dr. Richard Hart, president of Loma Linda University Health, to see if he knew of any mission opportunities for a radiologist. An option that best fit the skills of my future husband and me was to help bring the radiology department at a mission hospital in the Caribbean up to developed world standards.

When we arrived, construction was not as close to being completed as we had anticipated. I read only plain films, which were developed with wet film processing (ancient technology by today's standards) and viewed on a view box for at least eight months. My MRI technologist husband helped me with working on department policies since the MRI wasn't up and running for almost a full year. It felt like a great underutilization of our skills, to say the least.

We kept busy, though—started daily department devotionals, outfitting the radiology rooms with the equipment and furniture, writing department policies, figuring out departmental marketing to the community, organized with LLUH for a team to come teach BLS and ACLS to the whole hospital (many MDs and RNs hadn't renewed their certification in years), giving talks all over the island on cancer screening (emphasis on breast cancer) and cholesterol, and educating the local firefighters about safety in and around the MRI should they ever need to respond to a fire at the hospital.

Finally, the portable X-ray, ultrasound, MRI, and mammography rooms and PACS were up and running. Fluoroscopy and CT hit roadblocks that were not going to be surpassed in the time we had remaining. We ended up leaving a few months early of our original plan, since it seemed we'd accomplished as much as we were going to. We were disappointed and felt we had let God down.

A few months after we'd returned, I was preparing a slide show of our time at the hospital and all the things we did while we were there. That's when I actually realized that God had used us for much more than we had planned. Did it really matter that I didn't read as many imaging studies as I had thought I would? Didn't the long-term effect of the BLS and ACLS training to the hospital staff outweigh any CT interpretation I would've done? Not to mention the hundreds of women and men who now have a better understanding of the value of cancer screening. In retrospect we realize that our plan was not God's plan. He was able to accomplish so much more than we could have ever imagined.

Eva Ryckman Durbin, LLUSM and LLUSPH class of 2008, currently practices radiology in rural Ohio. She has a passion for the health message and using it to be a light in the community.

August 18

"Thus says the LORD: 'Let not the wise man glory in his wisdom, let not the mighty man glory in his might, nor let the rich man glory in his riches; but let him who glories glory in this, that he understands and knows Me, that I am the LORD, exercising lovingkindness, judgment, and righteousness in the earth. For in these I delight,' says the LORD."
Jeremiah 9:23-24, NKJV

I'm in my final year of residency at the time of this submission. I'm a fifth-year ENT (ears, nose, and throat) surgeon and a Black woman. Starting this journey, I knew that there would not be many other surgeons in this field who would look like me. However, it wasn't until the first month of my final year of residency that the significance of this really hit home. I was standing in the operating room after a case, when a fourth-year medical student—who was doing a great job on her subinternship—stared at me silently until the rest of our team left the room. She leaned in close and asked me, "Did you feel supported here as a Black woman? Would this program take care of me if I matched here?"

Thinking back to the four years of medical student applications to our program, and my time on the resident admissions committee, I could not remember a single Black female applicant for ENT at our program, in spite of the desperate need for them in this field.

Representation is a major theme throughout the Bible and beloved by the God I'm familiar with. So many stories hinge on people God desires to use to manifest Himself in our world. He chooses us to show people His kindness, His mercy, and His compassion. He often uses people to help demonstrate the depth of His support, sacrificial love, and trustworthiness. He uses people's hardships to show that through success and through failure He is with us always. During a time that questions how, we truly value Black people and Blackness, and given our country's history of slavery and widespread systemic oppression, representation, and authentic inclusion is part of our healing.

I know that I am called by God to do this work in otolaryngology (ears, nose, and throat surgery). The privilege to do it, while being a Black woman, is something that I cherish. I am empowered by institutions who value the entirety of what I can bring to the table, and individuals who are able to uplift all the parts of me through hardship and through success.

However, regardless of race, we all have something to bring to this particular table. We all can participate in the work to help heal the harms brought upon generations of Black people. There is a unique and special place for Black physicians and Black people throughout all layers of our health care system. There is work for compassion and self-reflection to check our implicit and conscious biases so that our interactions and care we provide to Black people is restorative. Data on racial disparity, specifically among Black people, demonstrates the adverse impact of bias throughout the health care system, compounded by societal structures designed to perpetuate division. This division adds to poor health outcomes. We see it, so we must act on it. Healing the Black community is "everybody's work." Let's get to work!

Tedean Green, LLUSM class of 2016, completed her ENT residency at Wayne State University in Michigan and is an otolaryngologist at Kaiser Permanente Antelope Valley, California. Tedean wants to emulate the example of principled leadership she respected so much from LLUSM's dean's office. She is married to her classmate Morgan.

August 19

> *"Then he put his hands on her, and immediately she straightened up and praised God."* Luke 13:13, NIV

Once known as "Paris of the Antilles," the dilapidated Old World charm of Cap Haïtien is a reminder of Haiti's tumultuous past. Life is hard in Haiti. People toil in the sun-beat streets and marketplaces day after day, grinding out the most meager sustenance. Without enough resources to plan for the unexpected, many treatable injuries end up causing permanent disability.

On this balmy afternoon in Cap Haïtien the orthopedic clinic was overflowing. Even though we had seen scores of patients, the large veranda outside was still full of people who had been waiting all day. No one was complaining; they were just waiting with hope and gratitude. Case after case of neglected injuries were seen. Ankle fractures, femur fractures, forearm fractures, kids with bowed legs, children with clubfeet, and others. Many operations were scheduled. In the midst of this busy afternoon one patient in particular brought me close to tears. Chantal was a 4-year-old girl who had been badly burned when a fire broke out in her family's shack a couple of years before. Her sweet face had thankfully been spared from the horrible burns that covered much of her body. The scars created webs that glued her right elbow to her thorax. She could not stand up or spread her legs apart because the weblike burn contractures kept her hips bent 90 degrees. She accommodated for this by hobbling around in a hunched-over position. I took some photos in order to get some advice from a plastic surgeon colleague. When Dr. Miles started discussing the complicated flaps and reconstructive techniques that would be required, I realized that I had better plan a trip for him to come take command of the operation. After all, a plane ticket to anywhere in the world is less costly than most operations stateside, and certainly a few days off work was a worthwhile sacrifice for the life of this girl.

After the first of three operations she was able to stand up straight and walk normally. Shortly afterward, the devastating earthquake that took the lives of more than 200,000 struck the capital, Port-au-Prince. Our efforts were immediately focused at Hôpital Adventiste d'Haïti in Port-au-Prince, a seven-hour journey from Cap Haïtien. In spite of all the life-threatening injuries calling our attention, I could not forget Chantal walking around with her right arm flexed up and glued to her side. Three more months passed, and then one day Chantal and her mom came to our clinic. They had found me! This time tears did come to my eyes, especially because coincidentally, Dr. Miles had plans to come to Port-au-Prince and help me with some patients suffering earthquake injuries! More successful operations were performed, and Chantal now has full use of her legs and arms!

She is now a beautiful 15-year-old girl whom I regularly see going to school and church. Her mother has been working for eight years at Hôpital Adventiste d'Haïti.

We might call it surgery, but for Chantal and her mother it was a miracle. In reality they are right. As surgeons, we merely make incisions, put things in, take things out, sew things, etc. This is the easy part. The real miracle comes from the Master Healer, who heals wounds and takes away pain. Without the miracle of healing, surgery would not be possible. Imagine if sutures had to be left in forever and the pain that patients have in the recovery room never went away. It is a sacred honor to take part in the miracle of healing and we must never forget where the real credit belongs.

Scott Nelson, LLUSM class of 1996, is an associate professor in LLUSM's department of orthopedic surgery. He and his wife, Marni, serve full time at Adventist Hospital of Haiti in Port-au-Prince, Haiti.

August 20

"So David said to Joab and the commanders of the army, 'Take a census of all the people of Israel—from Beersheba in the south to Dan in the north—and bring me a report so I may know how many there are.'"
1 Chronicles 21:2, NLT

The alarm went off, jolting me into wakefulness: 5:30 a.m., time to start my day. I sat up in bed and began to think about how I was about to start my second year of medical school. Self-doubt started to filter through my mind. It seemed as though all I had heard about second year was that it would be painstakingly difficult, the kind you couldn't describe and could only understand through experience. I reached for my Bible and felt a nudge to read from 1 Chronicles. As I flipped through the pages, my eyes landed on chapter 21.

It was the story of David taking a census of Judah and Israel. Even after Joab reminded David that God had multiplied his people and questioned the wisdom of the count, David went ahead with the census. I thought about it for a bit. Why would David feel the need to count his men? Hadn't God provided the victory in war many times? Then it clicked. David was looking to place his faith in the tangible things of this world, the same way that I was looking to depend on my own efforts in school. Satan had provoked David, convincing him to trust in the number of his men over the faithfulness of God to His people.

I looked back at the past year. I remembered all the times I was behind in studying and didn't know how I could catch up. A couple administrators even expressed doubt that I would pull through the year. Yet in the next few hours I was about to start the first day of my second year of medical school with full passes to all my first year courses. God had worked a miracle for me, but somehow throughout the summer I had begun attributing His miracle to the work I had put in to bring my grades up. I had counted my own talents and abilities over God's favor toward me.

It's so easy to forget the ways in which God has provided and to believe that I need to look to my own talents, possessions, or worth to make it through life's obstacles. Even David forgot God's favor toward him. But when he chose to put himself back in God's hands, God showed the depth and character of His mercy.

God led me to this particular chapter for a reason. He wanted me to know that my anxiety stemmed from relying on myself instead of Him, but He didn't want just to leave me there. He wanted to remind me that even though I'd messed up and forgotten Him, He was still there, and He would still be merciful. There is no reason to look toward the future as if we are walking alone, but rather know that we can always rely on Him.

Nilmini Pang, LLUSM class of 2021, was called to pursue medicine after a chance meeting with a woman who was impressed to tell her to become a doctor. God has since carried her through didactics and shown her the joy of caring for patients during clinicals.

August 21

"Only a life lived for others is a life worthwhile."
Albert Schweitzer (1875–1965): German Lutheran theologian,
physician, humanitarian, and Nobel Peace Prize Laureate

My dad, Ray Herber, was one of the last surviving members of the team of faculty that helped to consolidate the Loma Linda University School of Medicine onto a single campus. The school remained a lifelong passion for Dad, and each time we were together he would share new ideas for its support and success. When we lost him suddenly and unexpectedly, halfway through his eighty-eighth year, the outpouring of support was overwhelming. Stories were shared by colleagues, students, business acquaintances, neighbors, and friends. His children and grandchildren knew him to be kind, thoughtful, always interested, supportive, and unfailingly invested in their success. The breadth and depth of sharing, after our loss, demonstrated just how many lives he had touched. As one friend put it: "He didn't just care about others; he delighted in making a difference in the lives of people."

I am filled with gratitude when I reflect on the impact Dad had on my life as a role model, advisor, confidant, and friend. As I struggled to summarize his life and the accomplishments appreciated by so many, I came across something he had recently written in one of his many notebooks:

Creation:
We are created in God's image—what does that mean? Christ lives in us—what does that create? I look at the list of some of the endowments that I set up for Macpherson Society, Alumni Association, Union College, Loma Linda University School of Medicine, that will give help in the future even more than now, and all that comes out is: and it was good.

I look at the letters in my Book of Remembrance from administration, faculty, alumni, students, preachers, politicians, and patients, and all one can say is: it is good.

I walk through the house and see people who gave a blessing and some part of them left behind, and one has to shout: it is good.

I look at the dedication of three children, five grandchildren, and one has to say: it is good.

As one looks at created books, needlepoints, paintings of 80 years, and one has to shout: it is good.

My dad's life illustrates to me a true sense of calling. He was convicted that a Christ-centered life called him to serve others and the institutions carrying out the Lord's work. He was not content with mere good deeds, but was committed to making a difference for the people and projects on which he focused. Dad didn't desire for his efforts to be widely known. However, if you take away a little inspiration from life dedicated to following Christ's example, Dad would probably say, "It is good."

Steve Herber, LLUSM class of 1986, is the son of Ray (CME class of 1957) and Marilyn (CME class of 1958). He is a plastic surgeon by training, but responded to a call to move into hospital administration. He serves as president of St. Helena Hospital in California, but still cares for patients on a weekly basis. He is slated to be LLUSMAA president in 2023, an honor held by both his mom and dad. He and his wife have a son, Timothy, and a daughter, Helena (LLUSM class of 2023). Ray Herber died August 21, 2020.

August 22

> "We have nothing to fear for the future, except as we shall forget the way the Lord has led us, and His teaching in our past history."
> Ellen G. White (1827–1915): instrumental in the founding of Loma Linda University, one of the founders of the Seventh-day Adventist Church, and American author; in Life Sketches, p. 196

Annette had recently developed pain in her foot, followed by redness and swelling. She was seen in the ER and admitted for osteomyelitis of the foot and ended up sustaining a BKA* and being diagnosed with diabetes. She came to me when her stump became infected, and she was reluctant to seek help from her surgeon for fear that her BKA would become an AKA.[†] As an alternative to the typical surgical debridement, I offered her biological debridement therapy, more commonly known as maggot therapy. Annette agreed and was hospitalized for IV antibiotics and maggots. Out of whimsy she named each batch of maggots after The Beatles, but made it only through John, George, and Ringo before her wound was sufficiently clean to be discharged back home. Over the following six weeks her stump healed and was soon to be fitted for a prosthesis.

While surgical debridement is often a fast and effective way to clean a wound, it takes out good tissue along with the bad, but does allow the wound to be closed and hopefully heal. The maggots, on the other hand, take 48–72 hours to do their job, and often repeated treatments are needed. In reflecting on the above event, we are all victims of events that leave us traumatized with open wounds that are full of necrosis and infection. God in His wisdom has seen fit to use the Holy Spirit much as I used maggots to clean Annette's wound. It is never a neat and tidy process when it comes to healing wounds of the soul. We often try to resist the cleansing that comes before healing, much as many people are turned off by maggot debridement therapy. If we allow God to work, He introduces something into our lives that slowly works on the wound that Satan and the world have inflicted. Just as it took several maggot treatments for Annette's wound to be cleansed, through persistence and perseverance the Holy Spirit will make changes in our lives. Over time the dead, dying, and injured soul is slowly replaced with a vibrant, healthy soul.

As we heal, we see the love of God for His erring children, His wisdom in the laws that He gives, and maybe even a glimpse of why He allowed the injury to occur in the first place. In Psalm 51 David was able to see his need for cleansing and the need for a clean heart. We also need to seek cleansing and renewal from the Lord, and a spirit of forgiveness, when we are wounded by the world. We need to submit to His chosen method for our healing, remembering that He is the Master Physician and that "all things work together for good to those who love God, to those who are the called according to His purpose" (Romans 8:28, NKJV).

*BKA: below knee amputation
†AKA: above knee amputation

Kristy Crandell, LLUSM class of 1998, is currently practicing family medicine as a solo practitioner in Red Bay, Alabama. She enjoys providing wound care and teaching others about the benefits of lifestyle changes. Her parents are Donna Dunham Crandell (LLUSM class of 1966) and Merwyn Crandell (LLUSM class of 1967).

August 23

"Weeping may endure for a night, but joy comes in the morning."
Psalm 30:5, NKJV

I was 10 years old when my aunt and I secretly got on a boat and escaped from the ravages of the Vietnam War. We spent almost a year at Pulau Galang refugee camp in Indonesia. Eventually we were sponsored by the Canadian government, and we arrived in Canada in the winter of 1980. Life was improving but sometimes lonely in this new country. We knew that education was our ticket to success. I studied hard, and God led me to Walla Walla College (now Walla Walla University) in College Place, Washington, where I met my beautiful wife, Brenda, and discovered God's love for me through the Seventh-day Adventist message.

After Walla Walla we both attended Loma Linda University School of Dentistry and graduated in 1995 and 1996. After my graduation we got married and started our dental practice together in a small, rural town in Washington. God blessed us with one child after another. After our eighth child was born, Brenda started having pain in the lower part of her body and at first we thought it was just her body, recovering from the pregnancy. However, because the pain persisted, further examinations and tests were performed, and she was diagnosed with stage 4 cancer. This devastated our young family.

How could God allow this to happen when we had 8 young children from infancy to 16 years old. We were just starting out in life, and tragedy struck. We tried everything possible to cure her disease, but after two years of struggling with cancer, Brenda said her goodbyes and closed her eyes until the resurrection. It was an extremely dark time for our family. We pulled together and had to support each other. We questioned why God had allowed this to happen. Then one day I walked into church, and a dear friend handed me a package. In the package were a card and a book by Roger Morneau, *The Incredible Power of Prayer*. The card said, "I am praying for you and your family, and I found comfort from reading this book when I lost my husband." We received many cards and phone calls from our friends, but this card was different. It was from a stranger I had never met. Linda had lost her husband from cancer about a year before I lost Brenda. She had four young children to care for. At church one Sabbath, she saw an announcement about Brenda's memorial service in a town two hours away. Linda understood what we were going through and decided to pray for our family daily. A few months later she was inspired to send a sympathy card and the book to our family.

As I was still grieving the loss of my wife, I was lonely, and here was an understanding and supportive ear. We started communicating by email, which led to talking on the phone, and finally we met in person with our children. Linda was a godly woman who sincerely desired to follow God's will and be a blessing to others. As we spent more time with each other, we fell in love. Both of us never imagined this could ever happen after losing our spouses, but the Bible says in Psalm 30:5, "Weeping may endure for a night, but joy comes in the morning." It was a joyous day when we married and combined our families to have 12 children!

We live in a sin-filled world, and sometimes tragedy happens indiscriminately. But God is still in control! Our job, like Job, is to remain faithful to God. Sometimes He gives us answers, and sometimes we don't understand why. Hang in there; joy will come in the morning—if not in this world, then it will come at the resurrection.

David Reimche-Vu, LLUSD class of 1995, practices dentistry in Goldendale, Washinton, where he and his wife, Linda, are raising their combined family of 12 children. The birhday of his late wife, Brenda (LLUSD class of 1996), is August 23.

August 24

"Peace I leave with you, my peace I give unto you: not as the world giveth, give I unto you. Let not your heart be troubled, neither let it be afraid."
John 14:27, KJV

The little tugboat strained as it climbed to the top of each monstrous wave before dropping again in the storm the locals call a nor'easter.

I was not a local. I had never been on the North Atlantic during a nor'easter.

"You will take the tugboat to Portland and return after a nice day with your relatives in the city," my island summer host had told me. It all sounded pleasant and safe, but that was before the wind picked up and the clouds thickened. Alone on the open deck, I clutched the rail. Waves of nausea swept over me along with the spray and wind. I felt death was near. I was 10 years old.

Under a tarp at the bow a group of local kids laughed with hilarity. Being very shy, I hesitated to join them. I was trying to be brave and invisible.

A lad came out from under the tarp into the storm and led me to the pilothouse. He introduced me to the pilot, who invited me to sit next to him on the bench. I soon fell asleep in this place of safety with a person in command of the vessel.

We all experience storms of some form. Everyone is on a tugboat named life.

The thought has occurred to me that the main purpose in our life is to come out from under our tarp, to leave our cozy place and group of friends and lead them to the Pilot of their tugboat.

John E. Chen, CME class of 1960, practiced ophthalmology in Caldwell, Idaho, until he retired in 1994. His son David is a graduate of LLUSM class of 1990, and his grandson Justin is a graduate of LLUSM class of 2016.

August 25

> *"I will ponder all your work, and meditate on your mighty deeds."*
> Psalm 77:12, ESV

In August 2017 I began my second month as an emergency medicine intern. I entered the hospital and, like previous shifts, went to the hospital chapel for a brief moment of meditation. After five minutes of silence, I stood up and walked into the emergency department.

One hour into the day I hear over the telephone: "38-year-old male collapsed at the airport, seven rounds of epinephrine given in the field and patient shocked five times, coming in via EMS, 10 minutes out." My heart begins to pound, my palms get sweaty, my mind begins to race. Suddenly I realize I am not ready for any of this. I get up, prepare the room with equipment that I think will be needed to run a successful resuscitation based on what I studied. The nurses file in, the techs file in, the attending arrives, and we begin to assign our roles. We get to "team leader," and the attending looks at me and says, "You are running this today. You know ACLS, right?"

The patient is rolled in, and my mind goes blank, knowing that I am not ready for any of this. Twelve years of primary and secondary school, then four years of medical school later, all leading me to the realization that I am supposed to be ready to make life-and-death decisions. I clench my teeth, say a quiet prayer, and let my training take over. After running the code for 20 minutes, we get a pulse. During the next four hours, as we wait for a bed to open in the MICU, the team codes him another three times. Finally, after that fourth time of losing his pulse and no cardiac electrical movement, the time of death is called.

I remembered leaving that shift at the end of the night feeling drained. I thought that perhaps all the insecurities that I had were right and that I was simply not good enough. As I drove home, I heard an old hymn played from my post-shift playlist: "To God Be the Glory." It reminded me that the work that I do is not for myself, but for the glory and honor of God. I am merely a pair of hands that work toward His plan.

To this day I continue to spend time in the chapel before my shifts to refocus my mind. Meditating in the presence of the Lord has truly brought me comfort. I am reminded that God is the One that has the final say, and all I can do is meditate in His mighty deeds.

"To God be the glory, great things He hath done, so loved He the world that He gave us His Son."

Jerome Martin, LLUSM class of 2017, finished his emergency medicine residency at the University of Illinois in 2020 and is now a simulation fellow at RUSH emergency medicine in Chicago, Illinois.

August 26

"You will keep in perfect peace those whose minds are steadfast, because they trust in you." Isaiah 26:3, NIV

I arrived early at the HOPE Clinic in Cleburne, Texas, to volunteer for my afternoon of seeing patients. There were no cars in the patient parking lot. "Odd," I mused. The staff informed me that they knew I was coming but had failed to schedule any patients, so I now had an unexpected free afternoon. After running some errands, I spontaneously stopped (as is my habit when I have free time) to pick up trash by the road in my neighborhood. As I got out of my car, I heard a voice say, "The calm before the storm." I felt at peace. I picked up trash for an hour and drove home. I sat at my desk working on unfinished business.

As I sat there, my cell phone rang. It is unusual for me to pick up my cell phone when the caller ID does not clearly identify the caller and unheard-of for me to answer when the number is not even a recognizable U.S. number. For reasons unknown, I answered the call. It was my brother calling from the cruise ship's hospital. My mother had collapsed and was being coded. Her medical history was needed, which I had. During the time I was on the phone, the resuscitation was successful; the cruise ship (30 minutes from port) was then turned around, and she and my brother were off-loaded in Falmouth, Jamaica. After racing to a hospital board meeting and back home again, I spent hours tracking down the hospital my mom had been taken to. I downloaded a map of Jamaica and started at the hospital closest to the port. They didn't have her, and I struggled to understand their accent when they told me where she likely had been taken. At the second hospital I called, I found her, and talked to a very relieved brother. The hospital had demanded $10,000 before they would even start taking care of my intubated mother, and my brother didn't know how much more they would demand. I tried to talk to the nurses and doctor and got hung up on several times. After finally talking to the physician taking care of my mother, I knew I had to get her to the United States ASAP.

Numerous phone calls between the transport company, Texas Health Resources, the U.S. embassy, the Jamaican hospital, my brother, and the cruise line, and many sleepless hours later a plane landed in Jamaica 26 hours after my mother had arrived on the island. Thirty-three hours after her cardiac arrest, my mother rolled through the ED door in Fort Worth more dead than alive. I and the treating ED physician who were waiting for her arrival were shocked. The staff knew they had to work quickly even to keep her alive. After her initial resuscitation she was admitted to the ICU. In the morning a surgeon informed me that her CT showed an ischemic and perforated bowel, which had put her into septic shock. He wanted to know what I wanted to do. Without surgery, death was 100 percent; with surgery maybe less than 100 percent. I chose surgery. Just as the OR team arrived, she destabilized. They hesitated. Should they take her to surgery or code her? After a moment they grabbed her bed and raced toward the OR. Being a patient's family member was a different side of health care than I was used to. I was grateful the Fort Worth staff had let me stay at her side. Even through the stress and challenges of arranging transport, her critical care in the ED and ICU, and while making the tough decisions about surgery and aftercare, I had a sense of peace that defied the situation. I knew then, as I still know now, even though my mother ultimately died four months later, that God's promises are true. God is with us, even during difficult and dark times.

Delbe Meelhuysen, LLUSM class of 1987, is currently working as an ED physician at Texas Health Burleson and Cleburne. She is the mother of three adult sons and enjoys volunteering at HOPE Clinic and New Life Bible School.

August 27

"O Lord, how many and varied are Your works! In wisdom You have made them all; The earth is full of Your riches and Your creatures."
Psalm 104:24, AMP

I am a medical oncologist at the National Cancer Institute in Bethesda, Maryland. My academic area of interest is immunotherapy, and my disease focus is prostate cancer. I had been treating a patient with advanced prostate cancer for more than 10 years. He was no ordinary patient. He was a retired U.S. Army surgeon who was very involved in his care and willing to be aggressive with treatment. We had temporary successes with various medical management programs including several types of hormonal therapy and a chemotherapy regimen. Despite temporary improvements, his disease continued to progress, and eventually we ran out of the customary therapeutic options. By this time he was beginning to have symptoms from the cancer that were significantly affecting his life. He recounted that he could sense a rapid decline in his energy from being able to stand and sing in church one week, to having to sit and sing the second week, and by the third week having no energy to sing a single stanza.

I broached the idea of enrolling him in a clinical trial designed to have his own immune system recognize and attack the cancer. I felt that we had a narrow window to try this specific therapy. We agreed on a recently opened clinical trial of a vaccine and an immune checkpoint inhibitor. This would generate immune cells specific for the cancer (through the vaccine) and allow these cells the ability to kill tumor cells despite the stop signal often given by the tumor (immune checkpoint inhibitor). Using this approach, we hoped to harness the amazing immune system that God gave each of us to target his tumor effectively.

His PSA (prostatic specific antigen, a prostate cancer marker) was ominously doubling about every month. By the time he started the experimental combination treatment, the PSA was 55 ng/mL. Amazingly, three weeks later the PSA was less than 10, and his symptoms were markedly improved. The PSA was soon less than 1 and has been undetectable (less than 0.02) for more than a year. During the past year and a half, his energy has returned to normal, the disease known to be in his bladder base has decreased in size, and a biopsy of that mass has revealed no tumor cells.

He continues to come to clinic every two weeks for evaluation and treatment. At his last visit he told me that he was doing physically demanding jobs that he hadn't been able to do for at least two and a half years. To me, however, it wasn't the vaccine or the immune checkpoint inhibitor that eradicated the tumor—it was the amazing immune system that is designed to recognize up to a mind-boggling number of different targets and kill only the bad ones.

This complex system is just one of the incredibly marvelous works that God has made.

James Gulley, LLUSM class of 1995, PhD, is a medical oncologist. He is conducting cancer immunotherapy clinical trials and is the director of the Medical Oncology Service at the Center for Cancer Research, National Cancer Institute, in Bethesda, Maryland.

August 28

> *"Nothing is more honorable than a grateful heart."*
> Seneca the Younger (4 B.C.–A.D. 65): Roman philosopher

Note: The following was submitted as a heartfelt thank you from a grateful patient to her surgeon. It appears in its original, unedited form.

When i was born i had a pin sized hole in my heart but the docter said as i got older it would shrink and go away. When i was maybe 2 or 3 i was living with my aunt Evelyn and uncle Mike cause my mom was incarcerated and my dad worked too much to take care of me. When my mom got out i was with my parents for about 6 months when my mom got arrested again and i had to go back to my aunt and uncles. When i went back to my aunt and uncles house my aunt noticed that i havent grown at all in the past 6 months. I was 4 years old but looked 2 years old. She took me to a pediatrician to see what was wrong and we found out instead of the hole shrinking it grew. I had to have emergency open heart surgery maybe a day or 2 after that appointment. A Dr who told my aunt if she didnt take me into the Dr that day she wouldve found me dead in 4 months. It might have been Dr Bailey that told her that. I kind of remember the preparation and recovery of the surgery. I know one night which i asume was the night before my surgery i had and ultrasound done to make sure i havent eaten anything. I was so confused that night cause i couldnt see any of the foods i love to eat in my stomach. I kept asking questions. "Wheres this food? Wheres that food?" All i was able to consume was ice chips and the nurses put on "the jungle book" to help me fall asleep. It didnt work but i cant remember what happend after that. My aunt told me something about they needed me to go to sleep for a procedure but i couldnt fall asleep and they had me walked the halls for a while to get me tired. I think it was an x-ray i needed. I know one morning they let me go into a room and pick a toy to play with and nurses where confused cause i wanted the car and gas station toy instead of a doll. I know one night i really wanted a sip of my juice but i couldnt get in right away cause of some kind of emergency on the other side of the curtain. I know lots of nurses maybe about 5 had to hold me down to get a blood transfusion. The last thing i remember is going into Dr Baileys office for some sort of meeting. My grandma said i ran into his arms, gave him a big hug and said "Dr please dont hurt my heart." Not realizing the surgery was already over. I think my aunt didnt allow me to go into a Jacuzzi until i was 12. I had to go back to live with my parents and they never took me back for my follow up appointments for steroid treatments so im still very short. Im 22 gonna be 23 in September but everyone i meet thinks im 15. Other than that i graduated high school back in 2014. I got my second job. And im living with my aunt again. Id say im pretty healthy. Just a little chubby. But most importantly thanks to Dr Bailey im still alive!

Cheyanne Miller is a grateful patient of Leonard Bailey's (LLUSM class of 1969). Dr. Bailey pioneered infant heart transplants at LLUMC, beginning in 1984 with Baby Fae. Note: August 28 is Dr. Bailey's birthday.

August 29

> *"Give, and it will be given to you. Good measure, pressed down, shaken together, running over, will be put into your lap. For with the measure you use it will be measured back to you."*
>
> Luke 6:38, ESV

Lord, please don't let me be a "helicopter mom." Show me how I can be a supportive mama. I worked at Loma Linda University Health. I have seen 20 classes of students enter and graduate. When my son became one of those entering medical students, I was determined not to hover and smother.

My friend Sheila (who also works on campus) and I are two peas in a pod. Our biggest similarity, our sons, are away to college. We are each other's sounding board. After work we walk using the time to share our "empty" nest anxieties. One evening walk we took a detour passing through Centennial Complex where university students study. We were so surprised to find so many students (medical, dental, nursing, OT, and PT) studying everywhere; the study rooms were fully occupied, the whiteboards were covered with computations, notations, definitions, like a scene from *A Beautiful Mind*, and the halls were lined with backpacks. We both noticed students coming in with or going out to get convenient store snacks. We left that night with a plan in mind. Monday night snacks—homemade goodies to be passed out by two mamas who care!

We needed to recruit a few more team members for our Monday night adventure. Adding Jeanne as label designer to create labels with inspirational sayings and Brenda to take charge of packaging (labels on baggies and goodies in the baggies) completed our team.

Come Monday, 5:15 p.m. Two baskets packed each containing 50 beautifully designed goody bags filled with either a savory or sweet homemade item. Ready, set, GO! We were nervous; not quite sure how to approach students. Some students were apprehensive, they thought there was a cost. We began identifying ourselves as moms who care (who work on campus) passing out goodies "just because" and apprehensions disintegrated. We were welcomed with warmth and appreciation. We gave our last goody bag to a student who responded, "Thank you; you are a God-sent ANGEL." We haven't missed a Monday since. . . . We have gone from carrying baskets of 50 to pulling a wagon filled with 300 beautifully sealed and packaged goody bags. We have also received an outpouring of support from contributors to our cause.

The Lord answered my prayer. He showed me I am not a helicopter mom. I am a person with motherly instincts. Instincts to engage and nurture. He also provided the opportunity to use these instincts to bring smiles to others. Small acts of kindness can be the most JOYFUL. Today I pray, Lord, do not let me lose this Joy. I'm on FIRE. Guide me, show me more, so I may stay aglow.

Shari Haase worked for LLUH and LLUSM for a total of 34 years. Her son Tyler is a LLUSM class of 2021 graduate.

August 30

> *"For the* L{ORD} *sees not as man sees: man looks on the outward appearance, but the* L{ORD} *looks on the heart."*
> 1 Samuel 16:7, ESV

I was in the middle of a busy overnight shift in the ER when he checked in. As I was entering his room, his nurse snidely informed me that "another homeless addict" had missed his vein while trying to shoot up. He now had an abscess that needed to be drained. I was going to need about five minutes to complete the procedure. Everything about him displayed his inner feelings of worthlessness, pain, and defeat. As I began, I broke the ice by softly commenting that it looked as though he was having a rough night. It was easy to see that he was about to cry. I said a silent prayer asking the Holy Spirit to help me to see my patient the way that Jesus sees him. As I was numbing and incising his abscess, I reminded my patient that we are not defined by our biggest weaknesses and failures. That when God sees him, He sees a son that He loves. That God is not angry with him, but desires to help him step into a life of peace, hope, and joy—into wholeness. He began sobbing. I asked him if I could pray for him, and he nodded yes. As I was packing his wound, I said a short little prayer with him, and then I exited the room. I was with him for less than five minutes and was unsure if my encounter would have any positive impact on his life.

In emergency medicine we usually don't have the opportunity for patient follow-up. Usually. About nine months after treating him, an ambulance brought in a patient strapped to a backboard who had been in a minor car accident. As I entered the room, the patient cried out, "Doctor, I'm so glad it's you! I've been wanting to see you!" He was back, and he was overjoyed to tell me his story. He said his whole life had been changed after his last visit. He excitedly exclaimed, "I haven't used heroin since that night you saw me! I am no longer homeless, and I have a job, a girlfriend, and a car . . ." Laughingly he clarified, "Well, I had a car, until I crashed it tonight!" His joy was overflowing.

We know that God, because of His love, desires for us to partner with Him in helping our patients step into wholeness. He wants this even more than we do. This experience reminds me that while we may only be able to spend a few hurried minutes with our patients, the Holy Spirit continues to stay and minister to them long after we leave. Even our smallest efforts have big potential when God is involved.

Allen Patee, LLUSM class of 2010, practices emergency medicine in Redding, California. He is blessed to be able to get together weekly with 24 of his family members, who all live in town.

August 31

> *"Where no counsel is, the people fall: but in the multitude of counsellors there is safety."*
> Proverbs 11:14, KJV

One morning I was greeted at the hospital by the usual list of patients all requiring priority care. Whispering a prayer for strength and wisdom, I began triaging patients. After all of the family meetings, patient requests, pages, admissions, discharges, and paperwork pulling me in different directions, I finally came to my last patient. At the beginning of the day I had judged this patient to be the least critical, as she had been admitted to observation overnight, was young, and was experiencing minor abdominal symptoms and mild liver abnormalities.

On arriving at the patient's room, she complained of abdominal symptoms along with a headache. This wasn't surprising, as she had a history of migraine headaches and was already being followed by doctors. However, the patient's symptoms were somewhat puzzling, as she was declining despite the fact that all testing had come back negative except for mild liver enzyme elevation. I decided to order further imaging of the abdomen with repeat bloodwork and was considering ordering a head CT scan. Turning to the nurse, I asked her if she had any other suggestions. Given the patient's unrelenting headache, she encouraged me to order the head CT scan.

Quite unexpectedly, the new bloodwork now showed acute liver failure with liver enzyme elevation (AST/ALT) in the 1000s (normal is about 50). I immediately consulted gastroenterology (GI). While I was speaking with them, the nurse came to me and said, "Doctor, did you see the head CT results?" I pulled up the results, and was devastated to see a brain mass large enough to cause mass effect with midline shift. I contacted neurosurgery and the ICU while praying that God would save this patient's life.

The GI doctor indicated that given her acute liver failure, she needed to be transferred to another hospital for higher level of care. I shuddered because patients must be stable for transfer, and my patient was declining. Transfers can be very time-consuming and difficult to facilitate. My experience was that they could take up to days, and this patient didn't have days. Miraculously, within hours she was accepted and transferred in stable condition. In following up on the patient I learned that she had had successful brain surgery and that her liver function had returned to normal. God had answered my prayer. God saved her life.

God had orchestrated the people and events to save this woman's life. You see, previously that nurse was always stationed in DOU (step-down ICU) and never floated to other units. That day found her in the observation unit, where she was assigned to that patient. God also gave me wisdom to ask for and listen to advice from others. I thought about Solomon's words: "Where no counsel is, the people fall: but in the multitude of counselors there is safety" (Proverbs 11:14, KJV).

Teamwork, listening, and prayer saved this patient. I learned once again that life, including medicine, is a team effort with God at the helm.

Craig Seheult, LLUSM class of 2009, is an assistant clinical professor in LLUSM's department of medicine. He is currently a hospitalist at a local community hospital, where he enjoys practicing whole person care. He is married to Erin and they are blessed with two sons, Micah and Judah.

SEPTEMBER

ॐ COMPASSION ॐ

"I realized that 'Why is God doing this to me?' was not a question about God. It was a cry of pain, and the person asking the question didn't need my theological wisdom. She needed a hug."

HAROLD S. KUSHNER (1935–)
American rabbi and author of books on human suffering

September 1

> *"This is my command: Love each other."*
> John 15:17, NLT

For his last seven days I was the first face he saw in the morning. At age 69 he was a man riddled with cancer that had metastasized by the time of diagnosis. I was a third-year medical student on my internal medicine rotation at the time, and his case was complicated. He was fluid overloaded but intravascularly depleted with atrial fibrillation, diastolic heart failure, pulmonary edema and pre-renal acute kidney injury. Treating one problem just led to worsening of something else.

Every morning would start the same way.

"How are you feeling today, sir?"

"Fine, ma'am; just tired."

His severe back pain from the bony metastasis combined with orthopnea caused him to only be able to sleep sitting up in a chair with his head leaned forward over a table.

He was polite and soft-spoken, quietly complying with my morning physical exam. Next I would turn to his wife, having an identical conversation every day. I would inform her of the changes we made and what we were hoping they would accomplish. I stressed the complexity of his situation.

"We're stuck between a rock and a hard place," I found myself saying day after day.

We had run out of options, but our persistence made some headway, and as I left that Friday afternoon I felt a splinter of hope. When I returned the next morning, what I found instead was that he had been transferred to the ICU with severe respiratory distress after a failed procedure. I took a deep breath, and headed to the ICU.

When I entered his room, I saw him lying on his back for the first time. He was unresponsive, and gurgling sounds escaped as he struggled for air, using his accessory muscles of respiration. I stood somberly next to his wife. We exchanged quiet pleasantries, and it took a moment before she turned to face me.

"I'm going to tell the doctor that we're ready for comfort care."

She was crying, and I felt the tears welling up in my own eyes.

"I am so sorry; I was really pulling for him." My voice cracked.

She walked toward me with arms outstretched and wrapped herself around my waist.

"Thank you for being so kind."

He passed away later that afternoon.

This was the first patient of mine to pass away, and while so many things about him have stuck with me over the years, the strongest were his wife's words: "Thank you for being so kind." It wasn't our valiant efforts, medical knowledge, grand medications, or extraordinary measures that she thanked me for. It was the human connection that I made with them for about 15 minutes every morning. How easy it is to bury it underneath our medical knowledge and technical skills, but Jesus really said it best: "This is my command: Love each other." In the end, when all our earthly medical interventions fail, maybe kindness and love really are what matter most.

Tessa Lamberton, LLUSM class of 2018, is currently a general surgery resident at Harbor UCLA Medical Center in Torrance, California. She is passionate about traveling, exploring nature, and providing health care to the underserved populations of Los Angeles County.

September 2

A few years ago a group of friends cruised the Greek Isles and parts of the Holy Land. A good friend, Wil Alexander,* was with us—after two weddings and many Christmas Eves together, we called him our "family parson."

Wil agreed to lead out in Friday evening vespers on the two Fridays at sea. After the first, he gave us an assignment for the second get-together: to be prepared to explain what a certain Bible text meant to each of us personally.

That text, quite possibly the most popular and best known in the entire Bible, was John 3:16. I chose to do it as a poem—because that's what I often do. In the past 35 or so years I have written many things—some better than others, some published . . . but most not. They include some happy ones and some sad ones, though none about Bible verses.

And it's the poem on John 3:16 I would like to share with you, here:

John 3:16 at Sea

It's strange I've not done this before,
The verse is so powerful, eternal, and more.
It starts with a fact,
it speaks of God's love;
then ends with a promise,
life eternal above!
Wil made the suggestion
to answer the question
of what this text means
to us and others not seen.
I thought to do this all in rhyme,
I could with just a bit more time . . .
But the age-old prose is a perfect fit,
So I'll read the verse and not change a bit.
This might be slightly paraphrased
But the meaning is clear—the message unfazed.
"For God so loved the world
that He gave us His only Son.
that whosoever believed in Him
should not perish
but have everlasting life!"
To me, this power of God's love
is eternal, not evanescent.
To receive it, just ask;
it's always there . . . and it's incandescent!

It is my wish—better yet, my prayer—that the incandescence of God's eternal love will illuminate all of us. But not only that, may it emanate from us and touch the lives of those around us.

Oh, and that poem for the cruise vespers assignment? Wil liked it, a lot.

*For Wil Alexander's bio, refer to the devotional on January 18.

Hubert C. Watkins, LLUSM class of 1962, was an associate clinical professor in LLUSM's department of dermatology from 1968 to 2019. He was LLUSMAA president from 1984 to 1985 and an honored alumnus in 2019. He owns a private practice in Riverside, California. His wife, Dixie (LLUSAHP class of 1962), and he have four children, two of whom are graduates of LLUSM, and five grandchildren.

September 3

The Two Sides of Adventism

There have always been two unique visions for Adventism, producing somewhat contrasting statements of mission. One of these is the apocalyptic vision. It is grounded in the biblical books of Daniel and Revelation and the writings of Ellen G. White, such as *The Great Controversy*. This vision tends to be somewhat exclusive and world-denying. The other is the healing vision. It is based on the life of Jesus, as given in the Gospels, and in such books as *The Ministry of Healing*. The healing vision tends to be inclusive and world-affirming. It's not an issue of right or wrong, liberal or conservative, but two windows into how God looks at the world.

For many years I thought that Ellen White cast these two visions but never reconciled them. In *The Great Controversy* there is a strong focus on Daniel, Revelation, and the outworking of God's prophetic vision in history. There are few, if any, references to the healing vision of Adventism. In *The Ministry of Healing* you will look in vain for a single reference to the apocalyptic side of Adventism. It is as if God gave her two competing visions of His purpose for the Advent movement, allowing us to figure out how to integrate them.

Graham Maxwell, PhD, came to Loma Linda University Health in 1961 with this very issue in mind. He reasoned that a biblical scholar going to a center of healing might be able to integrate these two visions in a way that could not happen elsewhere. I believe he found that integration in Ellen White's book *Steps to Christ*. "Man was originally . . . perfect in his being, and in harmony with God. . . . But through disobedience, his powers were perverted, and selfishness took the place of love. . . . It was (Satan's) purpose to thwart the divine plan in man's creation, and fill the earth with woe and desolation. And he would point to all this evil as the result of God's work in creating man" (p. 17). At the root of all the suffering in this world (healing vision) is the cosmic conflict over the character and government of God (apocalyptic vision). The solution to that suffering lies not so much in God's judgment (apocalyptic) as in His loving, healing character.

"The enemy of good blinded the minds of men, so that they looked upon God with fear; they thought of Him as severe and unforgiving. Satan led men to conceive of God as a being whose chief attribute is stern justice—one who is a severe judge, a harsh, exacting creditor. . . . It was to remove this dark shadow, by revealing to the world the infinite love of God, that Jesus came to live among men" (*Steps to Christ*, p. 10-12). The mission of Loma Linda University Health and its School of Medicine is "to continue the teaching and healing ministry of Jesus Christ." "To make [humans] whole." Through caring and godly physicians, the infinite love of God is once more made flesh, and the world catches a glimpse of an even greater healing to come.

Jon Paulien, PhD, MDiv, is former dean of the School of Religion at LLUH and currently is a professor of religion. He is the author of more than 30 books and hundreds of articles. He loves golf, photography, and his family.

September 4

> *"And now these three remain: faith, hope and love.*
> *But the greatest of these is love."*
> 1 Corinthians 13:13, NIV

She was admitted on a weekday afternoon in the early 1980s to the UCLA Bone Marrow Transplant (BMT) Unit to undergo an allogeneic BMT for her acute myelogenous leukemia (AML), which had been diagnosed during the sixth month of her pregnancy. She had forgone active treatment until after her delivery a few weeks before.

She was a statuesque "All American" beauty in her late 20s, accompanied by her husband and parents. They were a very close-knit family unit. All were bright, well informed, warm, proactive, optimistic, and determined concerning her prognosis, but also fully aware of the risks and uncertainties of her treatment. The entire BMT staff rapidly fell in love with her and her family, who were reciprocally very appreciative of the tender care she was receiving. I was the faculty psychiatrist assigned to the BMT unit and collaborated with other team members in providing the patient and her family with support throughout her BMT stay.

She underwent the BMT, had early recurrence of her AML, and over the course of about six weeks had progressive development of multisystem dysfunction/failure, culminating in treatment-refractory pneumonia, requiring her transfer to the pulmonary ICU. She and her family were aware of her medical status and that she almost certainly would not survive the hospitalization. While she and they were appropriately sad, she and they continued to exhibit profound strength and resilience and genuine appreciation and warmth toward the BMT staff.

Shortly after her pulmonary ICU transfer, she fell into a moderately deep coma. It became clear that her survival prognosis was likely only a few days. Her family was informed and continued to hold vigil at her bedside.

About five days after her ICU transfer, I was urgently called by the pulmonary ICU team to help them manage the patient's family, who were very angry and hostile. We scheduled an urgent family/team meeting. Having known the patient/family well for two months, I was perplexed about this profound change in their reported behavior toward the ICU team.

It quickly became clear that the major source of the family's anger toward the ICU team was that the nurses were no longer applying eyedrops twice a day, which had been the initial routine. The family experienced not applying eyedrops as symbolic of the ICU team giving up hope and withdrawing care from their daughter/wife. The nurses did not believe that applying eyedrops was clinically meaningful, given the likelihood that she would die within the next couple of days, which she ultimately did. Once the source of the family's anger was identified, and the nurses understood the meaning to the family of their applying eyedrops, they resumed this care, and the family-team relationship was immediately improved.

Compassionate care of the critically ill often requires acts which demonstrate and preserve hope—the personalized equivalent of those eyedrops.

Deane Wolcott, LLUSM class of 1973-B, has spent his professional life leading the provision of comprehensive, multidisciplinary, psychosocial care services to patients with cancer and other life-threatening medical conditions. He and Elvina, his wife of 50 years, have two sons and two grandchildren.

September 5

> *"I have told you these things, so that in me you may have peace. In this world you will have trouble. But take heart! I have overcome the world."*
> John 16:33, NIV

I have seen a few thoracotomies now. I am never quite prepared for the moment a knife cuts across the chest wall to the thoracic cavity. Our senior trauma surgeon had just opened the patient's pericardial sac. A fountain of blood rushed out. She gave cardiac massage while two units were pushed in. She attempted to suture the large laceration in the right atrium. More blood, more attempted procedures, anything. After much action, he was declared dead, which was to be expected. But I did not expect what happened next.

The trauma senior asked for a moment of respectful silence. A room stuffed with moving people fell still. She grabbed the patient's hand and lowered her eyes. I was surprised when my eyes misted over as I looked at this young man. This moment was not about my education or experience. It was about a person who had expired in this room. The words of the Lord's Prayer flashed in my mind: "Your kingdom come; your will be done." Standing at the foot of the bed of a young man caught up in drug abuse and fatally stabbed in front of a cocaine house was not a manifestation of God's kingdom or His perfect will. I mourned for his story and so many similar ones where corruption, and not love, were at work.

The work of a Christian physician is so much more than seeing illness and prescribing treatment. A battle is at work that is bigger than a fight for healthy tissue. It is the opportunity for a meeting with the infinite and finding reconciliation with God, regardless of what happens to the flesh. This is why we pray the words of Jesus Christ and work toward something better. That in light of His grace, addictions, spitefulness, and disunity fall silent, and we can have peace with our failing bodies, our stories, and God. May the kingdom of heaven rush in.

Rachel VanderWel, LLUSM class of 2019, is "slogging through" her emergency medicine residency at Denver Health. She is grateful God placed her back in Colorado near family after living in Pennsylvania and California.

September 6

"That the world may know that You sent Me, and loved them,
even as You have loved Me."
John 17:23, NASB1995

The nearly full moon was still large and low in the sky as we walked through the empty parking lot. I tightened my jacket around me and shoved my hands in my pockets as the wind whipped strongly across the abandoned lot. A figure began to approach our posse, so a few of us went forward, with me at the front, as I was anxious to finally see her again.

"Hello!" I called out.

"Oh, it's you, little buddy!" she exclaimed with surprise as she grabbed me and hugged me tight against her. With just having finished interview season and a few away rotations as a senior medical student, I had not been out on the streets in several months.

"I've missed you so much, Millie! How've you been?" I asked.

"Oh, you know, still struggling, but I'm makin' it."

Yes, I knew. She had told me her sad story one evening when two other Street Medicine leaders and I met with her and her boyfriend at the public library. We had wanted to hear their stories and to find out how Loma Linda University Health Street Medicine could better reach the medical needs of the homeless community in San Bernardino. Years of abuse and life on the streets had taken their toll on her. Her hardened face and severe tooth decay were visible evidence of her many years of methamphetamine use, and the gynecological problems she'd whispered to us on one of our previous meetings with her were typical of a lady of the night.

She told us that Al, her boyfriend, and a main leader of the homeless community had been locked up for the past few weeks.

"What happened, Millie?" I queried.

"Oh, he just fell back into the same old stuff." She shrugged her shoulders and stared into the distance. "He should be out any day now."

Every time we go out on the streets, I feel the enormity of the need and my own inadequacy at filling it. We'd worked with Millie and Al for months now, and they were still on the streets, still struggling. I'm slowly learning, though, that God is the One to do the heart changing. I am only to go, to love, and to speak well of Him.

I took Millie's rough, nicotine-stained hands in mine, and we bowed our heads. "Dear God, we really need You...." Our tears hit the pavement beneath us.

After the Amen, I looked into her blue eyes and pleaded, "Take care of yourself, Millie."

She wiped her nose with her sleeve and mumbled "OK" as she turned around and walked back to her tent.

Sarah Belensky, LLUSM class of 2013, is currently practicing in Alaska. After completing a family medicine residency, followed by an additional year of OB training, she served for three years at Béré Adventist Hospital in Chad, Central Africa. She is married to Gabriel Silva and they have one son, Elijah.

September 7

First Corinthians 13: The Bible's Love Chapter
Translated for the Modern Doctor

1 If I use all the right medical terminology, but do not have love, I am only an annoying alarm because of a misplaced pulse oximeter.

2 If I can perfectly predict a prognosis and I can always give the right diagnosis and I can give all the healing modalities and medicines but do not have love, I am nothing.

3 If I give all I possess to the poor and give over my body to multiple residencies and fellowships that I may boast, but do not have love, I gain nothing.

4 Love is patient with the impatient patients; love is kind to the drug abuser. It does not envy the neurosurgeon's income or the banker's hours; it does not boast its productivity; it is not proud of patient satisfaction scores, but rejoices in the truth of where true life and spiritual health come from.

5 It does not dishonor other providers in order to boost one's image; it does not selfishly focus on one's own material needs; it is not easily angered when its ego or property is at stake; it keeps no record of how many times a patient ignores advice.

6 Love does not delight in the suffering of a "deserving" patient, but rejoices in the truth of the knowledge of God's love and His salvation of our souls despite our mistakes.

7 It always protects others' hearts, always trusts, hopes, and perseveres in God's system/kingdom of rule.

8 Love never fails. But where there are prophecies and prognostications, they will cease; where there are tongues and tongue depressors, they will be stilled; where there is medical knowledge, it will pass away when medicines are no longer needed.

9 For we know in part and we advise in part,

10 but when God comes, what is in part disappears.

11 When I was a medical student, I talked like one, I thought knowledge was most important, I reasoned like a computer. When I became a practicing doctor, I put those ways behind me.

12 For now we see only a reflection as in a mirror; then we shall see face to face. Now I know in part; then I shall know fully, even as I am fully known.

13 And now these three remain: faith, hope and love. But the greatest of these is love.

Thaddeus E. Wilson, LLUSM class of 2006, is an assistant professor in LLUSM's department of physical medicine and rehabilitation. As a pediatric physiatrist, he serves children with disabilities such as cerebral palsy, stroke, and spinal cord injury. He is married to April Wilson, his LLUSM classmate. He enjoys working with physicians in training, encouraging them to be compassionate, and hopes to continue spreading God's love in that capacity.

September 8

"Nobody cares how much you know until they know how much you care."
Theodore Roosevelt (1858–1919): twenty-sixth president of the United States and conservationist

I don't know what to do," the patient's mother lamented; "I don't know why he is acting this way." I have heard these words from multiple parents who seek help for a child, friend, or neighbor. I had persevered through medical school and training in order to be present at this very moment with this bewildered mother who was looking for guidance. The symptoms started slowly. First, there was the gradual decline in his grades. Then, he began isolating. He stopped showering. He ate little. He started hearing voices and seeing visions. He became paranoid of those around him.

I had seen this scenario so many times before. The agony of a parent watching as their child developed a psychotic illness. I discussed the diagnosis, prognosis, and treatment plan with the patient's mother. Medically, I thought I had done my duty. The session could now end with a plan in place. However, the patient's mother began sobbing. It was at this time that I recollected Colossians 3:12—"So, as those who have been chosen of God, holy and beloved, put on a heart of compassion, kindness, humility, gentleness, and patience" (NASB). These words of inspiration instilled within me the spirit of empathy. Through empathy we can give our patients a gift that many would not have received otherwise. Having empathy is hard. It can be draining. It is very easy to become jaded after seeing so much despair.

As physicians we have the unique opportunity to be with people at their most vulnerable moments. People entrust us with the most intimate details of their struggles. I knew that at this moment the greatest gift that I could give this mother was to be there for her. In psychiatry our patients are too often faced with stigma. The family and patient are blamed by society and blame themselves for the mental illness. Rather than having a medical model, patients, families, and society often view a psychiatric illness as a flaw in character.

The patient's mother cried for a bit more. She told me more about the fears she had for her child. At the end of the session she expressed gratitude because a light of hope was lit in her world. To impact someone's life with confidence and optimism gives purpose to a physician's practice.

Andrene Campbell, LLUSM class of 2010, is a child, adolescent, and adult psychiatrist in New York. She enjoys traveling and spending time with her husband, two daughters, and stepson.

September 9

> *"For she thought, 'I cannot watch the boy die.'*
> *And as she sat there, she began to sob."*
> **Genesis 21:16, NIV**

It was the fourth day of my internship year. I was assigned to the neonatal intensive care unit at the former Riverside General Hospital with Dr. Chul Cha, the chief of the neonatology division, as the attending neonatologist. A baby boy had been born the day before; at only 24 weeks of gestational age, his birth weight was 570 grams (1 pound 2 ounces), and his chest X-ray showed diffuse haziness. I had been up most of the previous night with my senior resident as the baby gradually deteriorated, blood gases showing worsening mixed acidosis despite higher and higher ventilator settings and the administration of saline, blood and sodium bicarbonate; his mean blood pressure dropping even though he was receiving high doses of dopamine and dobutamine. I had just finished medical school; I certainly had no experience in dealing with a situation like this.

Rounds began early that morning, but were quickly interrupted by bedside alarms, our team hurrying to the isolette, where the tiny infant boy lay, the heart rate dropping, and at the same time the latest blood gas was reported to have even worse values. Dr. Cha said, "There is nothing else we can do." He asked the respiratory therapist to turn off the ventilator and turned to me and said, "Let's go talk to this baby's mother." I had no idea what Dr. Cha would say to her; as we walked down the hall, I told him that I could translate since the mother spoke only Spanish. Would he tell her about the pH being 6.87? the persistent hypotension? the "hyaline membrane disease"? Would he say that we were using high ventilator settings? that we were giving her son many medications? Would he add that none of this had made any difference?

We walked into the mother's room, and Dr. Cha didn't say any of those things. He very unassumingly said, "I am your son's doctor" (so I translated *"Este es el doctor de su hijito"*), gently touched her shoulder, and followed with "I know you loved your baby" (*"Sé que usted amaba su bebé"*). He then quietly added, "We loved your baby also. I'm so sorry to tell you that your son died even though we did all we could." (*"Nosotros también amamos su bebé..."*). Empathy and compassion were evident in his tone and demeanor; the baby's mother didn't ask any questions; she just started to weep quietly. We stayed there at her bedside for a few more minutes, again said how sorry we were, and then left.

That little baby boy's death seemed to blend in with so many other events that month: long daily rounds, call every fourth night, writing orders and progress notes, dictating H&Ps and discharge summaries, and just trying to keep up with it all. And yet with the passage of time, having had on many occasions to give heartbreaking information to parents, I have grown to recognize and deeply appreciate the impact of that moment long ago when I learned from Dr. Cha the power of gentle words, empathy, and kindness.

Ricardo Peverini, LLUSM class of 1984, is an associate professor in LLUSM's department of pediatrics and a neonatologist. He is LLUSM's vice dean for clinical affairs, and president of LLU Faculty Medical Group. He loves family time, High Sierra hikes, palindromic prime numbers, and building Lego sets.

September 10

"Bless the LORD, O my soul, and forget not all his benefits, who forgives all your iniquity, who heals all your diseases, who redeems your life from the pit."
Psalm 103:2-4, ESV

The woman has been bleeding 12 years. Mark writes that she has suffered much at the hands of many physicians, has spent everything, and is no better but rather has grown worse.

How many patients have I seen that fit that description! Suffering, without improvement, broken from health care cost. Often the patient doesn't understand what the physician is trying to do and is mistrustful of the doctor because a lack of good communication is the most tragic fault of our profession—lack of connection.

The woman hears of Jesus. Hope springs again. Pressing through the crowd in her weakened, anemic state, she touches the hem of His cloak and instantly knows she is healed! Not wanting to make a scene, she starts to slip away. But although Jairus is trying to hurry Jesus to heal his dying daughter before it is too late, Jesus stops. He is not willing to heal without touching the soul of one He has healed. He is good at connecting. He asks who touched Him. This brings her trembling and fearful. She knows that by Moses' law her bleeding had rendered her ceremonially unclean and it makes anything she touches unclean, including Jesus. Preparing for chastisement, she hears only kind words: "Daughter, your faith has made you well; go in peace, and be healed" (Mark 5:34, ESV). She leaves in peace and health.

These lessons of connection and compassion have been made plainer to me as I stepped on the other side of the physician-patient relationship. After hesitatingly doing my first PSA, I was diagnosed with prostate cancer. Scans showed it to be localized to the prostate but the pathology following the radical prostatectomy indicated one lymph node had metastatic disease. It was a bit numbing to hear!

Fortunately, Dr. Herbert Ruckle, my urologist, was tuned in to my emotions, and as he described my pathology, he asked me to do something interesting. As he laid out his aggressive plan, he told me to get a piece of paper and write something. I thought he would tell me to write instructions. Instead he said, "I want you to write three words, and put them on your refrigerator so you will see them often." He asked me to write, "It's—not—hopeless." The words are still on my refrigerator and remind me daily of the hope that the surgeon handed me through connecting with me closely, compassionately. Those three words have guided my thoughts as I have suffered the treatment. The three words also remind me of Jesus, the one who is our hope, who has promised that whether we walk through the valley of the shadow of death or the mountain of cure, He walks with us, so we need not fear.

Bless the Lord, O my soul, and forget not all His benefits.

Jim McMillan, LLUSM class of 1986, is an associate professor in LLUSM's department of medicine. He is proud to be known because of his wife, Kathy McMillan, who directs employee spiritual care at LLUMC. He and Kathy have twins, Lisa and Mark.

September 11

> *"Finally, all of you, be like-minded, be sympathetic,*
> *love one another, be compassionate and humble."*
> 1 Peter 3:8, NIV

"Doctor! Doctor! Come, come!" It is our clinic employee, Barun, urgently calling my husband, Walter, to come outside just as we are finishing work in the dental clinic. It is December 1976 in Dhaka, Bangladesh, and dusk is overtaking the day. Walter rushes outside and crosses the busy avenue where a large, excited crowd has gathered. In the center is a small child, unconscious, now picked up like a hammock, with men pumping her arms and legs to see if anything is broken. She has just been struck by a speeding red car while gathering sticks in the deepening twilight. She is just 5 years old and wearing nearly nothing in her poverty. Walter immediately has the men put her down, then rushes back with Barun to get our car. He gently places the child in the back seat beside her mother, who has now been summoned, and they rush to the hospital. There we learn that little Bibi Honifa has severe head injuries and multiple broken limbs. Walter pays for her hospital expenses and for her first two surgeries. Eventually she will require more surgeries during her three-month hospital stay. And like a good uncle, Walter will visit her many times in the hospital, praying for her well-being.

The hit-and-run driver is never found. We live very close to the bazaar, and Barun begins to hear things there. He tells us that the merchants at the bazaar claim that Walter hit her, because why does he care? Why does he help? Barun says that he argues with the men, to tell them no, that Dr. Hadley's car did not hit her. But the rumor lingers. And I wonder: Is an act of kindness so hard to believe? Is life this cynical?

By early spring we are receiving visitors at the close of our workday. The visitors are Bibi Honifa and her mother. Bibi Honifa with her little shaved head, pronounced limp, disabled arm; her mother dressed nearly in rags. It tugs at our hearts and gives us lumps in our throats to see this little procession come to the clinic door. They come to say, "Thank you." They are sweet and shy and oh, so humble, but nothing can deter this mother from faithfully bringing her little girl to the man who helped them. Though Walter is fluent in Bengali, few words are spoken in their shared understanding of a child changed forever. This mother and child bear stoic testimony to their resilience and their gratitude. They will come once a month until we leave Bangladesh. They want nothing from us; they merely want to be near the man who helped them.

Over the years I have reflected upon this time, and hope and pray that the family is doing well. I think about the disbelieving merchants, how sometimes I am just like them in my relationship with God. I wonder how God can be so caring and so gracious with me despite my undeserving ways. I often sell Him short, projecting my human self-interests and limitations on a God who loves large. I am awestruck by God's greatness. I will learn that nothing can trump God's abiding love and care.

And I think about Bibi Honifa and her mother coming to see Walter on their faithful visits, finding a measure of comfort there. Like them, I also go to the place where I find safety and grace, kindness and compassion, in good times and bad, where love and acceptance await me. I go to God.

Beverly Hadley (née Van Auken) is a 1973 LLUSAHP physical therapy graduate. She and Walter (LLUSD class of 1974) served as missionaries in Dhaka, Bangladesh, at the newly founded Adventist dental clinic from 1974 to 1977. They reside in Pasco, Washington. September 11, is Walter's birthday.

September 12

"For the eyes of the LORD run to and fro throughout the whole earth, to give strong support to those whose heart is blameless toward him."
2 Chronicles 16:9, ESV

Loma Linda University Health is a training ground for training students how to give compassionate care. It was 1995; shortly after taking part I boards, I decided to join forces with SIMS (Students for International Mission Service) so that I could serve at one of our Adventist hospitals in Zambia, Africa. As we prepared for our trip, we were encouraged to obtain as many supplies as possible because the needs were so great. I collected many pens, pencils, erasers, sharpeners, staplers, paper, bandages, tape, gauze, cotton balls, alcohol wipes, and antibiotic creams. But just when I thought I had it all, someone decided to donate a piece of medical equipment—a heavy, bulky, cumbersome, impossible-to-pack piece of equipment called a chest tube drainage system. Not only was it difficult to pack, it was something that I would probably never use, because it is an apparatus that surgeons use to drain fluid from the lung cavity caused by chest trauma and inadvertent leakage of fluid or air around the lungs. I wasn't going to do surgery; I wasn't going into a war zone. I was just going to observe.

When I arrived in Zambia, I met Dr. Osario. He was a general surgeon who was filled with a heart of care and compassion. One day during our regular morning rounds we were faced with a new admission. It was a 12-year-old boy who was admitted with a chief compliant of malaise, shortness of breath, and fever. When I listened to his lungs, I could hardly hear any air going into the right side of his lungs. The chest X-ray confirmed a diagnosis of pneumonia with a large pleural effusion, which is fluid outside of the lung cavity. Dr. Osario, the supervising general surgeon, was really concerned. He expressed, "I haven't needed any equipment for this as long as I've been here, but a chest tube drainage system would surely help right now." By this time I started to feel the chills run through my body. Did he just say we needed a chest tube drainage system? In a voice that I hardly recognized as my own, I heard myself say, "I have one."

There was silence; then slowly all eyes turned to me. "You have what?" Dr. Osario asked.

"A chest tube drainage system," I replied, still in a state of shock.

"Well, thank God!" he said. "He is still working miracles in the mission field! He always provides what we need."

With a mixture of fear and excitement, Dr. Osario had me perform the procedure. Yes, Dr. Osario was right at my side, but it was our hands that God used to save that child's life, and I would be forever grateful.

Dr. Osario taught me lessons of compassion. Those lessons turned into acts of boldness and confidence. This resulted in healing and complete restoration for this young man. I saw him get stronger every day, and upon discharge his mother thanked us for saving her son's life—the feelings were priceless. I eventually learned that compassion is about taking risks; about going out on a limb to help someone in need. I learned that compassion transcends our fears and limited capabilities, and allows God's strength to be made perfect in our weakness. So let compassion send you to the ends of the earth, and do not shy away from opportunities that may help you grow personally and professionally.

Dexter Frederick, LLUSM class of 1997, currently practices internal medicine in Tampa, Florida, where he resides with his wife and two daughters. He has a passion for mentoring underrepresented high school students who aspire to be health professionals while extending the healing ministry of Christ to them.

September 13

> *"One of the essential qualities of the clinician is interest in humanity, for the secret of the care of the patient is in caring for the patient."*
> Francis W. Peabody (1881–1927): American physician

Most aspiring physicians begin medical school the same way—bounding onto campus, armed with thirsty brains and highlighters, ready to soak up every anatomy fact and devour each histology slide, and harboring a sincere desire to care for patients. The initial few years of medical training consist mostly of lectures, labs, and studying, with a bit of patient interaction tossed in here and there. Once on the wards, patients are everywhere, and we use them to develop the necessary tools of taking a thorough history, honing physical exam skills, and presenting information concisely. Further training in residency and fellowship provides additional training in efficiency, medical skills attainment, critical thinking, and medical coding and billing. With all this, our first love, our first desire, our earnest answer to the interview question "So, why do you want to be a doctor?"—all these too often fall to the wayside. We become so focused on keeping up with our clinic schedule, meeting deadlines, billing the correct ICD-10 codes, and documenting at least 10 review of systems, it's easy to forget about caring for the patient.

Since completing my fellowship, I have started to remember. I've begun to realize that if I am truly going to be a physician, a healer, an advocate, the only way is to care for my patients first. There will always be schedules and deadlines and meetings and Medicaid requirements, but if my patients are not my highest priority, my work as a physician will always be just that—work. If medicine is truly my calling, my vocation, my path, I have to care for my patients in order to care for my patients.

Recently a patient mentioned she felt overwhelmed with her diabetes management, and I listened—without charting at the same time. When a child came to clinic wearing a lovely new pair of pink glasses, I complimented her on her style. My patients are amazing—they are musicians, artists, chefs, physicians, nurses, teachers, homemakers, and entrepreneurs. One patient knows the secret to folding a fitted sheet perfectly. Another bakes the best chocolate chip cookies her family has ever tasted. These are my patients. Helping and caring for these exceptional people are what makes being a physician worthwhile. Today I love what I do, but in order to love it again, I had to remember—the secret of the care of the patient is in caring for the patient.

Lisal Folsom (née Stevens), LLUSM class of 2009, is an adult and pediatric endocrinologist practicing in Louisville, Kentucky. She provides endocrine and diabetes care for patients of all ages, and has a special interest in caring for transgender patients, as well as in easing the transition from pediatric to adult care for patients with type 1 diabetes. She enjoys spending time with her husband and their two rambunctious Boston terriers.

September 14

"After this I looked, and there before me was a great multitude that no one could count, from every nation, tribe, people and language, standing before the throne and before the Lamb. They were wearing white robes and were holding palm branches in their hands."

Revelation 7:9, NIV

During my thoracic surgery residency at LLUH I first met William Holmes Taylor, MD, FRCS (Eng.). Bill Taylor, CME class of 1947, devoted most of his professional life to medical mission service in isolated hospitals in Africa. Much of the time he was the only doctor available and had to do surgery to save lives. Recognizing that he needed additional surgical training (and because the countries where he worked were mostly British colonies), he trained in London, UK, and passed rigorous examinations to become a fellow of the Royal College of Surgeons of England (RCS).

Later in life he chaired the anatomy department of LLUSM and was greatly appreciated as an engaging and effective lecturer and demonstrator for the medical students' first semester human anatomy class. He had a great sense of humor and was a dignified and generous Christian gentleman with a distinctly Anglophile approach.

In the last years of his life he lost his wife, and became bedridden in a nursing home in Portland, Oregon. During my anatomy teaching sessions at the Western University of Health Sciences in Oregon, my wife and I made a habit of visiting him. He never complained about his difficult situation and was always cheerful and optimistic, even as his vital forces waned. It was during this time that he sent an unexpected and much-appreciated gift, delivered personally by a close friend of his.

Shortly before coming to LLUH, I had prevailed (an answer to prayer!) in the same competitive examinations in London to also become a fellow of the Royal College of Surgeons. The gift from Bill was his graduation robe with several College of Surgeons cords—all recently dry cleaned and in perfect condition!

It reminded me of the much greater gift of a graduation gown—sometimes referred to as "the robe of Christ's righteousness." But unlike the RCS gown, it's freely available to all simply by believing in the life, death, and resurrection of Jesus Christ.

Don Wilson, MB, BS, Sydney University, 1961, is a cardiac surgeon who trained in thoracic surgery at LLUH. He currently assists with cardiac surgery in Santa Rosa, California, and teaches thoracic anatomy at medical schools in Oregon and Mississippi.

September 15

"The time is always right to do what is right."
Martin Luther King, Jr. (1929–1968): American Baptist minister and civil rights advocate

In 2007 in a large metropolitan city in the midwest, a 16-year-old Black kid, on his birthday, might have shoplifted a pocketful of goods from a dollar store. As he and his friends left the store and crossed the parking lot in the early afternoon, a white man yelled for him to stop. He didn't. An off-duty policeman, who was not in uniform, pulled out his concealed service piece and shot that young man through the back.

A few minutes later that 16-year-old arrived at my hospital. He was dead on arrival, a Level 3 trauma. The ED attending physician and intern, as well as me, the second-year surgery resident, and my intern responded to the situation. No vitals, no signs of life, no heartbeat... there was nothing we could do. He had died before he arrived.

A single gunshot wound in the upper left back. No exit. We did a two-view chest X-ray and found a bullet lodged in the chest rib cage in front of the heart. It was a .38 hollow point. I know a lot about bullets. At that time, the majority of bullets we saw were 9 millimeter. We knew that .38 hollow points were the ones used by police.

Six hours after we declared the teen dead, I was called back to the ED. The family had found where their son was. And since ED does 12-hour shifts, the whole ED team was gone. I was the most senior person in the hospital who had been present earlier in the day when that young man had come to our hospital. So I was met by the ED charge nurse, a social worker, a nun from the spiritual care team, and a policeman. The nurse told me that I needed to break the news to the family that their son had died. The nun said she would be there with me. And the policeman said, "I'll be there too. Don't say anything about the injuries. It was an off-duty cop...."

We entered the room, and more than 20 family members were there, from grandparents to young kids. I had the difficult task of telling them their 16-year-old son had died before arrival, and there was nothing we could do to save him. There were screams and tears and utter despair. After several minutes, questions started flowing. Then an uncle asked, "Where was he shot?" I answered by pointing with my finger to my own back and said, "There was no exit." At that moment the policeman grabbed my arm and exited me out of the room, then said, "I told you not to say anything about the injuries."

That's all I remember about the day. I have racked my brain ever since.

I am ashamed that I didn't fight back against the cop, frustrated that I was not stronger. Whom should I have spoken to? What should I have done? Looking back, I'm sure the family never knew it was a cop who shot their unarmed son. There were no news crews, nothing said in the paper. There was no justice.

I remember thinking, *What a pathetic shame. He might or might not have had $5 of stuff in his pocket from a dollar store... and that plain-clothed policeman shot him in the back! He wasn't threatening. Wasn't endangering the police. He was moving away from the man who yelled "Stop!"* It made me sick, and still turns my stomach.

Today I march with my brothers and sisters of color because I now am strong enough to shout, "No racist police!" I've seen it. #whitecoats4blacklives

---

Ryan Hayton, LLUSM class of 2005, is a general surgeon and associate professor in LLUSM's department of surgery, program director of the LLUH Global Surgery Fellowship, and faculty member of Pan-African Academy of Christian Surgeons. Ryan served (2010–2019) as a missionary at Malamulo Adventist Hospital, where he started several programs in surgery education to help bring equity globally in access to safe surgery. One of his passions is integration of compassion and spirituality into surgical care.

September 16

*"Life is just a short walk from the cradle to the grave,
and it sure behooves us to be kind to one another along the way."*
Alice Childress (1916–1994): American author, playwright, and actress

I am awakened in the wee hours by the sound of rain. I usually leave the house by 5:30 a.m. with a target time of 7:15 for arrival at my workplace almost 70 miles away. The rainfall awakens in me a concern that I should depart even earlier.

As it turns out, I arrive at my destination about one and a half hours early. But better one and a half hours early than 15 minutes late.

The work queue is fairly heavy, so I am glad I can get a head start.

Around 8:30 I receive a phone call from a colleague, who thanks me for coming in early and lightening the workload. After I hang up, I think what a nice gesture on her part.

Two of the five procedures I perform that day are on a 20ish-year-old man who developed drenching night sweats not long before his admission. His physicians have requested needle biopsy of neck lesions and thoracentesis.

I have viewed his chest X-ray and CT scan. Among other things, he has bulky mediastinal adenopathy and pleural fluid.

I examine his neck and view the ultrasound images just taken. They confirm that the lumps I feel are enlarged lymph nodes.

After completing the neck node biopsy, I have the patient sit crosswise on the gurney, dangling legs, and ultrasound examine his chest. I decide to tap the right chest, where fluid is greatest.

I hold the small (5F), short (7 cm) sheathed catheter, as serosanguineous fluid flows into a glass vacuum bottle. I learn that he was contemplating matrimony before he took ill. He has other plans as well: travel, perhaps a new car. He seems sanguine, almost jovial, despite the gravity of his illness.

I think perhaps no one has told him. At this point I know nothing for sure. I have strong suspicions, however.

I wonder to myself why he got this (acute lymphoblastic leukemia as well as lymphoma, I later learn from a cytopathologist), but have no answers.

The flow slows to a trickle. He has not coughed or developed pain. I remove the catheter.

After I apply an oversized bandage to the puncture site, I tell him: "Good luck." But even as I say this, I know that what he needs is not luck, but a miracle.

The next day I view another chest X-ray. The fluid in his left chest has increased. His disease is aggressive. There may be no wedding, no travel, no new car.

I may not see him again, at least in this lifetime.

All die.

Some slowly, some less so. Time itself is relative.

I have an acute sense of mortality. Time becomes more precious with each passing day.

May we, in the time we have been granted, exercise as much kindness as possible.

Sam M. Chen, LLUSM class of 1965, is a diagnostic radiologist who retired in 2019. He is trying to connect the dots and discern the cracks (which let light in) and is a grateful recipient of grace.

September 17

> *"Could a greater miracle take place than for us to look through each other's eyes for an instant?"*
> Henry David Thoreau (1817–1862): American author and naturalist

How does one act compassionately in a busy hospital setting? My example came during my time at White Memorial Medical Center in Los Angeles. On the gynecology service, patients were admitted for a number of women's health issues ranging from ovarian cysts to pelvic cancers.

Our patient was in her early 30s, married with three children. She had presented with severe vaginal bleeding. She was admitted, then underwent a pelvic examination to determine the source of the bleed. Upon exam, the resident found a large mass extending from her cervix. A biopsy was taken for assurance, but this severity of bleed in this context screamed one diagnosis: cervical cancer. The pathology report confirmed our suspicions, and imaging showed it had spread to several pelvic lymph nodes. The chance of mortality was high.

Since we were her primary team, it was our responsibility to share the news. We shuffled into the hospital room. Our patient lay resting, watching the room's TV. I stood at the foot of the bed, my resident instead sat alongside the patient. "As you know, you lost a lot of blood yesterday," she said. "When we checked the source of the bleeding, we found a mass on your cervix. We took a biopsy to determine the cause of this mass. I'm here to inform you that the results have come back, and they confirm that it is cervical cancer. I'm so sorry."

I watched the patient as she received the news. Initially her eyes were locked on the doctor's, but as the diagnosis was shared, she seemed to enter a daze. Her eyes shifted to the television. It was only after the description was finished that she seemed to regain her senses, with tears flowing. Through her sobs she had such questions as "Is it bad?" and "How do we treat it?" My resident gently answered all of her questions, repeating points she had already addressed without any signs of aggravation. As she closed, she leaned forward and took the patient's hand, "Honey, I can only imagine how scary all of this is, but we're going to be with you every step of the way. Our radiation oncology team will begin treating you ASAP." Tears still streamed down the patient's face as she thanked us for being honest with her as we left.

I left the gynecology service several days later, so I never learned what happened. But what stuck with me was my resident's compassion for our intensely vulnerable patient. Throughout her training, she had developed an approach toward these situations. She set the stage for the diagnosis by recounting the illness narrative, then provided a clear diagnosis. This was expressed with compassion; she showed no impatience with having to repeat herself, assuring the patient that she wasn't alone, as well as quietly holding her hand as she wept. I'm honored to have witnessed this moment, and I hope to emulate her Christlike compassion.

Jonathan Goorhuis, LLUSM class of 2020, feels that he was incredibly blessed during his time at LLUSM. He currently is a family medicine resident at Adventist Health Ukiah Valley in California. He's hoping to find some time during residency to play his favorite sport, soccer.

September 18

> *"For God has not given us a spirit of fear, but of power and of love and of a sound mind."*
> 2 Timothy 1:7, NKJV

Mid-2017 I saw a young self-employed gentleman seeking medical care related to an accident that occurred while he was working. The patient was working with a diamond-tipped saw and, by accident, he carved a deep wound into his left forearm. My field, urgent care, is generally a place of medical work that focuses more on non-life-threatening illness. Seeing this man's arm having active bleeding and hearing his vocal indications of pain was out of the ordinary for all staff and medical personnel involved.

Having finished a family practice residency only one month prior, I was hesitant to take on the case because of my perceived lack of skills. As we were rolling him back, I told the patient that we could place a pressure dressing on him and order transport to the ER. The patient retorted, "Listen, I do not have medical insurance," and refused to leave. After we pressure-dressed him and gave him pain medicine, I proceeded to pray and had a strong sensation that I should get in touch with a friend who was a plastic surgeon. After a two-minute HIPAA compliant phone conversation, based on history and physical exam and my friend's go-ahead, I decided to take on the case. After placing 5 dissolvable sutures inside and 15 sutures on the outside in an hour of time, not only was I able to repair his wound, but also able to have him as a captive audience.

I distracted him from pain and discomfort by professing my faith, as well as giving him tips and tools to help him end his deadly habit of smoking. After the patient-doctor meeting was finished, I was able to pray with him. Even though I strongly recommended that he should not use his left arm for work until told otherwise by a medical professional and that he should seek medical care in two days for a wound check, he did not listen. Despite this, I was able to see him two weeks later for a follow-up visit, which is rare in the field of urgent care. Not only did he heal completely, including an uneventful suture removal; the Lord also blessed him by decreasing his desire to smoke.

I do not know how he is doing currently, but I know the Lord sent him into my life so that I could grow my personal faith, take care of his medical issue, profess my faith in God to him, and add tools to his toolbox to aid in his quest to quit smoking. God has a funny way of placing what seems to be too much for us to handle in our path so that He can show that everything is possible through Him.

Richard L. Elloway, LLUSM class of 2014, is a family physician who currently practices urgent care in Florida. He has a passion for praying with patients and listening to them despite a busy schedule, helping to spread God's love in that capacity.

September 19

"I will be your God throughout your lifetime." Isaiah 46:4, NLT

Loma Linda. The hill beautiful. My connection with this unique town had always been nonmedical, even though health care education and delivery define it. My memories take me there only through childhood visits to relatives who lived there. Although I've had many family members graduate from LLUH, it wasn't until 2016, when we proudly watched our daughter receive her doctorate in physical therapy, that we came to appreciate what takes place on this campus. Little did we know that just a few months later we would be back in Loma Linda with my husband's life hanging in the balance.

We live in a small town in central California where Kevin is a teacher. Five weeks into the school year he became extremely fatigued and was unable to finish out the week. He slept all day Thursday and continued sleeping until the next morning. He awakened Friday morning still not feeling well, only to realize he could barely walk. Our physician directed us to the emergency room. Prayers immediately ascended to our heavenly Father. The difficult time walking turned into losing reflexes in both legs and then worked its way up his body to where he was unable to use his arms. This deterioration was relentless and did not slow down. Soon his breathing was affected to the point where it was necessary to intubate him. Kevin's doctor told me that outside of a miracle, Kevin would not make it. My response: "Well, I believe in miracles." This wonderful doctor, who just happened to be the parent of a student my husband had taught many years prior, said to me, "So do I."

Through a series of events that I can explain only as God-directed, Kevin was airlifted to LLUMC. God used His earthly angels to make that happen. Waiting for us in Loma Linda were more of His angels and miracles. Although Kevin was extubated the next day, the physicians were still unsure of his prognosis. My daughters and I saw a bulletin board in the ICU that had pictures of hope—patients who had lived despite the odds. Another thing we noticed at the hospital is that there is scripture written on the walls and reminders of the hope God has given us. Such reassurance!

After much testing we received the diagnosis that had eluded the medical staff since the start—West Nile virus (WNV). A mosquito had changed our lives overnight! Besides the paralysis, Kevin's blood pressure was sky-high, his sodium and potassium were dangerously low, and he experienced nerve pain that he could hardly bear (we later learned that only 1 percent of WNV cases present with these symptoms).

In the days, weeks, and months to come, there were many more trials and setbacks, but matching those setbacks was peace and strength from God. We watched as our miracles unfolded: doctors telling us that Kevin probably would not live, to doctors telling us he would become a quadriplegic, to being so nauseous he was losing weight day by day, which seemed incompatible with life. Many nights I would leave the hospital to go to my niece's home not knowing if my beloved husband would make it through the night.

Just as God had led us to Loma Linda, He led the way home, where more wonderful doctors and therapists treated him. Kevin has worked hard, and now his upper body is strong. He continues to persevere so that someday he might walk again—God's timing. However, our greatest miracle is that Kevin is alive! Through the storm God gave us the strength and the peace that passes all understanding to make it through. And for that, we will praise His name evermore.

Connie Eller Thompson is the loving wife of Kevin; she watched these miracles unfold and is still witnessing God's hand in Kevin's journey. Currently, Kevin drives himself to Hanford, California, where he is a public defender. He has regained some movement in one of his legs and has been fitted for a brace for the other leg. Connie and Kevin continue to have complete faith in God.

September 20

> *"For to this end Christ died and lived again, that he might be Lord both of the dead and of the living."*
> Romans 14:9, ESV

In our profession we strive to master the art and ministry of healing, aiming to cheat death. But of course our best efforts are always temporary. Death, for now, always wins. I have learned, however, that my same efforts to provide healing are equally important when death is the final outcome.

As a fourth-year medical student at LLUH, I recall an after-hours code at the Jerry L. Pettis Memorial Veterans Medical Center, ending in the death of a veteran. I remember an intern, full of compassion, openly crying as the cleanup began. As Jesus wept with His friends, so we can grieve with our patients' families.

Once as a newly minted family doctor in rural Colorado, I realized the early-morning call for "patient found unresponsive, not breathing" was two doors down from my house. I ran out, meeting the ambulance, and commenced lifesaving, but obviously futile effort. How old was she? What was her name? I realized I had never met or spoken with this woman living so close to me.

During my residency I attended a woman suffering from end-stage kidney disease during her many inpatient stays. Near the end of her struggle, in the ICU, I watched a consultant refuse a requested hug from this dying patient, responding that it was "not professional." Do we appropriately comfort our patients in their time of dying? Are we present and available for their families?

Jesus' beloved disciple John carefully lays out Jesus' ministry in John 11. His friend Lazarus, whom He loved, takes ill, then dies. We often puzzle over His allowance of death and suffering, or the meaning of His grief, but throughout this chapter we see Jesus clearly engaged in loving care for His grieving and angry friends.

He responds to the consult (verse 9) despite the risks of going into a hostile area—He enters into their pain. He is kind but direct about the diagnosis (verse 14). He instructs and gives hope (verses 4 and 25). And He prays (verse 41).

However, perhaps the greatest example we take from this encounter is His immersion in their pain. He was not detached from this community, but had a history with them. They had spent time with the Great Physician as a friend and now turned to Him. Therefore, He "groaned . . . and was troubled"(verse 33, KJV); He wept, and He loved (verses 33-38).

Are we involved or exclusive of our community? Are we willing to enter into our friends' and patients' grief and pain, regardless of appearances or personal risk?

The template for our own "best practices" is here. We need only to follow Jesus' perfect clinical case study.

Richard Moody, LLUSM class of 1994, is a family physician in Chattanooga, Tennessee. In his senior year of medical school he found the love of his life, Nora (LLUSN class of 1993), while caring for a patient in the MICU. He most enjoys teaching medical students.

September 21

"A woman, when she is in labor, has sorrow because her hour has come; but as soon as she has given birth to the child, she no longer remembers the anguish, for joy that a human being has been born into the world."
John 16:21, NKJV

The call came from my resident that her continuity pregnant patient had come into the hospital after a soccer ball had hit her in the abdomen. Her uterus was contracting, but was dilated only two centimeters with borderline amniotic fluid. My first thought was that she was still in early labor, so hopefully we could send her home. Then we obtained another ultrasound to rule out an abortion, which also revealed intrauterine growth restriction. By then she had progressed to three to four centimeters, and was on the way to being admitted. When her exam was barely changed after a few hours, I drove in to see the patient.

Nothing that was said prepared me for what I would find once I arrived. The first hint I had that this was not my "normal" type of patient was the nurse asking, "Do you know about her?"

Well, of course I know about her, the dilation, her parity. "Do you know that she is from Haiti, and was in the camps, and that she is in treatment for PTSD?" These camps were set up after the earthquake and often had roving gangs. Soon I discovered that her sad affect, reflecting some unmentionable violence in the camps, was because of sexual assault, and that she had not even known that she was pregnant. The nurse mentioned that we would need to be extra-gentle with the examination to see how she had progressed. Confirming her lack of progress, the resident then broke her amnionic sac and inserted an IUPC for fetal monitoring. Still speaking little, she assented to these invasive procedures, possibly reminding her of some unspeakable violence she had endured. I thought of the courage or the cultural pressures she had endured in keeping this child.

She easily delivered a small baby boy. The reaction of many mothers on delivery is similar to what is described above in John 16:21. Would that be her reaction as well?

I waited. Her response was without emotion; then finally her face broke into a smile. Her host family from a wealthy neighborhood commented that the hardest part was over. I thought delivery was the easy part. Raising a child of dubious paternity, representing this dark time in her life, was to come. Would this be a constant reminder of that, or would the boy be the new joy or hope to rise out of the dark past? I prayed to myself that it would be the latter, that she would have some spiritual renewal or healing, and forgiveness that this child could bring.

Wrapped in the warm clothes that her culture deemed necessary, whether in the subtropics of Haiti or that of urban Los Angeles, she came for her follow-up appointment, the start of a journey. I prayed that, with God's help, joy would come from the midst of suffering.

Jack Yu is an associate professor in LLUSM's department of family medicine. He is triple-boarded in geriatrics, hospice palliative medicine, and sports medicine. His daughter Mary Beth is an MD/PhD student (LLUSM class of 2022), and his other daughter works at Disney.

September 22

"If we love one another, God lives in us and his love is made complete in us."
1 John 4:12, NIV

Since my childhood I felt intuitively aware of two apparently unrelated phenomena. One is the surprise and ongoing wonder of life, its overwhelming richness, its wanton opulence and sheer luxurious diversity. The other is the experience of love.

As children we instinctively gravitate to our loving parents, where we feel a sense of safety and a sense of home. In fact, our parents' love enables us to thrive. There comes a day, however, when we experience a sense of admiration and a desire to be near people other than our parents. Gradually we may discover that our thoughts wander more frequently over to the thoughts of others, as we rejoice and empathize with those who impressed us so unexpectedly. This develops into a mind-expanding vista of possibilities. We are no longer limited to the experiences of our own lifetime. Through love we gain access to visions from the perspectives of others, and this bestows on us new insights and freedoms. We are no longer limited to just our point of view. Instead, we begin to see ourselves as members of a greater community of life. A question presents itself almost implicitly: *How can I contribute something of value to this greater community?*

Christ's attempt to describe God's care for us by telling us about His knowledge of the falling sparrow, is an enormous understatement. Because God loves, He sees not only the sparrow but through the eyes of the sparrow. He feels the sparrow's joys and sorrows, hopes, and fears. And not only the sparrow but also the squirrel, the donkey, the eagle, every life form, and every individual. This implies that God sees reality from every perspective, because He loves. The greater the richness of life, the greater the range of perspectives.

There is a potential danger that could undermine a well-functioning web of life. Preoccupation with self, one's own goals and agenda, until the other begins to look merely like a means to some end. Our vision shrinks, as we no longer find someone else's perspective enjoyable. Progressively we become preoccupied with the idea of winning rather than seeing. Thus, we become blind, all the while laboring in pursuit of our own personal success. This leads us into conflict with others, which we conveniently rationalize as part of the presumably legitimate struggle, the competition, for success.

Fortunately, God did not leave us unprotected. He gave us a variety of hints, counsels, instructions, even commandments. To love God above all and to love our neighbors as ourselves. The genius of these commandments is that they enable us to learn and grow, literally thrive, while protecting us from selfish blindness. The more we are willing to care about God and His creation, the more we become able to appreciate glimpses of life as He sees it. Priceless!

Danilo Boskovic, PhD, is an assistant professor in LLUSM's department of basic sciences, division of biochemistry. His research interests: (a) perturbations in hemostasis, (b) neonatal intraventricular hemorrhage, and (c) recognition and treatment of neonatal stressors.

September 23

> *"Your life must be controlled by love, just as Christ loved us and gave his life for us as a sweet-smelling offering and sacrifice that pleases God."*
>
> **Ephesians 5:2, GNT**

My beeper rang. I thought I was dreaming. I had just fallen asleep after a long day. I looked at the table clock. It was 2:15 a.m. I had gotten home late at approximately 12:30 a.m.

I was wondering about the nature of the call. I hoped it was not one of those "disasters" from the emergency room. Half asleep, I picked up my phone and dialed the number that was flashing on my beeper's screen. It was indeed a call from the ER.

"Why are you paging me again?" I had received 17 calls from the ER that Sunday. The last call I had received from them was three hours earlier. I was becoming irritated.

"This is Dr. S from the ER. Are you on call?" came the answer.

"Of course I am on call. Why would you call me if I weren't? Look, you just woke me up, and I am not in a chatting mood right now. How can I help you?" I answered.

"Well, Doc, we have your patient Mr. H here. He is a 'frequent flyer' (meaning a regular ER patient). It looks like he was having one of his alcohol withdrawal seizures again. We have just given him a loading dose of phenytoin, and I am calling to let you know that he will be on your list of patients to see in the hospital this morning."

"Is he stable?" I asked.

"Yes. His vital signs are stable, and the EEG tech says that his electroencephalogram does not show any epileptiform activity."

I could not get back to sleep. At 6:00 a.m., I had a short devotional, read 1 Corinthians 13:4, 5, took a shower, had a quick breakfast, and headed for the hospital. I had to be in my office at 8:30 am. I planned on making rounds on the five patients I had admitted during the past 12 hours. I would start with Mr. H.

I must have popped in his room with annoyance written all over my face. He had awakened and was waiting for me. Before I could say a word, he said:

"Are you angry at me, Doc? I know you are. I have been trying very hard to quit drinking, Doc. It is not easy, Doc. Not easy.... The wife left me three weeks ago. Prior to her leaving, I had not had a drink for three months. After she left me, I began soaking my sorrow with Vodka for two weeks. Then I suddenly stopped, Doc." He started sobbing loudly. In between sobs he would say, "I am not a bad person, Doc . . . I am just messed up." "Don't give up on me, Doc."

His last words kept ringing in my ears when I finally left his room. It dawned on me as I drove toward my office that Jesus hired a thief (Judas), a terrorist (Simon the Zealot), and a cursing sailor (Peter) to be His disciples. He was so patient with them . . . so kind. And what was I doing? Getting angry at a struggling alcoholic?

E. Dan Udonta, LLUSM class of 1988, currently practices neurology and seizure disorders in Nederland and Port Arthur, Texas. He has a passion for teaching Sabbath School. He loves astronomy and high-end audio.

September 24

> *"I call out to my Creator for help, and he provides
> all that I need from his dwelling place."*
> Psalm 3:4, Remedy

The year was 1981, and an urgent call came for a doctor in Blantyre. Trusting God, we decided to make the move from Mwami Adventist Hospital, Zambia, to Malawi. As we prepared to transition to Malawi, we learned customs didn't have any record of our moving to Zambia five years earlier. We would have to take all our possessions hundreds of miles west to Lusaka for clearance—a huge waste of time and money.

"Let's pray and see if we can get bank clearance and do customs here in Chipata," my wife suggested. This is a three-month process when everything is in order—but we had no paperwork! Desperate, I went Monday morning to speak with the bank manager and explain our situation. Within 20 minutes we had our bank clearance papers and hearts filled with gratitude.

The next step was customs. We loaded all our earthly goods that afternoon. Tuesday morning I drove to the customs office in Chipata to complete the multiple copies of the required forms. The officer said, "Now, let's go out to inspect the load and seal the ropes that tie the tarp."

Just as we started to roll back the tarp, a huge thunderhead opened up on us, soaking us with giant drops of water as only tropical Africa can do. The officer ran for shelter, shouting above the roar, "Cover the load!" When I went inside, he was stamping the papers. Our goods were officially cleared for export to Malawi—no sealed ropes required!

Wednesday morning we were on the road early. At the Zambia side of the border, all six copies of those many forms were stamped again. At the Malawi border post we expected to receive "Report Order" forms for the customs office in Blantyre to clear our goods. "Is this your moving day?" the officers greeted us. "Welcome to Malawi." Again, I filled out itemized declarations of our goods. Then the officer searched 30 minutes to find the man with the key to open the stamp drawer. As I watched, he began stamping our papers "Duty Free," "Duty Free . . ." Graciously handing them to us, he said, "You are done; you may go."

Bewildered, I stammered, "What about the 'Report Order' forms?"

He repeated, "You are done; you may go."

As we left the border station, still trying to believe what had just happened, my wife commented, "We may need this experience in the future to be assured God wants us here in Malawi." At the mission office we were told clearance at the border had never happened before. In just three days God had accomplished a three-month process!

We spent three memorable years serving the people of Malawi. As we look back, we are secure knowing that God was leading and guiding in our lives. He truly provided for all our needs.

John R. Rogers, LLUSM class of 1974, is a family physician who served three years in Malawi, four and a half years in Zambia, and one year in Botswana. He has also practiced family and emergency medicine in Washington, Wyoming, and Nevada. He is board-certified in lifestyle medicine (2017). He is currently enjoying medicine too much to retire just yet. He lives with his wife of 52 years, Sue, in Caliente, Nevada.

September 25

> *"I call upon you, for you will answer me, O God . . . Wondrously show your steadfast love. . . . As for me, I shall behold your face in righteousness; when I awake, I shall be satisfied with your likeness."*
> Psalm 17:6-7, 15, ESV

She sat in the wheelchair, her French braid tight to her scalp, the rest of her in an oversized gray sweatshirt. Through a translator I learned she had diabetes, hypertension, overactive bladder, COPD, asthma, chronic back pain, sciatica, neuralgia, polyneuropathy, dyslipidemia, frequent falls, chronic fatigue, allergies, depression, anxiety, headaches, and intertrigo. She weighed 347 pounds; she was 45.

"I need my meds refilled," she told me.

I refilled 19 and withheld the rest. "We need records," I said.

And so the records came: 62 pages (pulmonologist); 35 (pain management); 58 (OB/GYN). She came back in, and we requested again from her endocrinologist, urologist, and psychologist. She came back, and we requested from her PCP (who still hadn't sent any), her optometrist, and her orthopedic surgeon (three back surgeries and one knee replacement). She came back, and we requested from her general surgeon (gallbladder removal); bariatric surgeon (placement of gastric sleeve); and allergist (currently testing). With growing horror I wondered what we as a medical institution had done to her.

Every visit she dug a gauze drawstring bag deep from within her purse and withdrew a three-centimeter stack of paper slips, each one neatly printed with one of her medications. She handed me the part of the pile with the ones she needed.

She lived by herself in her own house. Sometimes home health would come. She went to Mass on Saturdays and to her doctor appointments. Of course she used to work. Lately she had been tripping because her walker would get caught on narrow doorways.

There was just something missing, I felt, so I requested more records. As I read through the paperwork, it became obvious that what I was looking for just wasn't there.

"Did these things start at a particular time?" I asked. She didn't understand.

"Why do you think you have all these problems?" She couldn't think of anything.

"How is your mood?" It was fine.

The whole time she was agreeable and patient. When she asked for a refill on the Norco, I suggested another. She said that that would be all right.

She came in again, this time to talk about her headaches.

"How long have you had them?" On and off for years.

"Why do you think you have them?" They always seemed to start in the same spot. She pointed to a place on the top of her head.

"It's where my ex-boyfriend hit my head against the wall nine years ago."

And at last the pieces fell into place!

After he had repeatedly thrown her against a sofa bed's middle bar as he raped her, she began to have back pain. She had anxiety when she left him. Gained weight to stay hidden, developed irregular cycles from the weight, bladder problems from the hysterectomy.

No, she hadn't told her psychologist or her psychiatrist. They hadn't asked.

Why do we do this? Why does it matter to sit and hear these stories, sharpened and shadowed by the sheer force of their repetition?

Because there is a difference between compassion and simply watching suffering.

Because I am not and will never be a healer. I cannot fix this.

But I know the One who redeems. And compassion is sitting together, we three, visit by visit, pill by pill, tear by tear, and waiting for Him to make good on His promises.

Robin Hrdina completed her family medicine residency at LLUH in 2020 and now practices in San Bernardino, California. She loves to see the stories God has written flood through our "ordinary" things.

September 26

> *"We must learn to regard people less in light of what they do or omit to do, and more in the light of what they suffer."*
> Dietrich Bonhoeffer (1906–1945): German Lutheran pastor,
> theologian, and anti-Nazi dissident

Compassion. I did not realize just how pivotal my third year in medical school would be in helping me develop compassion for others.

One of the many patients who helped me was an elderly man named Mr. Rossi. He had dementia and was admitted to the hospital with a urinary tract infection. Very quickly his care became very difficult because he was thoroughly convinced that there was nothing wrong with him. At first, he simply refused all medications and as the first night of hospitalization progressed, he started to fight off any staff who tried to come into his room. When I arrived the next morning, I saw that he would be assigned as my patient. Since he had refused any treatment, I entered his room to ask if we could just talk. After a couple of questions, he began sharing his life story with me. I learned that he had been an actor in Italy, had traveled all around the world and now simply longed to return home to New York to be with his daughter. I shared some of my own experiences with some wonderful people I had known from Italy, and soon we had established a connection.

Though unsure of his response, I decided to continue our conversation and ask if he would spare a few minutes to explain his condition. He agreed, so I told him about his abnormal lab results, his ultrasound report showing damaged kidneys, and pictures from Google comparing his kidneys to normal kidneys. He was shocked! After some explanation of the medical care needed, he said he understood, and agreed to move forward with his treatment plan. The health care team rejoiced in this apparent small victory. However, the next morning I learned that he had become violent overnight and was again refusing all medications. I asked him what had happened, and again, he was adamant that there was nothing wrong with him. We were back to square one. So we talked. We talked about Italy, acting, and New York, and when the time was right, I again explained his condition the same way as I had the day before. By the end he once again agreed to treatment. We repeated this every day for several days. Although my team allowed me time to sit and talk with my patient, I knew I would be leaving for a new rotation soon.

It took time each day, and it took an even greater amount of patience. Though difficult, we didn't give up on Mr. Rossi. We tried to see his hospital experience through his eyes, and as a result he received the treatment he desperately needed and deserved.

This reminds me of the great compassion our God has for each one of us. Though Mr. Rossi could not help the fact that he did not remember, we often knowingly and willingly refuse to allow God to work in our lives. We convince ourselves that there is nothing wrong. Yet when we realize our need for God, His compassion and mercy are there, ready to receive us again. I am so grateful that I have a God whose love and patience are so great; He is willing to go back to square one with me as many times as necessary.

Rubicelia Perez, LLUSM class of 2019, graduated from Walla Walla University in 2012 with a BA in religion. She took a year off from medical school between her second and third years to fulfill a dream of completing a master's degree in theological studies. She is a third-year resident in family medicine in Richland, Washington.

September 27

"He has made everything beautiful in its time."
Ecclesiastes 3:11, NIV

While working as an intern in the LLUMC emergency department, I saw a 78-year-old woman with right hand weakness in bed 7. She had been accepted as a transfer to the emergency department from a nearby hospital, and her extremity weakness was secondary to a cerebral hemorrhage. As I cared for her, she remained stable, with no further bleeding on her repeat brain imaging.

Meanwhile, I moved past the curtain to bed 8 and began taking care of a 54-year-old homeless man with shortness of breath. My examination and the medical workup revealed multiple complicated medical issues, including a new mediastinal mass compressing his superior vena cava and trachea, as well as multiple intraabdominal masses. Despite his shortness of breath, he was still able to speak comfortably. Because of his complicated medical findings he was seen by multiple specialists—surgical oncology, cardiothoracic surgery, medical oncology, radiation medicine, to name a few—and it was determined he would need to be intubated and put on a ventilator for his planned procedures.

Oddly, these patients in beds 7 and 8—separated by a mere curtain from sight but not sound—shared a unique German last name. Curiosity piqued, I asked the patient and her husband in bed 7 if they had any children. Indeed, they had three boys and two girls. Where were their boys? Across the Midwest: one in Indiana, one in Ohio, and one who joined the circus more than 20 years ago, without further contact.

As we prepared the dyspneic patient for intubation, I discussed with the patient the seriousness of his medical condition. I thought he would need support, and asked him again if he had any kin he wished to contact. He responded that he had no one close for support, but gave family names and consented to information-sharing if I found his family. Upon discovery of his father's name I got goosebumps and marched back to bed 7 to ask the elderly husband his own name and his lost son's name. The names were the same! A divine match?

I delayed the planned intubation, pulled back the curtains between beds 7 and 8, and reintroduced parents to son after a 20-year separation. Wow! Mother and son clutched each other across gurneys. Tears flowed, from patients and staff alike. We delayed the intubation so that they could catch up on lost years of multiple Christmases and Easters. I shared the gravity of the son's condition and encouraged his family to keenly absorb these moments. Before the subsequent successful intubation, the family and I held hands and prayed together: We acknowledged God's dominion, delighted in His redemption, rededicated our lives to Him, and sought His strength and comfort.

In medicine we form assessments and plans. In emergency medicine we expedite those plans based on limited information. This wondrous family reunion reminds me to pause in the daily rush and to resubmit to the Holy Spirit's agenda for all my patients' care. Only the Great Physician, with His perfect timing, could plan for separated parents and son to land in the same hospital, at the same time, with the same physician, side by side, before their lives took the next turn.

Darren Brockie, LLUSM class of 2014, and LLUH emergency medicine residency class of 2017, is an emergency medicine physician in Kalispell, Montana. He is a lover of God, husband, father, skier, hunter, fisher, and servant.

September 28

"For I am not ashamed of the gospel of Christ: for it is the power of God unto salvation to every one that believeth; to the Jew first, and also to the Greek."

Romans 1:16, KJV

During residency an odd twist landed me platform chair of a section at a national meeting. The primary responsibility associated with this distinction consisted of introducing speakers. Details about each were needed. While approaching the first speaker for details, I noted he appeared younger than I. What a relief! I walked forward, extended my hand, and asked where he was training. Had he finished residency?

"Paul, I'm the dean of research at Johns Hopkins University" was his unemotional response. Apologies ensued. He was very gracious, feigning having been complimented for his youthfulness. The lecture was only memorable for the numerous references he made to me as his "young colleague."

Months later a flyer was posted in our department, advertising a lecture by the same dean of research at Johns Hopkins University whose introduction I had so socially mangled. Here was opportunity. I wondered what he studied, as I couldn't recall anything from the prior lecture I heard him give. Unfortunately, at the time of his lecture things were hectic, and I found myself sprinting down the hall to the auditorium 10 minutes late. No worries; I would duck into the back row, grab a seat, and miss only the lengthy introduction. I reached the large double doors of the unfamiliar auditorium. When I pulled the right door open, it seemed oddly heavy and very slow in opening. It was attached to a hydraulic system that opened and closed both doors in a slow and magnificently dignified manner. As they slowly glided open, I realized, to my chagrin, that I was at, not the back, but the front, of the auditorium, directly behind the speaker! There was no quick closing the door; the mechanism was doing its magnificently slow and stately task. Worse still, the faraway back of the auditorium was crammed. The only open space was a single seat, pinned against the wall in the second row. Reaching it required crawling over an 11-person gauntlet of crowded, glowering attendees. There was nowhere to run, hide, or duck.

Slowly the august dean of research for Johns Hopkins University turned. With just a glimmer in his eye he excitedly remarked, "Paul, I was hoping you'd make it. I was afraid you wouldn't. Hey, you folks in the second row, if you would all stand up, slide over one chair toward the wall, Paul will easily be accommodated." At that point his face broke into the friendliest grin I have ever seen. I took my honored seat. At the lecture's conclusion my fellow residents and even some attending physicians begged me to introduce them to the famous speaker whom I clearly knew so well!

As I reflected on the kindness shown me that afternoon, it seems embarrassment resides only in the mind of the embarrassed. Embarrassment melts away in the presence of genuine care. That care must be what the author of Romans felt when he penned, "For I am not ashamed of the gospel of Christ; for it is the power of God."

Paul Herrmann, LLUSM class of 2000, PhD, is a professor and chair in LLUSM's department of pathology and human anatomy. He and his wife, Sarah, have three sons. Their family enjoys outdoor activities, working on crafts and projects as well as traveling together.

September 29

"Blessed be the God and Father of our Lord Jesus Christ, the Father of mercies and God of all comfort, who comforts us in all our affliction, so that we may be able to comfort those who are in any affliction, with the comfort with which we ourselves are comforted by God." 2 Corinthians 1:3-4, ESV

It was the start of my third-year internal medicine rotation, and I was brimming with excitement as it hit me that I would finally be able to interact with actual human beings instead of just studying eight hours a day!

My first patient, 61 years old, had recently been diagnosed with stage 4 pancreatic carcinoma. This is a devastating diagnosis, as most patients survive only four to six months after diagnosis.

Why did I choose her, out of the 10-plus patients who were available to follow in their care? Honestly, it was because I wanted to witness a miracle of some type. I knew this was selfish, but my faith was already waning, and I needed something to reignite it.

Involvement with a person with metastatic stage 4 cancer and her care would be interesting and challenging in and of itself, but on top of that, her family was unwilling to let her begin hospice. They viewed hospice as a death sentence, and they believed wholeheartedly that she would be healed by a miracle. Because of this, they made her a full code. This resulted in the patient having to stay in the hospital for more than three weeks as her cancer progressed and invaded her GI system, which caused her to bleed. The bleeding required blood transfusions and was followed by an infection in her port-a-cath, which had to be removed. As she continued to deteriorate, she required intubation, and since she was still a full code, she could not go home. Sadly, she died in the hospital.

Yes, it was so frustrating, and emotionally challenging. Imagine coming in every day with your colleague to see her: She would grasp our hands with all of her strength. And day by day you could feel her grip lessen as she began to fade away. But she continued to reach out, hold our hands, and smile at us. After she was intubated and transferred to MICU, we no longer followed her every day; however, we managed to go in to the MICU and see her one more time. She was lying very still as we approached her and held her hands. Her eyes opened and then widened, as she appeared to recognize us: her grasp became stronger. However, being near her wasn't the same this time. She wasn't smiling anymore, and she began breathing harder and harder, although silently because of her endotracheal tube. After following her for three weeks, I could tell she was crying.

The one big "takeaway" message I gained from this experience wasn't about miracles, or whether or not families should be denying hospice to their loved one, or even about home PCA pump insurance policies; rather, it was from something the patient said earlier to us. "Having you around makes this so much easier."

Death is not an easy process. It's one of the most complicated inevitabilities we all have to navigate. Having someone nearby who truly cares is extremely important during a lonely time like this. And instead of focusing our time on all the necessary but time-consuming patient care management tasks such as charting, writing medical orders, and making phone calls, we need to spend a few more minutes at the patients' bedsides, talking to them, getting to know them, and giving them as much support as we possibly can.

Arlin "Larry" Bhattacharjee, LLUSM class of 2019, is a resident in psychiatry at Kaiser Permanente, Fontana, California. He was born in Bangladesh and, at the age of 1, moved to the East Bay with his family. He grew up mostly in Northern California and enjoys fishing, writing, investing, and Korean BBQ.

September 30

> "We are braver and wiser because they existed, those strong women and strong men.... We are who we are because they were who they were. It's wise to know where you come from, who called your name."
>
> Maya Angelou (1928–2014): American author and civil rights activist

One of the most enduring memories and important lessons that I have taken with me over the years since graduating from medical school at Loma Linda is something that took place on the very first day of orientation. As we filed into the large amphitheater, I was trying to take it all in. It was truly hard to believe. I was actually attending an Adventist medical school with 140 medical students in a single class. Nearly all had been valedictorians in high school and had excelled in math and science in the undergraduate years. I would later learn that a third of the students were also accomplished musicians and that many had remarkable experiences in mission service as well. There were some familiar faces that I recognized from my undergraduate years at Andrews University in Michigan, but the vast majority I had never met. We all knew that there was a clear expectation that each of us would process and learn a seemingly impossible amount of complex information at a frenetic pace for a sustained period of time. To make things worse, we would be ranked against each other again and again on every single exam until we graduated. I wondered if any of them shared my growing sense of impending doom.

As I scanned the room, I noted that some of my classmates were of African descent, so I was reassured I would not be completely alone, because I was not quite sure what to expect of my Adventist brethren in this regard. This thinking was an unfortunate legacy from my upbringing in a segregated farming community in the South at a time the country was going through the upheaval of the civil rights movement. Strangely enough, I had never lacked confidence that I would fulfill my dream of becoming a doctor. For reasons I cannot explain, I never experienced any angst about my career path. Even as a child, when asked what I would like to be when I grew up, I always answered, "I'm going to be a doctor." I don't know why this was the case, because at the time there were no doctors in my large extended family.

I was still lost in my thoughts when it suddenly dawned on me that someone I did not know had greeted me by my name as I had walked in. I had responded politely, but now I realized that I did not know who it was. I had never been in Loma Linda or even California before, and I certainly did not know any of the professors. I began asking if anyone knew who it might have been, and quickly discovered that it was Dr. G. Gordon Hadley (CME class of 1944-B), the School of Medicine's dean. The remarkable thing about Dr. Hadley was that his commitment to making each medical student feel like a part of the Loma Linda family went far beyond his call of duty. Each year he would greet each one by name on the first day of medical school. Though he never taught me a single class, each time he would see me in the following years, he would always greet me by name and would frequently mention a personal detail, such as the name of my hometown. It is nice to know that this special memory of Dr. Hadley is one that I share with hundreds of other physicians in practice today. He had the wisdom to realize that a simple act of kindness could make a stranger feel at home. This memory serves as an enduring reminder that our heavenly Father also knows each one of us by name and can hardly wait for us to come home.

Wayne B. Harris, LLUSM class of 1988, is an associate professor of hematology and medical oncology at Emory University in Atlanta. He is currently serving as a member of the board of directors for LLUH.

OCTOBER

○₃ WHOLENESS ℰ○

"Wholeness does not mean perfection;
it means embracing brokenness
as an integral part of life."

PARKER J. PALMER (1939–)
American author, educator, and activist

October 1

> *"Far from being simply the absence of disease, health is a dynamic and harmonious equilibrium of all the elements and forces making up and surrounding a human being."*
> Andrew Weil (1942–): American physician

From my many years of experience as an addictionologist, these are lessons I have learned from impaired physicians: I think all of us can benefit from knowing about these under the heading of whole *personal* care:

1. We all have some kind of personal, emotional, relational issues, as we are all human. None of us has things "all figured out." We can all use help at various stages of our lives and that does *not* mean we are weak, flawed, stupid, or deficient.

2. If we choose to experiment with a mood-altering substance, even for infrequent and sociable reasons, the mind does not know we are doing such with perfectly reasonable motives. The substance still affects our neurochemistry. Some with genetic predispositions can have different, seemingly beneficial effects that lead to ongoing use. Some with traumatic experiences have a beneficial effect that "teaches" the user to keep using. And some by just trying to fit in with their peers and to not seem rigid, moralistic, or unreasonably religious might then develop an ongoing problem because of our genetics or environment. Others begin by taking prescribed benzos or opiates for legitimate reasons then develop tolerance and eventually habituation and difficulty stopping.

3. All physicians (and other professionals) at some point become overwhelmed with the demands of our jobs. We feel we don't know enough, we aren't capable, we're too tired, and we make errors of judgment.

4. There is always a beginning, small at first, undetectable to the self, sometimes quickly, sometimes slowly, progression. One can be in the thrall of the disease and still be a good doctor. Eventually the doctor feels desperate, trapped, and helpless. The overwhelming fear and shame hinder them from asking for help.

5. Help *always* comes from a concerned other. If we wait until they learn their lesson, we wait until their death. Someone other than the afflicted has to make the first move. We are "our brother's keeper," both as colleagues and as protectors of our patient's safety.

6. There is a "state of the art" in dealing with this issue. It is not a black box. There are the mechanisms of a well-being committee at some hospitals, diversion programs at the state level, and treatment programs that treat professionals.

7. The test of when to act is when you are having the internal debate *Should I say or do something? I could be wrong.* Your uncertainty is the proof that the time is *now* to get help—don't agonize or procrastinate!

8. My sickest patients have been professionals and also the recipients of the greatest miracles of recovery of self-respect, safety to practice, regaining others' respect, and having a genuine spiritual renewing experience.

Mickey Ask, LLUSM class of 1979-A, practiced as an addictionologist for 37 years with a special interest in physician well-being. He did not choose to go into this field but rather felt that he was called into it. "I had recently completed an internal medicine residency in 1982 and was wanting to be used in the reorganization of all the preventive medicine entities at LLUH into the Center for Health Promotion. I was asked if I would like to be the medical director of the addiction treatment program. I mused to myself, 'I could do that; I know all there is to know about alcoholics already as all I have to do is give them Librium for 3 days and then discharge them home.' Little did I know back then . . ."

October 2

Our mom was hours away from death on the fifth floor of the west wing of a local hospital on Sabbath, October 30, 1999.

The unique events of that day were recalled and interpreted to me two days later around 3:00 a.m. in a dream by an old American Indian elder after I had prayed for the words for an Indian theme poem for our mom's "going away" (funeral) service. In that dream this elder spoke to me: "Billy, do you remember that day, immediately after your mom told you she loved you, a hawk in a tree outside her hospital window screamed once, at which point she lapsed into a coma? That hawk brought you and your mom a message in the Indian way to let go.

"Your mom obeyed, but you did not, trying to hold on to revive her. Then, Billy, do you remember later that early evening, a faint light was on your mom's face, originating from the now dark western sky? Everyone in that room witnessed that as soon as your mom took her last breath, that light vanished into the evening sky. That light was sent by Grandfather (Creator) to guide your mom's spirit to heaven for safekeeping. Now, wake up and write that poem!" I immediately awoke and wrote the poem as it appears below, based on the actual events of that day that our mom "walked on," as death is sometimes referred to in American Indian culture and as interpreted to me by that elder in my dream.

It Was My Time

It was my time to die; do not feel sad.
I do not feel any more pain, for this be glad.
Today I heard the voice of the eagle in the sky:
"Sister, do not be afraid of death; be brave; do not cry."
Tonight, as I took my last breaths, did you not all see
A light from heaven shining on my face, sent specially for me
To guide my spirit upward for Grandfather to keep.
He felt it was time that I had a long well-deserved sleep.

My frail body will now return to the warm loving arms of Mother Earth,
For I will now complete the circle from where all life has its birth.
So my people, weep for just a little while, for it is true:
Someday soon we will meet again re-created in bodies made new.

That poem represents the circle of life from which we all have in our origins (birth) and our departures (death) from this life here on earth, and also that someday we have that hope to be reunited in immortal, unblemished bodies at the second coming of the Lord.

E. A. "Billy" Hankins, LLUSM class of 1964, PhD, is a retired dermatologist. He is the curator of vertebrate zoology and chief preparator at the World Museum of Natural History, located on the La Sierra University campus in Riverside, California. October 2 is his mother's birthday.

October 3

> *"Life is like riding a bicycle. To keep your balance, you must keep moving."*
> Albert Einstein (1879–1955): German-American physicist

"Holism" and "whole-ism": These are the words I saw and heard from the beginning of medical school in 1978. I often heard from Dr. Wil Alexander* the difference between those two words, his spiritual history-taking, and how some internalize spirituality while others have it as part of the outward "costuming" of their lives. He didn't address how one practices this motto when one's own spiritual rituals are "outward costuming" and not internalized the way most of my classmates and mentors seemed to take for granted.

Exit Loma Linda and enter the real-world practice of medicine as a general internist. Much of it is spent constructing a coherent whole with patients, who have received partial advice from multiple specialists, coming up with a plan that juggles the needs of individual diagnoses to an integrated life. A lot of it is spent listening to patients who in time tell one what's important to them, what needs to work the best, touching them, sharing the fabric of their lives.

Continue to motherhood, where another juggle is balancing the needs of family with the needs of practice, where life is defined as giving urgent attention to the thing that needs it most while queuing up the other urgent things that can wait just a little.

Continue to the love of one's life diagnosed with pancreatic cancer and compressing all the need-to-do, need-to-say things into a few short months while still trying to be there for the practice.

Continue on to reconstructing a solo life that was never wanted. And in this process, I find that the goal, "To make man whole," comes to my aid.

There is nothing that happens to me that hasn't happened to a patient with whom I have shared that challenge in his or her life. Their words come back to me; support me; sustain me. The complex web that is humanity has talked, sung, written, carved or painted the hope that I need to get through the days, weeks, years. "To make man whole"—an ideal yet practical motto for everyday life.

*For Wil Alexander's bio, refer to the devotional on January 18.

Ruth B. Woolcock, LLUSM class of 1982, practices wholistic general internal medicine in the hospital, office, and nursing homes in Indiana, Pennsylvania.

October 4

"See God in every person, place, and thing, and all will be well in your world."
Louise Hay (1926–2017): American motivational author, publisher, and activist

I would like to begin this story with something that everyone who has ever attended a faith-based educational institution can relate to: religion homework. I didn't think long and hard about one of the assigned tasks for "whole person care," one of my favorite medical school classes. A classmate and I were in the hospital looking for a patient who would be willing to talk to us about their life and sources of support, spiritual, or otherwise.

This is how we found Mrs. H, loving wife and mother of two children, who was currently hospitalized for colitis. She was sitting upright in bed, propped up with her massive tote bag, mesmerizing sparkly Christmas-themed manicure, wide awake and happy to talk to us despite being confined to her bed. It didn't take long for us to discover that Mrs. H was not quite as happy as she appeared and that her journey to our hospital was a rocky one. Mrs. H's life revolves around her children. One child struggles with ADHD and depression; the other was born with hypoxic brain injury and has severe neurologic deficits requiring full-time care. Her husband's job requires near-constant travel and she is the linchpin keeping her family together. She had even delayed seeking medical attention for fear that no one would be able to care for her son properly. Then she collapsed at home, and her daughter called for an ambulance. All of her fear and anxiety was completely focused on her children; it was a much heavier burden than her physical pain or any fear she might have for herself. When Mrs. H was finished with her story, she took our hands and thanked us for coming.

We couldn't offer her anything; we didn't have resources to help her situation, we didn't have a cure for her illness, we couldn't bring her children to her, and yet she felt that just by listening to her story and praying with her that we had helped her in some way. We as physicians have the privilege of being permitted into the lives of strangers. It is incredibly humbling to walk with them and to share their burdens for even a short time. I have had many opportunities to see the face of God. If there is one thing that I can say beyond all doubt, it is this: I have never seen the face of God with more clarity than in the faces of my patients.

Victoria "Tori" Burghart, LLUSM class of 2020, is a resident in psychiatry at LLUH. She was born and raised in the Pacific Northwest, where most of her family still live. She is also an artist that runs a medical education instagram @minipsychmd.

October 5

> *"By judging others we blind ourselves to our own evil and to the grace which others are just as entitled to as we are."*
> Dietrich Bonhoeffer (1906–1945): German Lutheran pastor,
> theologian, and anti-Nazi dissident

I remember the first time that I was made aware that I was Black. It was my first year of secondary school in my home country, Trinidad and Tobago. As a former sugar-producing British colony, Trinidad's population is divided evenly between the descendants of enslaved Africans and indentured Indian laborers. The majority of the students at my school were of Indian heritage with Afro-Trinidadians representing 10 percent of the school. One lunch break a few of my classmates thought it necessary to highlight that I had a darker skin tone, a wider nose, and were inferior to them in every way imaginable. My parents weren't doctors or lawyers, so they made it their duty to persuade me that I wasn't good enough to make it—I was Black, poor, ugly, and stupid. Sadly, they made it clear that this was all linked to my being Black.

Years later, during graduate school, I found myself in the midst of racial tension and turmoil in the great USA. This is a part of the U.S. dream that everyone omits; although everyone was created equal, everyone isn't treated as equals. In the wake of the killings of Philando Castile and many others at the hands of police officers sworn to protect them, I found myself once again facing my Blackness. One particular November night I recall having a late night at the laboratory. When I finally finished my tasks, I took off my lab coat and replaced it with a warm hoodie as I braced to face the 50-degree weather. As I walked up to the glass door of Mortensen Hall, my heart broke as I saw my reflection.

For a moment I didn't see the MD/PhD scholar who had spent the day isolating mitochondria from the hearts of transgenic mice in order to explore the mechanism by which my overexpressed protein was protecting the mitochondria from oxidative stress. I didn't see the religious director of the Black Health Professional Student Association who had planned several outreach programs with neighboring churches. I didn't see the church member who had been volunteering with the San Bernardino Community SDA Church and trying to provide the community children there with a positive male role model. Nope, I saw a 6-foot, 200-pound Black man with a hoodie on. And I knew in that moment that anybody who saw me would see that too. That night as I walked back to the student dormitory, I braced the cold night with my hood off, hoping that I could appear less threatening.

It took me several years to accept myself as a Black man. Time spent in God's Word has assured me that I too am fearfully and wonderfully made. My big eyes, wide nose, and broad shoulders are the product of the Master's design, and when He was finished with me, He proclaimed that His creation was very good. I long for the day that everyone who looks at me sees me for who I am—a child of God. I pray that as you interact with others today, you remember that many of our differences are only skin-deep, and while we may be drawn to focus on outward appearances, the Lord looks at the heart.

Shaunrick Stoll, LLUSM class of 2023, earned his PhD with the LLUSM class of 2019. A native of the Caribbean islands of Trinidad and Tobago, Shaunrick spends his free time exploring the lakes and beaches of Southern California. Upon completion of his training, he hopes to serve internationally at one of the Seventh-day Adventist affiliated medical schools.

October 6

"Seek ye the LORD while he may be found, call ye upon him while he is near: Let the wicked forsake his way, and the unrighteous man his thoughts: and let him return unto the LORD, and he will have mercy upon him; and to our God, for he will abundantly pardon." Isaiah 55:6-7, KJV*

My late husband, John, grew up in China during World War II, where the horrors of war plagued him with nightmares and phobias his entire life.

In 1936, when John was just 2 years old, his father had an unusual opportunity to come to America to pursue higher education, so leaving his young family behind, he immigrated to the United States. Shortly thereafter, the Sino-Japanese war broke out. Whenever the siren rang, John's mother would rush John and the rest of the family to the closest bomb shelter. When it was safe to go home, they would walk home along the roads and see dead bodies of young and old that had not made it to the shelter.

John immigrated to the U.S. in 1949. After finishing high school, he attended Emmanuel Missionary College (now Andrews University) in Michigan. While in college he was fascinated with the stories of medical missionaries—David Livingston, who dedicated his life to Africa, and Peter Parker, who served in China during the Qing Dynasty. Most inspiring to him was the medical work of the "China Doctor," Dr. Harry W. Miller. Shortly after completing his medical training at age 23, Dr. Miller went as a medical missionary to China. His patients included indigents on the street as well as famous dignitaries like Generalissimo Chiang Kai-shek and his wife, Madame Chiang (Soong Mei-ling). Dr. Miller was responsible for building 19 hospitals and sanitariums in China, Taiwan, and Hong Kong. He was the hospital director where John's mother and my mother were student nurses. These physician stories inspired John to apply to the College of Medical Evangelists (now LLUSM) to become a physician. After finishing college, he drove from Michigan to California, discovered a new word, "smog," and learned to cope with the summer heat of Loma Linda.

Four years later John received his MD degree, and we were married. Once married, I wondered why he had so many nightmares. One night when I was asleep, we were awakened by an ambulance siren blaring outside. John panicked, pulled my arm, and said, "Quick, run to the bomb shelter. The siren is ringing!" John then hid under the bed. The next morning I noticed that his arms had several scratch marks. I asked him how he had gotten hurt, but he refused to answer me. A few days later he said that when he was under the bed, he couldn't find his way out. He kept crawling toward the wall in darkness and bumped onto the bedposts, which gripped him with fear. The ghosts of war . . .

On October 6, 2016, John took his final breath on this earth. Only Christ's promise of His soon coming gives me the strength and courage to live each day (Psalm 147:3). He heals the brokenhearted and binds up their wounds. I look forward to seeing my dear husband restored completely, where he will be at peace forevermore. And I look forward to hearing John's melodious voice sing in heaven. Even so, come, Lord Jesus!

*This verse was set to a song that John would sing.

Betty Hwang Wang, BSN, RN, and her husband, John (CME class of 1960), raised four children, all of whom became physicians, two of them LLUSM graduates (Marilene Wang and Waylene Wang-Swenson, both LLUSM class of 1986). Two of their grandchildren, Sasha Swenson and WayAnne Watson, graduated from LLUSM class of 2020, and another granddaughter, Shaelyn Swenson, matriculated into the LLUSM freshman class in August 2020. Betty and John made 10 trips to China supporting health centers, nursing homes, and schools.

October 7

> *"Look carefully then how you walk, not as unwise but as wise."*
> Ephesians 5:15, ESV

Originally given to young medical students, these principles hold true for medicine and beyond.

1. Take care of yourself. Sleep. Exercise. A few times a week, do activities you enjoy. If you aren't healthy, your study time won't be efficient, and you will have little to offer patients. Take one day off per week if you can. God didn't do it because He was tired; He did it to exemplify a rhythm that we are to emulate. That one day will change your other six. You will study and work your tail off, but do one thing each day for your physical, relational, and spiritual health. Seek professional help for your mental health if you need it. Many medical students and providers do.

2. Stay positive. There is always something to complain about. Yes, you have to study and work a lot. You know who else works hard? Tons of people. You chose to be here. You are lucky to be here. If you have food in your stomach, a roof over your head, and caring people in your life, then you are ahead of most. Be thankful.

3. Resist comparison. Many of your compatriots will be talented and driven. They've earned their place in medicine. Just like you. Don't be intimidated by the number of publications they have or their 5:00 a.m.-to-midnight study Sundays. Comparison is the thief of joy. Do not look to your left or your right with envy or anxiety. Look up to heaven and fix your eyes on His beauty and grace; then appreciate Him all around you. Recognize your strengths and weaknesses and become the best, most loving version of yourself. The only person that it is helpful to measure against is Jesus. You will realize that you are not perfect, and that's OK, because He is. This will drive you to worship and humility.

4. Beware the aggregate depression. Every medical school in America is hard. Being a doctor is hard. And that's good. It's supposed to be hard. And while grumbling about it is the easiest thing to do, it is neither helpful nor productive. Don't whine.

5. Set boundaries. The work is never done; you will never know all there is to know about medicine. Commit to a time that you will stop studying or working every night. If you do not take precaution, your work will find its way into every part of your life, always demanding more of your attention. Do not grant it such authority.

6. Take moments every day to meditate on the good news. Now, through the Son, you can have a personal relationship with the God of the universe. You are not defined by your successes and failures; you are defined by your kinship with the King of kings. Enjoy that freedom! Love God. Love people. The rest will fall into place.

Kory Markel, LLUSM class of 2021, is incredibly grateful for his time at LLUSM. In his past life he was a whitewater rafting guide and rock climber with his beautiful adventure partner/wife, Paula.

October 8

"Beloved, if God so loved us, we also ought to love one another."
1 John 4:11, ESV

There are experiences that stay with you throughout your life. I remember an encounter I had during my second year of residency training. We had been taking care of a patient who had advanced cancer but was admitted because of an infection. As we treated the infection with antibiotics, it became clear that our patient's body was weak and ravaged by his underlying disease. Recovery was slow and complicated by a process beyond our power. After many discussions with the patient and his family, it was decided to shift our focus toward comfort care. We would no longer focus on the infection or the underlying malignancy. Rather, we would make quality and comfort our goal.

In some cases patients who choose to proceed with comfort measures only are able to go home and spend their remaining time in the company of friends and family in the setting in which they are most comfortable. On some occasions they are too sick, and succumb to their illness in the hospital. This particular patient was in this latter group. After choosing to focus on comfort and quality of life, he soon passed away in the hospital, surrounded by his loved ones.

After receiving the page notifying me of this patient's death, I went to the room for the final death exam. As I stepped into the room the patient's brother noticed me and stood up. He met me halfway across the room and stood right in front of me. Unsure of what to expect, I paused and made eye contact. My gaze was met with a full embrace from my patient's brother. And as his arms hugged me, he whispered, "Thank you."

It took me several years to fully process the events of that day. Initially I was cynical. Thank you? Why would he thank me? I felt like a failure. I had failed to help him fight through the infection. I had failed to get him home to his family. I had failed.

But as time passed and I continued to replay that day in my head, I realized that I was being too myopic. In examining myself as a physician, I was too focused on the disease and the illness rather than on the patient. Throughout my training, from medical school through residency, I had been taught about whole person care—about treating the person and not the disease.

Finally I realized that in that encounter, I was applying whole person care. I was taking care of the patient. I was there for the family. And more important, the family felt I was there for them. They felt cared for. While I couldn't fix the problem, I was able to remain present and walk them through their darkest of days.

If I am "to continue the healing and teaching ministry of Jesus Christ"—"To make [people] whole"—then whole person care needs to be the tool that helps me communicate Christ's love and compassion to each patient I see.

Jeffrey Wonoprabowo, LLUSM class of 2012, is an assistant professor in LLUSM's department of medicine. In his free time he enjoys photography, writing, and exploring locally and abroad with his wife, Allison, and their two children, Faith and Jedidiah.

October 9

Beauty, like a flower on a weed,
like none I had ever seen, met me unexpectedly in the ER today.
She made me uncomfortable
as she talked rapidly, with pressured speech.
I could barely breathe—she reeked of smoke.
One by one she introduced me to her problems,
as if they were each one of her very own children.
None would go missing.
And most frustrating—every "review of system" question I asked
awoke a lengthy story from her distant past.
But I escaped her needy grasp,
back to the safety of my doctor's area to place orders, at last!

Oh, Lord, how often have I missed You . . .
A meeting with God Himself, Almighty, Magnificent.
By my impatience, by shallow judgments?
A benign workup emerged,
and I went back to report great news of discharge.
I mentioned briefly the benefit of smoking cessation.
And to my surprise, something opened up in her . . .
She began to overflow with tears,
crying, even weeping, then smearing her face with an overused paper towel.
"I know I need to quit. It's so hard.
"And I am so weak. I pray every day for the Lord to give me the strength."

In this moment the Lord showed me the beauty.
He is near to the brokenhearted.
Blessed are the poor in Spirit:
for though she had not yet quit, her weakness, like a thorn in her flesh—
it was through this that she knew the Lord,
with a tender intimacy that had me reexamining my own relationship with God.
Through peaceful streams I have carefully navigated my boat
where the water is calm and shallow.

But You, Lord, are well known also,
in the churning storm of illness.
Tossing and turning us until we unquestionably know
the grace of a mighty, undefeated Savior.
And You hear the cries of those stranded in the windless doldrums,
held captive by a merciless addiction:
those who are suffering, and long waiting for Your deliverance.
Oh, how responsive these may be to the slightest of Your winds . . .

My judgments of her fled, and I sensed the Lord's compassion.
We held hands and prayed together. Overwhelmed by God's love, I wept with her.

Continued on lower half of October 10 . . .

October 10

"Come aside by yourselves to a deserted place and rest a while."
Mark 6:31, NKJV

When morning gilds the skies, my heart awaking cries: May Jesus Christ be praised." If anyone else had been nearby in the hills behind Loma Linda, they might have heard me singing these words. But as far as I know, it was just Jesus and me. Each step on the familiar trail led me farther from the frantic pace of life that threatened to squeeze every ounce of peace out of my heart. Up, up, I climbed. Above me stretched a masterpiece of the Creator's beauty—exquisite hues of tangerine, rose, and robin-egg blue, blending into another unprecedented sunrise. The fresh morning air was invigorating. Climbing a little higher, I reached the point where the sun just peeked over the distant mountains, flashing its golden light across the desert slopes. Not too far away the traffic still rushed and the exams still loomed, but in this quiet space with Jesus my heart received peace.

Talking daily with Jesus, claiming promises in His Word, and taking time to listen, I found recharge, refocus, and renewal. During my years in medical school it is this time apart with Jesus that sustained me the most. In this space I received a preparation for each day's challenges and a mindset to share Christ's healing love with my patients. "Amidst the hurrying throng, and the strain of life's intense activities, he who is thus refreshed will be surrounded with an atmosphere of light and peace. He will receive a new endowment of both physical and mental strength. His life will breathe out a fragrance and will reveal a divine power that will reach men's hearts" (Ellen G. White, *The Ministry of Healing*, p. 58).

What about you? Do you need some quiet space with Jesus?

Jonathan Sharley, LLUSM class of 2020, is a family medicine resident at Cahuba Medical Care in Alabama. He looks forward to working as a team with his wife, Melissa, to unite medicine and evangelism and to carry on the legacy of his godly grandfather Dr. Paul Smith (CME class of 1958).

Continued from October 9 . . .

But not for long, for tears made way for healing and laughter.
She flung her arms wide, and we embraced in a hug . . .

My brother, my sister, family of the same Great Father,
I learned never to be led to condescend—
we, who have been so keen to avoid sin.
For Christ came for sinners.
Mercy and compassion must flow from us,
for we don't know, and we must not judge.
That very addiction, illness,
their points of weakness
(which frighten us),
is where His power is made perfect,
and where grace is most abundant.

Christopher Peoples, LLUSM class of 2012, practices emergency medicine in Memphis. He spends his days off eating his wife's delicious homemade cookies and praising the Lord for her great baking skills.

October 11

> *"In the end nothing we do or say in this lifetime will matter as much as the way we have loved one another."*
> Daphne Rose Kingma (1942–): American author and speaker

I sat in the conference room of Megan Hall in a meeting for a newly formed diversity council at Loma Linda University Health, wondering what would be different this time. As an Hispanic female administrator, I had participated in a diversity council several years before remembering that only a few people vented their frustrations but nothing else was accomplished. The chair, Dr. Richard Hart (LLUSM class of 1970), began the meeting with prayer and then led with "LLUH needs to become a place where all individuals feel welcome, accepted, and loved." He proceeded to share the story of his college roommate who is transgender and now lives as a woman. He asked that each council member share their background and why they felt it was important they serve on this diversity council.

As others shared their stories, my mind raced through my various experiences I could present. When my turn came, I said, "I am a third-generation Seventh-day Adventist. My father was an SDA minister, and I grew up knowing that being LGBT+ was not acceptable in God's eyes. When my son was in junior high, he turned to me one day and asked, 'Mom, would you still love me if I told you I was gay?' A few years later my daughter announced she was gay." I sat with this reality as an SDA administrator on the LLUH campus wondering if I could admit this truth to anyone at work. *Would I lose my job? Would I lose friends?* I had been silent for long enough, and that day, sitting on the diversity council and thanks to Dr. Hart, I found the courage to share my realities with a group of 20 leaders.

During the following weeks Dr. Hart wrote a powerful statement about the LGBT+ community and our need to learn all we can. It falls on us to shape our campus in a way that will communicate love and respect for all persons, not just certain groups. Through this experience I have discovered many individuals within the university who have a relative or a friend who are part of the LGBT+ community. I have also learned that secrets separate us and lead to loneliness, sometimes with dire results, while transparency unites us and helps us feel connected and supported. I discovered that the LGBT+ community does not want to be considered a lifestyle; they don't consider it a choice. According to them, they don't choose who they are attracted to any more than heterosexuals do. Instead of sitting in judgment, we need to learn all we can about the LGBT+ community, and more important, we must listen to their stories and get to know them on a personal level.

So when my son asked me so many years ago, "Will you still love me?" I knew at that moment that I could never turn my back on my child. I responded, "There is nothing you can do or say to cause me to love you less; if anything, I will love you more."

Esther Forde, LLUSN class of 1980, held administrative positions in nursing at LLUH for 12 years. In 2006 she transitioned to LLUSD, fulfilling the role as assistant dean for admissions and student affairs. Esther is motivated by encouraging students to pursue their dreams and to find joy in serving others.

October 12

"Ask and it will be given to you; seek and you will find; knock and the door will be opened to you."
Matthew 7:7, NIV

He didn't like seeing doctors, and hadn't seen one in years. The last time he saw one, he was told that he had high blood pressure, diabetes, high cholesterol, and kidney problems, and was advised to go to the emergency department right away for management of his uncontrolled blood pressure. He never went back to see that doctor—or any doctor, for that matter. Yet here he was today, brought in by family because of slurred speech and leg weakness. They were worried he was having a stroke. He confessed that he had been feeling quite poorly for the past few months, with progressively worsening nausea, vomiting, hiccups, itching, fuzzy thinking, generalized weakness, metallic taste, and now slurred speech. He had been taking Advil/Aleve every day for the past 20 years, and felt that it did help a little with his body aches, but finally was starting to realize that his own efforts to manage his health by himself were insufficient. He was found to have profound renal failure and was started on emergent dialysis. Within minutes of being connected to the dialysis machine, he felt immediate relief, and all of his symptoms started to fade away.

Why didn't he seek help sooner? It's true that he didn't have any health insurance, but he was aware of the low cost/no cost county health programs for individuals such as himself who didn't have insurance. The truth was that he didn't feel the need to seek help. He felt that he was able to manage adequately on his own.

Why don't we as imperfect humans seek help from the Great Physician sooner than we do? Pride? Self-sufficiency? Lack of awareness of our situation? We have all the resources we need right in front of us. "Ask, and you will receive; seek, and you will find; knock, and the door will be opened to you" (Matthew 7:7, GNT). The sooner we ask and seek, the better it will be for us.

Aimee Hechanova Rivera, LLUSM class of 2009, currently practices nephrology in Texas, and is associate program director of the Internal Medicine Residency program at Texas Tech University, El Paso. She is married to Donovan Rivera, who graduated from LLUSPH's MBA program.

October 13

> *"I will also give You as a light to the Gentiles, that You should be My salvation to the ends of the earth."*
> Isaiah 49:6, NKJV

I met Watheq on a warm Thursday in my small office in the Northern California town of Grass Valley. Nevada County, where my office is located, is very racially homogenous; largely white. Meeting an Iraqi refugee was quite unexpected.

When I first walked into the room, immediately noticeable was a large scar across the left side of Watheq's face. The scar, however, quickly seemed to disappear behind his warm smile, the kind of smile I'd expect to get from a close friend after a long absence. Watheq was warm, friendly, and extremely polite. However, Watheq had an urgency in his mannerisms. I could tell he was uncomfortable.

It turned out that Watheq had severe reflux because of a moderately large hiatal hernia. We discussed surgery with a sterile clinical focus. Because of his friendliness and politeness, I sensed that Watheq would be an interesting person to get to know. I asked him about his background. He told me that he fled his home country of Iraq around the time of the fighting in Iraq after the September 11, 2001, attacks on the U.S. He told me of the violence there and how he got the scar on his face, but only in vague detail. He left Iraq as soon as he could. In the United States he came to Sacramento to work in the radio business and has a station for Iraqis, or those that speak Arabic.

The day of surgery arrived. In the preoperative area things began as usual—and my usual is to offer to pray with patients before surgery. But something was different this time. I knew that Watheq was Muslim, so I hesitated before offering to pray as I considered whether I, praying to God as a Christian, might offend Watheq. I had decided I wouldn't pray with him, but as soon as I decided against prayer, a very strong voice came into my mind that I must pray with him. I resolved to at least offer prayer. If he declined, I'd immediately drop the idea. I proceeded as usual to explain to him my custom and asked if it would be all right if I prayed. Instead of him refusing, something surprising happened. He immediately became emotional as tears welled up in his eyes. He breathlessly and enthusiastically said that he would love prayer, and that this was the most amazing thing a doctor had ever done for him! We prayed and he immediately expressed the relief he experienced because of the prayer.

The surgery went well and immediately relieved his symptoms—it was the first thing he mentioned the next day when I rounded on him in the hospital. He again expressed that my prayer was one of the most meaningful things anyone had ever done for him. We talked for a while about his faith journey and mine, and he questioned many times how a doctor could also be a "pastor."

And isn't that what medicine is all about, beautifully intertwining the spiritual along with the physical healing? I delighted in telling Watheq of the Great Physician Jesus, who alone can bring true healing to our lives. That Great Physician has given us a high calling, not only to minister to the physical needs of our brothers and sisters, but to offer them so much more: a spiritual ministry. So as we model Jesus, may we be a bright light to all, and pray that we all may be grafted in by His grace.

Stephen Waterbrook, LLUSM class of 2004, is a general surgeon in Kettering, Ohio. This story was written in honor of his wife, Katie, and those affected by breast cancer.

October 14

> *"Three words take on their true meaning when we see them as verbs more than nouns: volunteer, love, God."*
> Sue Vineyard: contemporary American author

It was early evening as I parked and made my way to LLUMC. As a volunteer for the NODA (No One Dies Alone) program, I was familiar with the usual circumstances—a vigil for an elderly patient who has no friends or family to be with them at the end of their life.

I introduced myself to the nurse, who told me that she didn't think the patient had much time left. The sun was setting, and the room was dimly lit as I entered and reached out to touch his weathered hand. "My name is Dale, and I'm going to sit with you for a while," I began. There was no response; no flicker of eyelids or even a twitch of the hand. I continued talking with him as I pulled up a chair and sat down. I knew it was possible that he could hear me, even though he couldn't respond.

The nurse joined me in the room to let me know that it was nearing the end of her shift. In about 30 minutes she would give her report and then head home. She explained to me that the patient's family was on their way from the East Coast but wasn't likely to make it in time. I asked if there was any information about his religious background on the chart, and she shared that he was of the Jewish faith.

Not knowing a lot about this faith, I did a quick Internet search and found an article by a Jewish rabbi explaining the prayers and rituals that are sometimes performed at the time of death. I showed the instructions to the nurse and she printed a copy for me. "Let me give my report, and I will come back. We can do this together."

The first was a prayer to be said by the patient, but since he wasn't able, I said the prayer for him. The patient's breathing was shallow and irregular. According to Jewish tradition, during the actual dying stage no one is allowed in or out of the room. The patient's feet must point to the door and a candle lit and placed near his head. The nurse made sure no one entered the room, and we positioned the patient accordingly. Since we didn't have a candle, we used a picture of a candle on our phone. While the nurse and I read the second prayer that was listed, the patient quietly took his last breath. We covered his body with a sheet in accordance with the rite, and we said our goodbyes.

I gathered my things and headed for my car, grateful that I had been able to be on holy ground once again.

Dale McGrosky is the vice president of Satori Seal Corporation. In his free time, he enjoys giving back to the community through volunteering. He started as a youth counselor and then became a teacher for the next 18 years. In 2008 Dale started volunteering at LLUCH in childlife on the oncology unit and as a NICU snuggler holding many of the unit's special babies. In October 2009, when the NODA (No One Dies Alone) program began, he signed up immediately as one of LLUMC's first volunteers. In his off time he can be found on the trails mountain biking, hiking, or camping.

October 15

> *"Behold, I will do something new, now it will spring forth; will you not be aware of it? I will even make a roadway in the wilderness, rivers in the desert."*
> Isaiah 43:19, NASB1995

"And what if a thousand sleepless nights are what it takes to know You're near?" (Laura Story, "Blessings").

On the evening of October 14, 2013, I went into labor with our first child. Excited, scared, and nervous, my husband, Nick, and I drove to LLUMC. Twelve hours later my precious little girl, Emily, lay on my chest, looking up at me with dark steel-blue eyes. But I couldn't focus on her. The physician and resident worked at the end of the bed for what seemed like ages, sewing up the third-degree tear I had suffered. In much pain, physically and mentally spent, I remembered the events from the night before.

Emily's heart rate dropping at 2:00 a.m.
Emergency team arriving.
Flying down the hallway to the surgical suite.
Ultrasound on my belly.
Listening to Emily's heart rate stabilize.
Nick in a yellow "bunny" suit, standing outside the door.
Waiting.

And then it was over. After wheeling me back to my room, the emergency team trickled out until it was just Nick and me, and the familiar whoosh of our baby girl's heart.

This experience became a major cause of the postpartum depression I suffered for a year and a half after Emily's birth. During this time I struggled to stay alive, let alone take care of Emily. I blamed much of how I felt on my husband, but mostly I blamed God. I pounded my fist into the floor of our daughter's room, feeling abandoned and alone.

"We cry in anger when we cannot feel You near.
We doubt Your goodness, we doubt Your love..."

I abandoned God in return, avoiding church and discussions of His love and mercy, ultimately letting my spiritual life fall by the wayside.

It wasn't until the summer of 2016 that I saw God again for who He really is—loving, kind, gracious, and beautiful. I realized He had walked beside me through my entire experience. He never abandoned me; never left me to flounder. I finally began to understand that God uses our difficult experiences to bring us toward Him, if we let Him. Now when I hear the song again, the last line turns my experience around completely:

"What if trials of this life,
The rain, the storms, the hardest nights,
Are Your mercies in disguise?"

I may doubt His love in the future. In fact, it's probably a given. But I will also cling to the promise in Isaiah 43:19, HCSB, where God says: "Look, I am about to do something new; even now it is coming. Do you not see it? Indeed, I will make a way in the wilderness, rivers in the desert." He is working in my life, and He is working in yours. Do you not see it?

Ruth Will is a stay-at-home mom of two very beautiful and silly children, Emily and Peter. She lives in Vancouver, Washington, with her wonderful and handsome husband, Nick (LLUSM class of 2015). Ruth enjoys doodling, perusing fine literature, and wrangling the kids on a day-to-day basis. She feels blessed to have survived postpartum depression and makes it her mission to regularly check in on new moms.

October 16

"Therefore humble yourselves under the mighty hand of God, that He may exalt you in due time, casting all your care upon Him, for He cares for you."
1 Peter 5:6-7, NKJV

Urgent care is not a place for chronic conditions. Nowhere in the name is the word "chronic" found. Occasionally, however, chronic conditions need urgent care.

At 30 years of age, Esteban has chronic sinusitis and chronic anxiety, and the two conditions make a real acute couple. He lacks the health insight to understand his symptoms or stick to a treatment plan.

When Esteban feels good (no panic attacks, no sinus symptoms), he stops all his SSRIs and his nasal steroid spray. Then he is soon alarmed as his symptoms spiral out of control. The nasal congestion triggers panic attacks and insomnia and racing fears of strokes or heart attacks, and Esteban "casts" about, searching urgently for care.

An urgent care.

MY urgent care.

My colleagues groan when his name pops up on the schedule, but he doesn't worry me. I've dealt with Esteban for years; I'm familiar with his tactics and fears, and we've built a decent "connection," of sorts. It definitely helps that I can speak Spanish with him, interpreter-free. (¡Mil gracias, madre!) So I always pick up his chart with a smile as my colleagues visibly wilt with relief.

I don't mind our predictable circular 20-minute conversations: me advising ENT evaluation and medication compliance, him regaling me with WebMD search results. During these wandering encounters, I've explored Esteban's social support network (lousy), his living situation (impoverished), and his spiritual beliefs (flickering but alight). At his last visit, we even prayed together. (Rest well, Wil Alexander,* your legacy lives on....)

But today's chief complaint is ... unusual. Even for Esteban.

"Not feeling sick, wants to discuss upcoming surgery."

(My initial reaction? "Somebody tell him this is an urgent care, not a 'surgent' care.")

In the exam room Esteban stammers and delays, anxious but with purpose: "I'm going to get that sinus surgery next week, just as you recommended, Doctor. I'm just ... nervous about it. And I remembered how you prayed with me before, and that really calmed me down. So, I was hoping that ... you would ... you know ..."

We pray together—for his courage, the surgeon's skill, outcomes and recovery, and pain control. I pray for Esteban to rest in God's will. He smiles, shakes my hand, and leaves. My colleagues are in shock—a five-minute visit with Esteban? Inconceivable. The urgent care is not a place for chronic conditions. But everywhere should be a place for whole person care.

And today, in my urgent care (and through my mother, Wil Alexander, and myself), God cared for Esteban.

*For Wil Alexander's bio, refer to the devotional on January 18.

Austin Bacchus, LLUSM class of 2004, completed his residency at LLUH family medicine, and now works in urgent care in Wisconsin. He operates a free Christian book ministry (RXF1888.com) with his wife, Marie-Lys. They homeschool their two boys.

October 17

> *"Iron sharpens iron, so one man sharpens another."*
> **Proverbs 27:17, NASB**

Proverbs 27:17, ERV, says, "As one piece of iron sharpens another, so friends keep each other sharp." It reminds me of my three very best friends from Washington Adventist University in Maryland. We met while playing in the university orchestra, and traveled around the world together with the group. I often wonder what brought us together. We played different instruments, we came from different parts of the country, and we had never met before college. Then I read Proverbs 27:17. One of best things about my friends is that they are intelligent and challenge me; they keep me sharp. We love spending time together on an intellectual and creative level. Since college, for more than 20 years now, we have dedicated spending time with each other at least once a year. We call it our annual "beach week," since that is where we love to spend most of our time.

This verse also reminds me of *The 7 Habits of Highly Effective People*, by Stephen Covey. According to Covey, it means having a balanced program for self-renewal in the four areas of your life: physical, social/emotional, mental, and spiritual. Examples he lists are:

Physical: beneficial eating, exercising, and resting

Social/Emotional: making social and meaningful connections with others

Mental: learning, reading, writing, and teaching

Spiritual: spending time in nature, expanding spiritual self through meditation, music, art, prayer, or service

This sounds a lot like Loma Linda University Health's focus on whole person care! He goes on to say that feeling good doesn't "just happen." Living a balanced life means taking the necessary time to renew yourself. I thank God every day for my amazing friends, who help me sharpen my saw in this manner and who dedicate at least one time a year to connect.

One of the most important things you can do to live a great life is to surround yourself with friends who will sharpen your saw. I hope that you will continue to challenge yourself intellectually, take time out to practice whole person care, connect with others and seek to become more like God every day.

Excerpts taken from https://www.stephencovey.com/7habits/7habits-habit7.php.

Karen Studer, LLUSM class of 2010, LLUSPH MPH 2003, MBA 2017, is an assistant professor and residency program director in LLUSM's department of preventive medicine. She also teaches in LLUSPH. She enjoys spending time with her family and continues to meet at least yearly with her best friends from Washington Adventist University.

October 18

*"He will cover you with his wings; you will be safe in his care;
his faithfulness will protect and defend you."*
Psalm 91:4, GNT

One of the most humbling aspects of medicine is caring for patients who are at the weakest and most vulnerable times of their lives. While this may be just another septic shock admission in the eyes of the overworked medicine intern, this is the scariest infection ever in the eyes of the sick patient. It is easy to lose sight of these patient perspectives in the midst of long days on a medical service.

As a third-year medical student I cared for an elderly woman who was hospitalized in inpatient psychiatry for electroconvulsive therapy (ECT) for her major depression. She was a frail, withdrawn patient who didn't often interact with the medical staff and never had any visitors. After prerounding on her every day for several weeks, she took a liking to me and we had awesome conversations on topics ranging from dream vacations to hero dog stories. I looked forward to seeing her every morning, but unfortunately she remembered me only on days that she was not receiving her ECT treatment, because she had severe postictal amnesia. Despite this, I patiently introduced myself every day and watched as her mood and anxiety slowly improved with each treatment.

As my month-long psych rotation came to a close, my amnesic patient was still hospitalized, so I warned her on a nontreatment day that I will no longer be checking in on her every day. She was sad, but she understood and wished me well. My last day on the service was an ECT day, and I checked on my friend one last time, hoping by some miracle she may remember me. She didn't, but at the end of our conversation I mentioned once again that I was leaving, and her eyes immediately filled with tears as she whispered, "Will I be alone then?" I quickly assured her that she is never alone, that Someone is watching over her every second of every day.

Our patients need more than medical healing; they want to be unafraid in a life that often is scary and lonely. We must not forget to share these promises of love and hope with each and every one of our patients.

Jennifer Pauldurai, LLUSM class of 2018, is an adult neurology resident at George Washington University Hospital in Washington, D.C. When she is not working, she enjoys meeting different people, exploring new countries, and playing with her pet Pomeranian.

October 19

> *"Joy does not simply happen to us. We have to choose joy and keep choosing it every day."*
>
> Henri Nouwen (1932–1996): Dutch Catholic priest, professor, writer, and theologian

He wasn't a religious man, that he made clear, but he seemed to have what he needed. His wife, his son, an unbroken sense of humor: three pillars of strength, a refuge from which he faced the unknown time ahead. It could be months, weeks, perhaps days now. The doctor said, "Two weeks," if he left the hospital untreated, and that was four days ago, but maybe the chemo would offer more time. So he sat, with all the tubes and wires that had been jabbed inside him, on the top floor of the cancer ward.

His hair was a grizzled gray, matted into locks that fell diagonally down his forehead. His skin was worn but still colored with life. I could see he had been here awhile, more than just a day or so, and he confirmed this. It was Friday, and he entered Monday after feeling progressively weaker for two months.

"I got a big three-story house"—he became wide-eyed and waved his hands to emphasize its great height—"and I knew sumthin' was wrong when I couldn't get up those stairs."

He told me the story of his illness. The weakness began on Thanksgiving, but soon left him nearly motionless. He felt unable to move, as if he were cinched tightly to his bed by some invisible belt or strap. There was also his warm skin and the feeling of burning at one moment and freezing the next. He had a fever, yes, but this one felt different. Maybe he needed a doctor. It was the day after his hospital admission that he learned this was different, and he did need a doctor. This was leukemia.

As we talked, I was increasingly intrigued—this man spoke without worry or grief or frustration. Sadness and confusion, of course, but none of the previous. He spoke more of his pillars. The presence of his wife and son, and the sweet time he still had with them. Also the hospital staff, a group of whom he said was "professional and nice, with a great sense of humor."

A great sense of humor—important at a time like this? I was baffled. I knew I'd be told to understand him by putting myself in his shoes, but slipping into his shoes led only to more confusion. Would I be willing to laugh with only weeks to live? I didn't know the answer.

Some of my perplexity must have come from the knowledge that this man was not religious, while I was. For him there were no pearly gates, no Deity, no loved ones awaiting him. All that he had, or ever would have, was with him presently. But maybe this was why he could laugh—his pillars. Maybe he didn't need religion, or at least religion as many people think of it, because he already possessed much of the truth it offers. He had community and love in his wife and his son. Joy and laughter, despite fear and pain, in his commitment to stay humorous and lighthearted. He had what he needed, what each of us need, to begin to let go.

"Have any favorite jokes or comedians?" I asked before leaving.

"Nope, just love bein' difficult." He chuckled and said goodbye.

Zachary Reichert, LLUSM class of 2020, is an emergency medicine resident at LAC+USC Medical Center in Los Angeles, California, and continues to be motivated by the opportunity to meet and interact with the many patients he sees daily.

October 20

"I counsel you to buy from me gold refined by fire, so that you may be rich, and white garments so that you may clothe yourself and the shame of your nakedness may not be seen, and salve to anoint your eyes, so that you may see."

Revelation 3:18, ESV

The air was piercingly crisp, the trees were exquisitely green, the sky was serenely blue, the sun was terribly bright, and I had been awakened from a deep slumber.

It was during the second year of medical school that I reached the lowest point of my life. I cried long and hard, but did not shed another tear for three years. I did not understand that I was losing the ability to feel. And with that loss went my hope for anything I had ever wanted in life: a family, a fulfilling career, and a vision for the future. Instead, I was a prisoner of the present: long days of endless studying, subpar exam scores, and fading hopes and dreams.

The last thing to go was my belief. While I continued to attend church and even to lead worship, my mind and heart began to accept that God did not exist.

After the battle of USMLE Step 1 and a long-anticipated outward liberation, I began to perceive an inward emotional captivity. My body deeply felt this confinement, but would not accept it as a permanent sentence. As it desperately struggled for life, I experienced an acute vertigo attack that left me incapacitated for three days and seasick for a month. I took no time off of my rotations, however, because I was determined to stay on a one-track academic train with no stops.

It was in this valley of despair that I wrote the following words: "In Your arms I rest. Give me new eyes, renew my mind, take my life. I want to know Your heart."

A year later the words became a song I wrote with my close friend, Adam Bussey (LLUSM 2019). And although my heart did not believe them, it wanted to. Two years later, during my first year of residency, I experienced a life-changing event that brought unforeseen yet overwhelming victory to my life. I was emotionally set free and delivered from a lifelong struggle with anxiety. It felt irrational but was profoundly transformational. My outer and inner worlds were now united in a frightening yet ravishing existence.

Paradoxically, it was at this point that things started to make sense. I realized I had come to think that faith and feeling contradicted each other. What I had not previously considered was that faith could literally become a new way of feeling. It was only when my heart and mind were united in admitting their captivity that they were able to be delivered.

The complexity here is that this spiritual captivity is not readily apparent. It is unseen. But it is only as I recognize that I am wretched, pitiful, poor, blind, and naked that I can experience the hope and love that is offered by an infinite Beauty.

My prayer is that our faith would become a feeling that can be experienced, embraced, and cherished for eternity.

Joshua Wendt, LLUSM class of 2018, served as chief resident of the family medicine residency program at LLUH. He is currently an attending physician in the LLUH family medicine department. He is from Modesto, California, and enjoys music production, classical guitar, cycling, basketball, running, hiking, skiing, and beatboxing.

October 21

> *"But as for you, be strong and do not give up, for your work will be rewarded."*
> 2 Chronicles 15:7, NIV

Why would she keep seeing me? During my second week back from maternity leave, already 45 minutes behind, I quickly reviewed the next chart, a breast cancer survivor. She had been seen for shoulder and hip pain three times in the past four months, prescribed opiates each time. She was coming in today for the same concern.

"Knock, knock, I'm so sorry. Thank you for waiting for me." A carefully honed entrance, she was no longer annoyed about the wait, especially since we had some catching up to do. She told me about her grandson and the experiences she won from radio contests; I showed her a half dozen pictures of my baby, all in the same pose. She then started to tell me about her concerns and I quickly realized that this was not a chronic opiate visit, but one that was much more alarming. I refilled her medications and, as a parting gift, X-rays and a hug. The results came back at 4:58 p.m., just 17 minutes before I was due to pick up my son from day care. Wondering why these things happen to good people and, selfishly, why I returned to work, I said a silent prayer asking for the strength to make a difficult phone call. I told her the news. I told her I ordered further imaging. I told her she needed to see her oncologist. In the end, she thanked me for calling and listening to her concerns.

She returned a couple of months later to update me with her diagnosis—recurrent breast cancer, metastatic. She told me that she would not proceed with chemotherapy. She was taking the palliative route, focusing on living life to its fullest. I told her that I would support her in any decision that she made and that if she needed anything, all she had to do was ask. I gave her a hug and told her that she could follow up with me as needed. I did not see her again for a couple of months. I sent a couple of messages here and there, asking how she was doing; I just wanted to let her know that I was thinking about her. But one day she was on my schedule for a physical, a wellness exam.

A wellness exam in a patient with metastatic breast cancer? Counseling her on osteoporosis and colon cancer screening seemed like a moot point. I am not an oncologist. I am not a radiation oncologist. I'm not a surgical oncologist. I am family medicine. "Knock, knock, I'm so sorry. Thank you for waiting for me." We started our visit with a hug; she said she did not have any concerns. She just wanted to have a reason to see me and update me about her cancer journey. We talked about her pain control and upcoming trip to the Grand Canyon. She asked about my son. It was a lovely day that focused on emotional wellness. We wrapped up the visit with well wishes, her giving me parental advice and me giving her reassurance that I will always be here for her.

The struggle of balancing medicine and motherhood can be overwhelming. Medicine wins some days; motherhood wins the others. But I remember this patient, and she is the reason I continue to do this dance. I try to give my all to patients because on those days, when I cannot be the all for my son, I need to be able to tell him that it was for a good reason: to care for others. I am a mother, and I am family medicine.

Van Nguyen is assistant professor in LLUSM's department of family medicine. She is married to Larry Ngo, a neonatologist at LLUCH. They have their hands full with an energetic 3-year-old son, Liam, and sweet 1-year-old twin boys, Connor and Nolan.

October 22

"The person who has seen me has seen the Father!"
John 14:9, NET

Stepping into the exam room, I saw an elderly couple. She met my greeting with silence, but her silence opened the door for her husband to share his concern for his wife, whom he obviously adored. He was worried about her increasing despondency and depression. She continued to sit in silence as he talked in spite of my attempts to engage her in conversation. Finally I asked, "Marion, when did you last feel happy?"

"Once last year," she said with the hint of a smile and eyes brightening.

"What happened last year?"

"I went on a hot-air balloon ride!" As she described a harrowing sideways landing in unexpected high winds, she was giddy with excitement. It was the first sign of a breakthrough in our visit.

Trying to reach another level of understanding about her life I inquired about her interests, family, and whether faith had ever been part of her life. She talked of activities she really didn't enjoy anymore, and then announced that they had been churchgoing people earlier in their lives, but had become disillusioned. "We just could not believe in a God that would want bad things to happen," she said, reliving the common response after tragedy that it was God's will.

"I don't believe in that kind of God either," I replied. "What about Jesus?"

"Jesus was real! He was loving and did good things." This strong perceived separation and contrast between an arbitrary God and a loving Jesus was at the core of her disbelief. She was now obviously engaged in our conversation, so when I reminded her of the text in John where Jesus told His disciples that if they had seen Him, they had seen the Father she thoughtfully responded, "I've never thought about that before. If God is like Jesus, then I could believe in Him."

Our visit ended with standard medical diagnostic assessments and treatment recommendations, but with the added benefit of having addressed something perhaps even more important for her. It was a privilege to pray with this precious couple to a God who was made known through His Son, Jesus, whom Marion already appreciated. She was visibly more pleasant and open. Her husband was obviously feeling some relief. I was grateful once again for my medical training in a place where addressing the whole person is at the core of medical practice—where presenting the beauty of God's love is what we do! I'm thankful that they received this added and essential spiritual dimension of care as we dealt with her medical diagnosis of depression.

When the disciples questioned Jesus about the Father, Jesus responded, "The person who has seen me has seen the Father." His response continues to echo down through the ages through human hands led by Him to touch the lives of hurting people today. Marion felt that touch!

Roger D. Woodruff, LLUSM class of 1981, is an associate professor and chair in LLUSM's department of family medicine. Through teaching and example, his mentors and faculty at LLUSM showed him the power of integrating spiritual care with excellent medical diagnosis and treatment, a practice that has enriched his life and the lives of his patients over the years.

October 23

> *"The LORD is near to all who call on him, to all who call on him in truth."*
> Psalm 145:18, ESV

There are few other days young eye surgeons in training look forward to more than the day they perform their first cataract surgery from start to finish. Many ophthalmology residents will tell you that witnessing that first cataract surgery was the moment that sparked the desire to pursue an ophthalmology residency.

I spent many hours practicing to prepare for that first case. Yet despite all those hours in the lab and despite the calm voice of my attending guiding each step while I operated, those first dozen surgeries working inside a real human eye were relatively terrifying. Every resident knows what stands between a successful result and a more tenuous outcome is their ability to dissect the cataract out of the membrane that encapsulates it. At only four micrometers thick, it can easily be torn. I had never felt the need to elicit divine help more than I did for those first few months of performing surgery inside the eye.

What was less certain to me, at first, was if I should tangibly involve my patients in that divine petition by offering a word of prayer with them prior to surgery. I was no longer in a faith-based hospital system like Loma Linda, so how would folks respond? Would they take offense? I ultimately decided that I couldn't afford not to pray, and it has now become part of my pre-op routine. Leaning over the bedside after I've finished the consent, I ask each patient, "Would you mind if I prayed with you before surgery?" I usually get a big smile, a nod, and frequently I will feel their hand clasp mine as I bow my head. I ask that God will guide the hands of all of us in the operating room, that the surgery will be successful, and that the patient will have a smooth recovery. The nursing staff and anesthesia personnel, unprompted, pause to gather around the bedside and offer a few soft amens. Then we are off, and the procedure is shortly underway.

Anyone involved in eye care knows how rewarding it can be to remove that eye patch after surgery and celebrate improved sight with your patient. What I didn't anticipate, however, was how frequently patients thanked me for that bedside prayer. "Doc, I was so nervous before surgery, but as soon as you prayed, I felt peace" has been a common theme. One patient, after successful surgery, confided in me that he had been so nervous about any procedures that he had prayed for several years that God would miraculously remove his cataracts. He told me that because I had prayed, he knew God had sent him "one of His doctors" to help restore his vision in a direct answer to his prayer of the past few years. I've begun to pray before trauma cases, too. I prayed with a large family surrounding the bedside of a 4-year-old boy whose right eye had been badly damaged during a car accident. Following repair of the large ocular laceration, I gathered the family again, admitting that I didn't know how much vision he might regain. With tears in his eyes the father gave me a big hug and said, "As soon as you prayed, I knew we had come to the right hospital. Our boy's sight is in God's hands now." I am continually amazed at the faith of my patients and how prayer gives me a glimpse into the depth of that faith.

No, prayer doesn't ensure a perfect outcome. I've certainly had some imperfect results. But Psalm 145:18, ESV, says that "the LORD is near to all who call on Him." Prayer ensures that His presence draws near to us as we strive to make men and women whole again. I know I'll need that presence in my clinic and my operating room for the remainder of my career.

Matthew Hartman, LLUSM class of 2015, completed an ophthalmology residency, followed by a cornea fellowship. He lives in Nashville, Tennessee, with his wife, Elisabeth, and two boys. Connecting in meaningful ways with patients and helping improve their vision keeps him challenged and motivated.

October 24

"But when Jesus heard that, he said unto them, They that be whole need not a physician, but they that are sick. But go ye and learn what that meaneth, I will have mercy, and not sacrifice: for I am not come to call the righteous, but sinners to repentance."

Matthew 9:12-13, KJV

When I started my week on addiction medicine at the Jerry L. Pettis Memorial Veterans Medical Center as part of my junior psychiatry rotation, I was told I would be spending the week attending counseling groups for those undergoing intensive outpatient treatment for long-standing addictions. Initially I didn't know what to make of sitting through hours of meetings. However, it was extremely educational and a great opportunity for me to reflect as I came face to face with the horrors many of our veterans have gone through defending our country. Many of them had unthinkable stories of trauma they had seen and experienced. For them, alcohol and drugs were the best coping mechanism they could find to escape these horrors. For others, it was a distraction from the boredom of military life. Many of them were traumatized by combat experiences, and the resulting drug and alcohol abuse often caused them to do other things they later regretted. Hearing the struggles that so many of my patients were going through was very revealing, as I began to see the underlying issues and stories that had caused these addictions we were treating.

During the same week we were also asked to attend an Alcoholics Anonymous meeting, Narcotics Anonymous meeting, and an Al-Anon meeting for relatives of alcoholics. What struck me from these meetings was the supportive atmosphere for listening to people's stories. Many of the attendees stated that their addictions and resulting behavior had caused loss of relationships and stigmatized them. However, they loved the fact that no matter what their past was like, they could go to a meeting and feel supported and loved and not judged. Initially, I felt awkward sitting through these meetings since it was obviously geared for recovering addicts and I don't know personally what it is like to suffer from severe addiction, but the attendees made us feel extremely welcome. One of the attendees told me that when he was undergoing inpatient addiction treatment at our facility, he really appreciated our team's empathetic and nonjudgmental care for him despite his past life and addiction.

From my experience I realized that what my patients suffering from addictions really need is someone to listen to their stories and see them as humans, just as we are. Jesus during His ministry spent much of His time with tax collectors, prostitutes, and other marginalized people of society. Despite their past and how they were perceived by the world, He saw every person as an individual deserving of His grace and mercy. People who suffer from addictions need the same love, support, and compassion that all my other nonaddiction patients deserve. By dining with tax collectors and sinners, Christ showed us that these people had value to Him and that He was willing to show it to everyone around Him. As Christian physicians we have the opportunity through our actions and words to show God's healing love toward people who are in brokenness.

David Eng, LLUSM class of 2019, served as a class senator his junior and senior class years of medical school. He currently is an internal medicine resident at University of California, Irvine Medical Center. He is the oldest of 10 homeschooled children, all of whom are entering health care related fields. His dream is to go on medical mission trips with his family, using their skills to further Jesus' healing and teaching ministry.

October 25

> *"So we fix our eyes not on what is seen, but on what is unseen, since what is seen is temporary, but what is unseen is eternal."*
> 2 Corinthians 4:18, NIV

In Michael Rosen's and Helen Oxenbury's children's book *We're Going on a Bear Hunt*, five children along with their dog go out to hunt a bear. In order to reach the cave where the bear lives, they must face tall grasses, a river, and even a snowstorm. When encountered with each daunting task, the children recite the following phrase regarding the obstacle before them: "We can't go over it. We can't go under it. Oh, no! We've got to go through it!" One after another, the children manage to overcome the challenges and make it to the cave.

Like the children in the story, we all come across obstacles of varying degrees that need to be dealt with on this journey we call life. For me, one of my biggest struggles to date began shortly after commencing medical school.

A few weeks into our fall quarter I began to experience symptoms of anxiety, burnout, and depression. Unfortunately there is a stigma associated with mental health, which made it harder for me to deal with the situation when it came into my life. Instead of reaching out for help, my attitude toward those around me changed as I slowly began to push away the people I once confided in. I tried to go through the motions on my own by putting on a facade that masked my private anguish for the months to come. In my isolation, I ended up benching God to the sidelines while I attempted to be my own savior.

My moment of realization came one sleepless night when I reached for my phone, searching for a distraction. There was one notification on my lock screen from the Bible app containing the verse of the day, 2 Corinthians 4:18, NIV: "So we fix our eyes not on what is seen, but on what is unseen, since what is seen is temporary, but what is unseen is eternal." It was at that moment, when my defenses were down and I was the most vulnerable, that I heard God whisper: "You are not alone." All this time I had attempted everything in my power to get through this circumstance to no avail. I'd tried going over the problem; I'd tried going under the problem. And there was only one way left. With courage from above, I reached out to the school administration and received the help I desperately needed, at just the right time.

We all have those challenges in our life that need conquering. When faced with such tasks, we take a step back and attempt to come up with a brilliant solution for our problem. "We can't go over it. We can't go under it." Stumped and distraught we focus on our past failures and accept defeat, forgetting the existence of a third option that will get us to the other side. It is often at our most vulnerable moment that God comes along, lovingly takes our hand, and says: "Well, looks like we've got to go through it!"

Randy Sanchez, LLUSM class of 2022, enjoys spending time with close friends and family while also attempting to pick up new musical instruments; he's currently learning to play the guitar.

October 26

"Trust in the LORD with all thine heart; and lean not unto thine own understanding. In all thy ways acknowledge him, and he shall direct thy paths."
Proverbs 3:5-6, KJV

In 2017 my husband of nearly 29 years passed away suddenly from a rare reaction to his targeted therapy for stage 4 lung cancer. When he first responded to his targeted therapy, he was able to continue enjoying life with our three kids. So when we discovered that his cancer had spread three years later and he was changed to a newer drug, we never thought that two months later his lungs would react so violently to his medication that I would have to hold his hands and hug my children as we said farewell to each other.

As a physician losing my husband to illness, I questioned everything. I had thoughts of why I had not been able to pick up on his various symptoms. I prayed all the time, but I was not sure I could really hear God through all of this.

One month after my husband's death, I was in clinic when God came to me. My first patient of the day was a man I had treated for a few years. He expressed his condolences and asked how I was holding up. I told him that I was OK—that I was thankful I had God to lean on. He told me that his sister had lost her husband to cancer recently and that she had struggled with why God had taken her husband. He said that she had found a book, *Through the Eyes of a Lion*, that helped her accept his passing as part of God's love. I read it from cover to cover the next week, and it brought me peace and understanding.

My second patient was an older man who was solemn and expressed his condolences. I told him I was OK and trying hard to heal. He then proceeded to tell me that a year earlier he had lost his sister to lung cancer. At the end the lung cancer had spread to her brain, and surgery had been performed. After coming home from her surgery, she never recovered. Her first weeks were extremely difficult, but she was able to communicate. By the third week she was in and out of consciousness, and finally passed away. He said that he realized that the surgery had not worked. What he told me was an answer to one of my questions: Should we have been more aggressive? Should we have tried surgery, or more medicines? God sent this patient to answer my burning questions.

My third patient was a woman I had seen once. She expressed her condolences and said that she had lost her first husband to cancer that had spread to his lungs. Her husband had become oxygen-dependent, and it had been difficult on her younger son, a high school senior. Her husband had asked their son to attend a local college so he could look after my patient after his passing. My patient wished that her younger son had gone away to college, because by being home he had been unable to grieve completely. Her other son had attended an out-of-state college and had been able to grieve. God had heard my prayers. Part of my anguish was whether we should have pushed for more treatment and maybe my husband could have been home on oxygen. My patient's words told me that that would not have been my husband's wishes. During this time my younger son, who was at college, had been asking me if he should attend a local school. I had struggled with what to tell him except that I didn't think it was a good idea. Now I could tell him that it would not have been a good idea. God had sent my patients to heal us. He heard my cries, prayers, and questions, and answered them in a way that a physician would hear.

Bonnie Chi-Lum, LLUSM class of 1991, is an associate professor in LLUSM's department of preventive medicine and chief medical officer at SAC Health System. She was married to her physician husband, Daniel Lum (LLUSM class of 1987). They have three children, Geoffrey (LLUSM class of 2023) and twins, Joshua and Kalisa (LLUSM class of 2025).

October 27

"Come to me, all you who are weary and burdened, and I will give you rest."
Matthew 11:28, NIV

In 1974, shortly after starting at LLUSM as a new freshman, I had the opportunity to shadow a senior student nearing graduation. He took me with him to a SAC clinic in Redlands. One patient we saw that evening was a middle-aged female still in her clinical garb from work. She presented with abdominal pain. After history and exam, the senior clinician advised an antacid for an upper GI tract linked epigastric pain. Later in the evening another "clinician" from the department of religion, Dr. Wil Alexander,* gave us quite an "expanded" history that we had failed to obtain. He reported how her son was hooked on street drugs and her husband was incarcerated, and it was insightful to me how the sympathizing ear he offered revealed more of what was likely the crux of her physical problems.

Harrison Evans (CME class of 1936), former chair LLUSM's department of psychiatry, in his lecture to us on depression, opened the lecture sharing from the classic on whole person care, *The Ministry of Healing*, by Ellen G. White (published in 1905), from the chapter "Mind Cure." "The relation that exists between the mind and the body is very intimate. When one is affected, the other sympathizes. The condition of the mind affects the health to a far greater degree than many realize. Many of the diseases from which men suffer are the result of mental depression. Grief, anxiety, discontent, remorse, guilt, distrust, all tend to break down the life forces and to invite decay and death. . . . Courage, hope, faith, sympathy, love, promote health and prolong life" (p. 241).

A perennial favorite pathology teacher, Carrol Small (CME class of 1934) and his wife, Lucile, were also a great inspiration to me. Lucile's small book *Not by Prescription* delineated clearly a crucial role that spiritual care provides for patients. She pointed out that if we are connected to God's Spirit and are willing to make spiritual care a priority, we will be presented with daily opportunities to share promises from the Scriptures that will be a real blessing to people. Matthew 11:28 (see above) was one Bible verse she called the "Master Prescription." I saw this in an article by Mrs. Small published in the LLUH publication *Scope* many years ago. Since then I have incorporated giving this "Master Prescription" to many patients in my practice. Through the years many patients have been blessed with that verse, printed on an Rx, from the Master Physician, Jesus Christ. Refill: prn. Dated: Anytime. Office hours: 24/7. And no copay!

Everywhere people are hungry for this kind of refreshing spiritual care that so much of the traditional medical model fails to provide. May God give us all the ability to be the salt and light and help people realize there is someone big enough to assist them with the overwhelming challenges of life's great struggles.

*For Wil Alexander's bio, refer to the devotional on January 18.

David K. Miller, LLUSM class of 1977-A, maintained a general practice through the years to include a strong focus on healthy living, wellness, and whole person care in a lifestyle center, medical clinic, and hospital. His present mission field is in Tulsa, Oklahoma, doing in-home health and wellness evaluations. He has a passion to share not only healthy living but also spiritual encouragement and literature for those weary souls that need to know they can have life and have it more abundantly.

October 28

"There's an opportune time to do things, a right time for everything on the earth:
. . . A right time to shut up and another to speak up."
Ecclesiastes 3:1, 7, MSG

If there is a time to be silent and a time to speak, it has taken me some time to figure out which is which. Early in my life silence served me well. An introvert by nature, I remember a high school classmate telling me that she respected my quiet demeanor, saying, "Still waters run deep." That moment stuck with me. I learned that silence was good.

As I grew older, my relationship with silence evolved. The summer before college, I admitted to myself that I was gay. Having grown up in the church, I sensed that this would not be accepted and that my realization would lead to the loss of everything I knew. I considered my options and decided upon an uneasy truce with the church: "I will keep silent, and you will let me stay."

For a while this worked. I could live with the illusion of belonging. But over time my resolve wore thin. Having hidden behind my own silence for years, I became resentful when I noticed it in others. I grew frustrated at my church's silence about homosexuality and at my school's refusal to support the LGBT students on its campus. I realized then that silence was not always good and could at times be a barrier to acceptance. I decided to come out by writing a letter in the school newspaper. I started the letter with a quote about silence.

During my medical training, I watched the church finally start to break its silence on LGBT issues. For the first time in its history, the School of Medicine included language in its orientation materials affirming that LGBT students would be protected there. With only a few words, these students could now feel welcomed and accepted. The wall of silence was starting to come down.

Times change, but the need to speak up remains. Since joining the UCLA faculty, I have learned that I must now use my voice to protect others. Recently a resident in my program encountered a patient who didn't want her as his doctor for no other reason than the color of her skin. When this resident looked for someone to protect her, to stick up for her, to put their foot down, she heard only silence. It was the same silence that she had experienced too many times before in response to racial slurs from patients and prejudice from colleagues. In response to this silence, she did what she needed to do: She spoke up. She wrote a letter to the department, asking faculty never to accept hatred and to create a space where everyone can feel safe, protected, and welcome.

Silence has its place, but when it acts as a barrier to belonging, it can and should be broken. Sometimes we must challenge the silence of institutions and organizations. At other times the silence we must break is our own. In all of our lives there are times to keep silent. Maybe now is a time to speak.

Jonathan Heldt, LLUSM class of 2014, is an assistant clinical professor at UCLA's David Geffen School of Medicine and an associate program director of UCLA's psychiatry residency training program.

October 29

> *"There is a season for everything under the sun—even when we can't see the sun."*
> Jared Brock: contemporary Canadian author and PBS documentarian

As far back as I can remember, my dad was the first person who said I would become a physician. Various snippets of memory from when I was about the age of 4 and beyond consist of my dad telling members of extended family, family friends, and church members that I said I wanted to be a doctor—even though I don't actually recall saying this myself! Even during times (such as in the act of sitting for the MCAT) when I wasn't so sure medicine was right for me, he stood by his conviction; and, fortunately for me, this path seems to have been in my heavenly Father's plan as well.

There are so many things I could share with you about my dad—how he was a good man and a good father; how much he loved God, family, and his home church; how kind and generous he was; how much he sacrificed for others; and how he had a great sense of humor, which came through even amid intermittent clouds of dementia in his latter years.

The 2017–2018 flu season was terrible. I would come home, and my husband would be listening to the evening news while preparing dinner; there seemed to be daily stories about the rising death count, especially among children and seniors. Although my dad received his influenza vaccine every fall, the vaccine seemed to fail him this year. Even though the sad and painful details of what he suffered are still so fresh in my mind that I can't rehash them all, I still feel that it would be helpful for me, and possibly for others, to share at least some parts.

It begins with the antagonist of the story, Influenza A. Halfway through, this monster powers up and transforms into Guillain-Barré syndrome. When the protagonist is a 79-year-old man who had never fully recovered from a stroke that three years prior had caused left-sided weakness, it is somewhat difficult to convince neurologists to start a relatively expensive treatment for a condition that clearly doesn't meet the diagnostic criteria. Prayers center on recovery; hope is contingent on a cure delivered by way of an infusion pump. IVIG becomes the Holy Grail, or possibly Excalibur—the sword to slay Guillain-Barré, the evil foe.

The treatment is started, given daily along with antibiotics for sepsis, parenteral nutrition, and medication for pain. As a family we discuss possible long-term plans, rehabilitation... thinking there would be weeks and months ahead, not knowing it would be a matter of days. The conversation changes from long-term care to hospice; then much too quickly the phrase becomes "comfort care."

And now as I slowly and finally get closer to acceptance, I find my solace from various sources—family, friends, colleagues, music, and the Bible. "'For I know the plans I have for you,' declares the Lord, 'plans to prosper you and not to harm you, plans to give you hope and a future'" (Jeremiah 29:11, NIV). Father knows best.

Elizabeth Endeno-Galima, LLUSM class of 1998, currently practices pediatrics with the Wesley Health Centers in Los Angeles County. She has recently been baking a lot of banana bread for and with her family.

October 30

Where Have the Stars Gone?

Mom, your eyes used to hold
a map of the constellations;
> why go camping to see the legends
> in the sky
> when I could see the stars from
> the couch—
>> just sitting and talking with
>> you?
>>> **But I**

haven't seen them lately.
Where have they gone?

Are they hidden beneath dark clouds
of impenetrable confusion?
> "Mom, it's me, your daughter,
> remember?"
> Silence. Wonder if they're
> even there.
>> **Want**

so desperately to see the stars again.
God, why would You let them burn
out?

Mom, your mind used to hold
marvelous ideas
that could stretch the universe a little
past infinity;
> why take a trip to outer space
> when I could see the strings that
> fuse the cosmos—
>> just sitting and talking with
>> you?
>>> **To see the stars**

shimmering on a night clear like
glass—that's all I need.
So why won't the clouds go away?

Are you listening when I
hold your hands and say,
> "Mom, it's me, your daughter,
> remember?"
> I know you'll remember. But
> perhaps not until
>> the Maker of the stars comes
>>> **again.**

—Ellie Ito

This poem written by my daughter, reminded me of an unforgettable encounter with an elderly Alzheimer's patient at a board and care facility. I was a hospice physician making a house call in order to recertify the patient for continued hospice service. "Mrs. M is bed bound, and can neither feed herself nor communicate. She is nonverbal." The nurse's report described Mrs. M impeccably. Her eyes were open, but she lay silent, gazing at a single point on the ceiling. Although I knew that she would provide no palpable response, I introduced myself and asked permission to perform a brief physical exam. As I packed up my stethoscope, I said, "Goodbye, Mrs. M. God bless. I'll be praying for you."

"Uhhh," Mrs. M muttered. I turned around in disbelief! Mrs. M, who was apparently out of touch with her surroundings, was looking straight into my eyes. I walked to her bedside, held her hand, and said, "Mrs. M, you heard me. You must know God. I do, too." She continued making indistinct sounds. Her facial muscles relaxed, as though she were smiling. "Dear Jesus, thank You for being with Mrs. M. Please give her comfort and peace." This was my first and last prayer at her bedside. Mrs. M passed away a few weeks later. But on that day I witnessed a miracle that could have gone unrecognized had I neglected the faint sound that escaped her lungs. I have since been more cognizant of life's small miracles.

Shiho Ito, LLUSM class of 2001, is currently on the faculty at the University of California, Irvine, specializing in palliative care. Ellie Ito is an aspiring premed student at Washington University in St. Louis. Note: This poem is not about Ellie's mother. Rather, Ellie was inspired by stories she had heard of individuals losing touch with their parents due to dementia. The structure of the poem was requested by its author.

October 31

"Your eyes saw my unformed body; all the days ordained for me were written in your book before one of them came to be." Psalm 139:16, NIV

He couldn't have had worse timing. We weren't ready for him. He was still breech, and we were doing everything we could to spin him. My wife stood on her head. We did myofascial massage and chiropractic. I even took the advice of one of my acupuncture friends involving burning mugwort near the pinky toe. My evidenced-based medicine professor, Dr. Lawrence Loo, would not be proud. Just not something you do for a breech baby.

We ultimately decided on doing an external cephalic version—a maneuver during which the obstetrician manually turns the baby. The procedure was scheduled the very day the baby would be term at 37 weeks. But he never gave us a chance. Kevin Schultz (LLUSM class of 2009), who was incredible in walking us through the nine months of the pregnancy, works one day every two weeks in Kellogg, Idaho, 90 miles away. Unfortunately, my son would break my wife's water bag the day Dr. Shultz was not in town. Another obstetrician would have to deliver. We were grateful for Dr. Shultz's partner, Andy Henneberg (LLUSM class of 2002), who delivered our son.

Because my son came just 12 hours shy of 37 weeks, he was technically premature. He would require heel pricks every three hours to check blood sugars and additional newborn screens. Prior to discharge he had to do a car seat challenge—a test involving hooking electrodes to his body and placing him in his car seat for two hours while in the NICU. He was even evaluated by a developmental specialist and a speech therapist. That's right. Our newborn had to be evaluated by a speech therapist! However, some incredible things unfolded on my son's birth day.

I texted my close friend Nathan Brinckhaus (LLUSM class of 2011) the morning we found out that we were going to have a baby. He texted back immediately. His wife, Eurides Brinkhaus (LLUSM class of 2012), was going into labor too. In fact, our firstborns came into the world 77 minutes apart, even though their due dates were three weeks apart!

That's not the only incredible thing. October 31, 2017, marked the dawn of the Protestant Reformation 500 years ago. An unknown German monk nailed 95 criticisms on the church door of Wittenberg, laying the foundation for religious liberty, and ultimately democracy and scientific reasoning. Later, in the mid-twentieth century, a Black man named Michael King would study the life of Martin Luther. Inspired by the German monk, Michael King would change his name to Martin Luther King, Sr., and his young son' name to Martin Luther King, Jr., who would become one of America's greatest civil rights leaders.

As I reflected on these events, I've learned one important lesson: Whatever plans I have for my son, God has better plans. I don't know why Melanie had to undergo a C-section despite my prayers, fasting, and effort. But I do take comfort in Psalm 84:11: "No good thing will he withhold from those who walk uprightly" (ESV). Perhaps my son was spared from harm. Whatever the case, I don't know what the future holds, but I know who holds the future. And that future is a good one.

As a result of these events we changed course with our son. We changed his name from Joshua Andrew Roquiz to Joshua Luther Roquiz. Why?

Because whatever plans I have for my son, God has better plans.

D. Andrew Roquiz, LLUSM class of 2011, is married to Melanie and practices family medicine in Florida. He blogs about whole person care at www.thechristiandoctor.com.

NOVEMBER

GRATITUDE

"Gratitude bestows reverence . . . changing forever how we experience life and the world."

JOHN MILTON (1608–1674)
English poet

November 1

> *"Gratitude, like faith, is a muscle. The more you use it, the stronger it grows."*
> Alan H. Cohen (1950–): American author, radio broadcaster, and columnist

We all talk to ourselves. Not usually out loud, but silently in our heads and continually throughout the day: *What should I do next? Why is this taking me so much time? I'm glad that went so well. I can't believe I said that! I'm fortunate to have this job. Won't it be great when . . . ?*

Studies on the ways we talk to ourselves vary in some of their outcomes, but they agree that most of what people say to themselves is negative rather than positive. Self-talk tends to have a negativity bias. As psychologist Barbara Fredrickson observed: "The negative screams at you, but the positive only whispers."

Martin Seligman, the founder of the field of study known as positive psychology has developed and tested, along with colleagues, an array of specific practices that have been empirically demonstrated to promote resiliency and flourishing. One of the earliest and most popular of these tools is known simply as "three good things." This exercise consists of taking a moment before going to bed to write down three good things that happened that day along with an explanation of why they went well. It is important to actually write them down, rather than simply spend a moment in positive reflection. The act of writing has the effect of sealing the positive thinking, making it linger in our memories.

Seligman and his colleagues published the initial results of this intervention using randomized subjects and controls in the year 2005. Measurable results continued for up to six months after as little as one week of practice. Today a common prescription is to practice the activity for two weeks with the recognition that people often find it so beneficial that they choose to keep it up. Writing down three good things at the end of every day has been shown, in numerous studies, to have long-term positive effects in mood and outlook, reducing symptoms of depression and other health problems. Type "three good things" into your Internet search engine, and you will find an abundance of information about the efficacy of this and other positive psychology practices.

When I started this exercise, I was sobered by the fact that thinking of three things to write down wasn't always easy, especially at first. My experience is not uncommon. "Memories are tricky," notes psychologist J. Bryan Sexton. "Good ones are like Teflon, they slip away, while the bad ones stick like Velcro (especially when we are tired)." We tend to remember irritants, even when they are minor, but take positive things for granted.

This tendency may be especially true of the good things that come from God. It is not surprising that the authors of Scripture repeatedly call us to give praise and thanks to God, to remember His blessings, to think on things that are, in the words of Philippians 4:8, true, lovely, pure, admirable, of good report.

Why does this activity work? As Seligman puts it: "From ancient scriptures to the latest science, gratitude is known to be good for us and those around us. Yet it isn't always our automatic response. . . . So we have to consciously learn to get into the habit of being grateful." When we begin keeping a record of positive experiences, we start to notice things that we can write down at the end of the day. We see and remember what would have otherwise gone unnoticed.

More than 100 years before the three good things exercise was formalized, Johnson Oatman, Jr., wrote these words as part of a hymn you may have learned to sing: "Count your blessings, name them one by one, and it will surprise you what the Lord has done."

Henry Lamberton, PsyD, MDiv, is the associate dean for student affairs at LLUSM. He has served in this role since 1994 and has provided counsel to more than 4,000 medical students. His father, Harold Lamberton (CME class of 1946), and father-in-law, Philip D. Spechko (CME class of 1953-B), are both alumni. He and his wife, Elaine, have two daughters and four grandchildren.

November 2

"He profits most who serves best."
Arthur F. Sheldon (1868–1935): American businessman, author, founder of a correspondence business school, and author of the secondary motto of Rotary International, quoted above

I was only in my second year practicing as a primary care physician when I found myself asking what I could do with a medical degree that didn't involve practicing medicine. Perhaps it was the constant inundation of patients being double-booked in my schedule, or maybe it was the pressure of maintaining a high patient satisfaction score in order to keep my job. It could have been the forms, emails, refills, meaningful use, quality metrics, or the micromanaging clinic chief that crushed my perseverance. The increasing mountain of student debt also was a strong contributor to a feeling of futility. Regardless, I was facing my biggest identity crisis with being a physician.

To become a physician, I had to survive. I made it through the initial cut to get into medical school. I survived numerous exams to pass medical school, and I worked obscene amounts of hours during internship and residency to obtain the designation of board-certified physician. The culmination of my resilience was being disenchanted about how medicine was practiced in real life. I thought my feelings were internal, but when I inquired with my other colleagues, I found my feelings and perception of modern medicine were validated.

I never felt so much anxiety and fear about the future. I knew I wanted to be a physician, but I was not thriving in my environment of corporate-style medicine. My entire adult life was dedicated to becoming a doctor, and I thought I was following God's will in my life. I kept praying to God for guidance and deliverance of my seemingly helpless situation. Who knew that I could be saved by noticing a small, obscure advertisement for a position in a small, rural town in South Dakota? I had no desire to move from beautiful sunny Hawaii to frigid cold South Dakota. As I searched the Bible for guidance, I came across the story of Abraham, who by faith had listened to God's command to move to a foreign land with a promise of an inheritance. The doors of this opportunity were swung open. I just had to have faith to move with my family to the unknown.

In this community I definitely work more hours, but the shackles of corporate medicine were broken. I enjoyed a broader scope of practice, which taught me to be a more well-rounded physician. The community saw me as a vital part of society. The distractions of city life faded away in the simplicity of a small rural town. I slowly became invigorated and found my love for medicine again. I am glad that I listened to God's solution. He helped me get back onto my feet and planted me back on the ground with a new resolve to continue my calling as a physician.

Eric C. Chow, LLUSM class of 2009, is currently a practicing hospitalist in South Dakota. He and his wife, Irene, have three children.

November 3

"But the fruit of the Spirit is love, joy, peace, patience, kindness, goodness, faithfulness, gentleness, self-control; against such things there is no law."
Galatians 5:22-23, NASB

We believe that addressing spiritual health is as important as a thorough history and physical examination. That's why we've incorporated this spiritual wholeness assessment as an integral resource to whole person care—every patient, every visit. Upon completion of this intake form, our medical assistant reviews the responses with each patient, adding appropriate narrative, then flags the chart for the provider's benefit, highlighting all "No" and "Not Sure" responses for the provider's attention.

Instruction to patient: Please highlight your response to each of the following questions.

1. Do you have religious beliefs that influence your medical decisions?
   Yes / No / Not Sure

(It's OK if a patient declines to answer one or more questions. But it's important to note that most of us hold beliefs that impact our medical choices. Sometimes these have to do with diet or hygiene. Or it may be more about treatment, choice of medication or a surgical procedure. More commonly, most of us hold to certain beliefs concerning the edges of life—serious illness, birth, and death. Documenting these deeply held beliefs is good clinical practice and important information for each medical record.)

2. Do you have someone who loves and cares for you? Yes / No / Not Sure

No. (Abrupt torrent of tears.) My spouse died last year ... and I'm estranged from my children. I live alone and rarely get out of the house. I don't have anyone I can depend on—no one close who really cares about what's going on with me.

3. Do you have a source of joy in your life? Yes / No / Not Sure

Yes. I belong to a book club that meets once a month. A half dozen of us get together for brunch and conversation about what we've been reading. I wouldn't say we're close friends, but it's a pleasant diversion and a time that we all look forward to.

4. Do you have a sense of peace today? Yes / No / Not Sure

Not really. That's why I'm here. I'm afraid these headaches mean something bad, and I don't know how I'll manage if this turns out to be serious or complicated.

Along with routine clinical evaluation and treatment, the provider sensitively explores the "love, joy, and peace" responses. A comforting word or touch may bring hope; sometimes an offer of prayer is gratefully accepted. Before departing the office, the patient is referred to our telephonic spiritual care center for follow-up and scheduled for a return visit to the office.

That's the process. That's how we practice whole person care. Against love, joy, and peace, there is no law.

Ted Hamilton, LLUSM class of 1973-A, family practice and practicing at family. He works at AdventHealth in Orlando, Florida. He now walks rather than jogs, and is thankful for hearing aids, contact lenses, dental crowns, and other fine replacements for worn-out originals.

November 4

"My friends, you were chosen to be free. So don't use your freedom as an excuse to do anything you want. Use it as an opportunity to serve each other with love."
Galatians 5:13, CEV

Late on a Friday afternoon an elderly gentleman came to the emergency department (ED) after having had an angiogram earlier that day. He and his family were worried about possible bleeding at the angiogram site. In addition, there was concern for aneurysm . . . and he was unsure if he wanted surgery.

The patient was a distinguished man who was retired from the military. It was apparent that he was used to giving rather than receiving orders. Since he was used to being in charge, he did not take kindly to any advice—expert or not! His wife and two adult sons appeared to be used to carrying out his orders rather than giving him advice. His frustration from being in a situation he could not control was apparent and continued to grow.

When I discussed potential treatment options for his concerning prognosis, he became angry. He yelled, cursed, and accused me of trying to make money off him by suggesting additional stabilizing care. His family didn't know what to do. I repeatedly tried to reassure him that I wanted to give him the best care possible as well as provide potential options that he could choose from. The afternoon and evening were long, and he continued to be challenging to communicate with. While his attacks were personally directed to me, I did recognize that he had the right to make his decisions, whether bad or good for his overall health. His family wanted him to make what they felt were clear decisions, but they were reluctant to intervene.

As the evening wore on, the patient became more unstable and ended up being admitted to the ICU. Prior to the patient leaving the ED, I went to talk to his family. His son—a tall, well-dressed attorney—had observed but not said a lot during the ED visit. As I walked into the room, he broke into tears and said, "He was a jerk to you for hours. He was such a jerk to you . . . but he is our jerk . . . and we love him. So thank you."

I remain so grateful for this experience. Patients dealing with so many things are not always easy. It is something that has stayed with me when dealing with varying degrees of humanness. This is someone acting badly whom many people—including Jesus—love.

Tamara Thomas, LLUSM class of 1987, is a professor in LLUSM's department of emergency medicine. She is an executive vice president of LLUH and dean of LLUSM, a position she has held since July, 2019.

November 5

> *"The mediocre teacher tells. The good teacher explains.*
> *The superior teacher demonstrates. The great teacher inspires."*
> William Arthur Ward (1921–1994): American author

Dear Dr. Wood,

I just received our alumni journal today and saw you on the front cover. I was having a salad with my beautiful 88-year-old mother, and pointed you out to her.

It was then that I told her the story that began in 1973. A story you know well. A story etched vividly in my mind. It was winter. It was cold. You were searching for your young daughter. Unable to find her, you went to your swimming pool to see if by some chance she could have fallen into the water without anyone knowing. And there she was, to your terror, at the bottom of the pool.

I was a young pediatric intern at Loma Linda when we got your little daughter in as a "near drowning," rushed from the depths of your cold swimming pool. I'll never forget your words. You were staring past me at the tiny form of your little girl, practically whispering, "It was the hardest decision I ever had to make... whether to try to resuscitate my daughter when I found her at the bottom of the swimming pool.... I didn't know how long she had been there."

I remember caring for your precious little girl. Each of us watched and worked and prayed, hoping she would be OK. We were lowly interns and residents, and you were attending staff. We knew you knew the battle to be waged. And fight she did. A valiant fight. And she won! What joy it was when we realized she would survive!

Having two toddlers of my own at the time, I went home and promptly had a tall, green-vinyl-coated chain-link fence built around my little pool on Van Leuven Street.

My mother listened intently to each word of the story. Her brow furrowed; I could see in her eyes the great concern for your little girl. She was eager to know the "rest of the story." Finally I told her that your little girl made it and that she was whole. Her brain was healthy. Oh, how fortunate that the pool water was so cold!

Later, during my anesthesiology residency, I gave many anesthetics for your cases as well. Thank you for your mentoring during my learning years of internship and residency, Dr. Wood. May God continue to richly bless and keep you and your family.

With Aloha,
Linda

Linda Harsh Dixon, LLUSM class of 1972, resides in Hawaii and Sun City West, Arizona. She is retired after 33 years as an anesthesiologist. She is grateful for the faculty at LLUSM who lived what they taught and served our Lord Jesus Christ. Note: For Virchel Wood's bio, please refer to the devotional on February 13.

November 6

> *"All the gold in the world has no significance. That which is lasting are the thoughtful acts which we do for our fellow man."*
> Adolfo Prieto (1867–1945): Spanish humanitarian

In 2013 I had major reconstructive jaw surgery at Loma Linda University Medical Center. I had 48 screws and eight plates surgically and expertly placed in my maxilla and mandible by Dr. Alan Herford (LLUSD class of 1994, MD) and his team from the oral and maxillofacial surgery department. This complex procedure piqued my interest in human anatomy. Even after enduring excruciating pain for the nine days during my postoperative recovery, my fascination with the human body and medical procedures grew.

During this time of recovery my mouth was wired shut so I could not eat. I was sleep-deprived, suffered agonizing pain at the surgical sites, and had an extreme, unrelenting headache. Thankfully, on the tenth day my recovery unexpectedly progressed from intense pain to having no pain at all. Feeling better, I found myself continuing to research vasoconstriction, platelets, coagulation, and osteogenesis to satisfy my newfound curiosity with the human body and the healing process.

After I recovered, I started volunteering in the emergency department at Loma Linda University. I also began to explore career and educational options in health care. In 2015 I earned my certified nursing assistant (CNA) license. I practiced as a CNA at a local nursing home for two years before working in my current position as an emergency services technician in the emergency department at LLUMC. I can proudly say that I am now a nursing student and will graduate with a BSN and earn my RN license in the summer of 2021!

I am forever grateful for my Loma Linda experience as a patient. I am appreciative of the competent and skilled physicians who performed my surgery. And I am especially grateful for the nursing staff who cared for me with so much love and compassion while I was hurting and recovering. I credit the skilled and compassionate care that I received as a patient as the reason I chose to pursue a career in nursing. Thank you all!

Jesse Gomez is currently enrolled at West Coast University in Ontario, California, as a nursing student. He would like to thank his lovely wife, Janelle; daughter, Jaclynn; son, Jayden; his parents; and other family members who have been so supportive and generous during this time of his life. Without all of them, this dream would not have been possible!

November 7

"The LORD your God is in your midst, a mighty one who will save; he will rejoice over you with gladness; he will quiet you by his love; he will exult over you with loud singing."

Zephaniah 3:17, ESV

I'm used to children not talking; some of them because they have cerebral palsy and their brains have sustained enough damage to limit their ability to speak. Others are infants soaking in the world of language, not yet able to communicate with words. Some are older and have speech delays from developmental disorders.

Sitting in front of me in silence on my clinic exam table was 7-year-old Kathy. Kathy was recently adopted from another country by her mother. With that came a litany of tests that needed to be ordered and vaccinations that needed to be administered. What she lacked in words she made up with a radiant smile.

That entire first visit she didn't say a single word. While her adoptive mother spoke lovingly to her, Kathy was unable to tell me what was going on, where she hurt, what she experienced, what she looked forward to. At the end of that visit I offered to pray with them. We prayed that God would give wisdom to the physicians taking care of her and that Kathy would know how precious she is in God's sight.

As the ensuing months continued, Kathy came back often as she had multiple medical concerns. On one such visit she was back in my office after I had treated her for yet another infection that we had found, a vestige from her home country. Yet still no words.

Toward the end of that visit, as I was walking out the door, I felt a prompting to remember that each patient encounter is sacred ground. I turned around and said to the adoptive mother and Kathy, "Would you find prayer helpful at this time?" The adoptive mother said yes.

To my surprise, Kathy indicated that she wanted to pray first. She proceeded to say, "Dear God, thank You for Dr. Wai." I was shocked to hear words coming from her, much less a prayer! I realized that God had used her to speak a blessing to me on a busy clinic day. I concluded with a prayer thanking God for Kathy and her mother.

I sometimes reflect on that day. It stands as a reminder to me of someone I had never heard speak, but who now spoke, and spoke in such a way to bless others.

Her words are a precious encouragement to me.

For this mother and every parent that I know, there is this deep abiding love that they have for their children filled with powerful emotion. And yet I am reminded that there is a Father with an even greater love. God the Father stayed silent when His own Son, Jesus Christ, was hanging on a cross, so that we could experience adoption as His children.

Sometimes we do not think that God speaks, because we do not hear anything audible. But God does talk with us. Today I pray that we would hear from God often that we are deeply loved and precious in His sight.

Andrew Wai, LLUSM class of 2011, is an assistant professor in LLUSM's department of pediatrics. He serves as the pediatrics clerkship director and is excited to continue the tradition of training and equipping Christian physicians to heal in Jesus' name.

November 8

"At the end of life, what really matters is not what we bought, but what we built; not what we got, but what we shared; not our competence, but our character; and not our success, but our significance. Live a life that matters. Live a life of love."

Anonymous

As you read this, it's several years after Northern California's deadly Camp Fire, which started on November 8, 2018. But as I write, it's barely eight weeks after the fact. By now you will have heard many more stories than I have, told much more dramatically. I have no idea where we'll be, physically, in 11 months. I have no idea where I'll be, emotionally, in the next 10 minutes. So the only thing unique I have to offer is a fragment of a reflection.

What I can say with reasonable certainty is that one emotion, strangely, is relief. I no longer need to worry about the dry rot in the posts holding up the porch roof. Or the tendency of the root cellar to flood during heavy rain. The downsizing project is done, without a lot of difficult decisions.

I am occasionally overcome by a sense of loss. Often it comes as I seek to solve a problem: "Oh, I've got a . . . uh . . . no, I don't." And it's not the loss of the "stuff," as inconvenient as that may be. It's the "stuff" that has memories linked. My grandfather's carpentry tools, for example. I can still buy a good century-old Stanley #6 plane that can be sharpened and adjusted to work just as his did, but I won't see his big farmer hands holding it and working a rough board smooth. I won't be able to unroll his canvas roll of auger bits and wonder if my grandma stitched the webbing loops in it that hold the bits secure.

I can buy another copy of the *Messiah*, but it won't have my father's elegant signature on the front cover, and it will cost a lot more than the $1.25 he paid for it.

So it's not the "stuff" I miss; it's the memories it engenders. And for a few more years, anyway, I can maintain them unassisted. Hopefully I can honor the past by remembering to execute my projects with the skill and care that my grandfather, or my father-in-law, would have used. Maybe I can put my heart and voice with skill and care into future performances. And maybe, just maybe, I can pay it forward by sharing these skills and interests with my grandchildren, so that the legacy can continue irrespective of the physical implements. Stuff just doesn't matter. People do.

As I reflect further on "fire," I realize that it has beneficial functions as well. I think of the refiner's fire, liquefying metal to release the impurities, and consuming them. Maybe to some extent the "stuff" in my life was, if not an impurity, at least a distraction from the relationships around me. Maybe God is using the fire to refine me to be a better reflector of His character.

Fire also permits the blacksmith to forge steel into tools. I think I'm beginning to see that among some of my church members and the town's people. We may be seeing the forging of a stronger community. I hope so.

Wally Schmidt used his media skills to support LLUMC's educational mission for almost 30 years. He is married to Donna (LLUSN class of 1971). After the Camp Fire they relocated from Paradise, California, to Oregon to be closer to their two daughters and grandchildren. Watching the West Coast burn in 2020 only intensified their desire for Christ's soon return. Note: Approximately 15 LLUSM alumni were affected by the Camp Fire in Paradise and surrounding communities.

November 9

> *"He determines the number of the stars; he gives to all of them their names."*
> Psalm 147:4, ESV

My family and I recently took a camping trip with friends to Joshua Tree National Park in California. We set up camp in the shadow of massive, golden boulders. For dinner we ate haystacks while a gentle breeze kept us cool. My kids, Maya (then age 5) and Bode (then age 2), loved being outside with minimal oversight. They crawled over rocks, piled sand into indecipherable formations, and named every lizard they encountered "Lizzie."

As the sun set, my wife and I laid Maya and Bode down in our roofless tent for the evening. But the darkness is when Joshua Tree is at her best. With each passing moment, more and more stars came into sharp focus until we were lying underneath a vast sequin tapestry.

Bode rocketed to his feet and yelled, "Stars!" He pointed. "Daddy! Stars!" Because we live in a densely populated area, my son had never really seen stars. Until tonight.

"I see it!" he shouted.

"Mommy! Can we take stars home?" There was a wondrous seriousness in his voice.

For the next 20 minutes (yes, 20 minutes!) my son stood beguiled by the stars. He continually waved at them, called to them, and asked my wife and I if we saw them. I have never heard wonder in someone's voice as I heard it in my son's slurred English that evening. Which is what made the next event all the more bizarre.

After my kids fell asleep, my wife and I rejoined our friends around the campfire. We all leaned back and took in the stars, and shared stories about the highs and lows of parenting. Less than 10 minutes into our conversation/stargazing experience, our neighbors in the campsite next to us pulled out an array of lights (yes, an array of lights!), and projected rapidly shifting lights on the stony mountains all around us. Forty-five seconds after the lights began, our neighbors added loud music to their lights, and my friends and I assumed that their dance party had begun. Their music blared, and the lights shone disruptively for one hour and 45 minutes.

At 10:45 p.m. the party crossed our tolerance threshold. My friend headed over to their campsite to request our neighbors bring their party to a close. But when he arrived, he was stunned to find that no one was dancing. Instead, he found a handful of middle-aged men who were wholly indifferent to the lights, the music, and the world-class display of stars overhead. Instead, all of these men were staring at their phones! What I find fascinating about this story is the contrast between these men and my son. Something happens to us as we grow into adulthood.

One of the strongest temptations adults face is to become calloused to the overwhelming beauty and grace of God and Creation. Which means the work at hand is not to point at these men and say, "These guys are what's wrong with the world today!" Instead, the work is to be aware of and understand this temptation to take grace for granted.

This awareness inspires us to look inward and ask, "How have I become apathetic to the grace of God around me?" Today, may you and I strive to have the eyes of a child so that we might see the beauty and grace of God's work that surrounds us.

Craig Hadley, La Sierra University MDiv class of 2011, is the lead pastor at Paradox church in Redlands, California. His wife, Kimi (LLUSD dental hygiene class of 2007), works part-time as a dental hygienist. They live in Redlands with their two kids, Maya, age 7, and Bode, age 4.

November 10

> *"'When, Lord, did we ever see you hungry and feed you, or thirsty and give you a drink? When did we ever see you a stranger and welcome you in our homes, or naked and clothe you? When did we ever see you sick or in prison, and visit you?' The King will reply, 'I tell you, whenever you did this for one of the least important of these followers of mine, you did it for me!'"*
>
> Matthew 25:37-40, GNT

The patient was an 83-year-old male who was terminally ill because of metastatic pancreatic cancer, and I was assigned to admit him to the Veterans Affairs Loma Linda Healthcare System (VALLHS) hospice program. I entered his room, introduced myself, and began to assess him.

My work in hospice has confirmed what I was taught at the Loma Linda University School of Medicine: It is imperative to address the physical, psychological, spiritual, and social needs of patients.

After my assessment revealed that he was too weak to perform any activities of daily living, I asked him, "Would you like me to help you contact your family?"

He turned slowly, looked me in the eye, held out his hands toward me, and said with a soft voice, "I don't have any family. You are my family."

His response astonished me. I was speechless. Although I had just met him, he considered me to be his family. After I composed myself, I thought, *What an enormous responsibility and privilege it is for me to care for those who are terminally ill.*

I collected my thoughts and responded, "I am honored to be your family. Thank you for your service to our country. You deserve the best health care, and we will provide it for you." He answered by smiling and nodding his head.

The VALLHS hospice team did its best to address his physical, psychological, spiritual, and social needs. He consistently responded with a quiet "Thank you, thank you" each time we exited his room. He died peacefully three weeks after being admitted.

Gratifying experiences, including this case, remind me why I went to medical school. I am blessed to be an alumnus of the Loma Linda University School of Medicine, a medical school that taught me the importance of addressing the whole person.

Russell E. Hoxie, LLUSM class of 1988, is an associate professor in LLUSM's department of medicine. He has been married to his wife, Danielle, for 32 years. They have three children, including a daughter, Dana Michele Hoxie Brockmann, who graduated from LLUSM in 2019.

November 11

Veterans Day

> *"This is the confidence we have in approaching God: that if we ask anything according to his will, he hears us."*
>
> 1 John 5:14, NIV

The sun filtered gently through the oak trees in the healing garden at Ochsner Clinic in New Orleans, where I sat praying with my mom. We had all been living in the "unknown" since January 2013 when Mom was first diagnosed with cryptogenic cirrhosis and we learned that she would require a lifesaving liver and kidney transplant. My doctor eyes told me she had days left to live at this point with hepatic encephalopathy and requirements for daily paracentesis, thoracentesis, and dialysis. She had no quality of life and was suffering which was extremely hard to witness. Her time was running out, and I prayed to God to ask Him for a miracle.

I had come to New Orleans to celebrate my mom's seventieth birthday on November 11, 2013, which I feared would be her last birthday. I am a medical hematologist/oncologist, yet this was the first time in my life that I really began to understand what my patients and their loved ones suffer on a visceral level. Cancer patients live from CT scan to CT scan, and often in this "unknown" territory where we are hopeful (but not certain) if a therapy will be effective or not. Waiting . . . waiting . . . for pathology results, imaging results, prognosis, etc. It is very easy to lose hope in these times of waiting while living under the dark cloud of the "unknown."

A thought came to my mind as I sat holding my mom's hand in the healing garden, where birds, butterflies, and beautiful flowers surrounded us. I was in this peaceful location but was in agony, fearing how I would ever be able to bear losing my precious mom. Her time was quickly running out, and, truthfully, I had lost my hope for this miracle over time. Then the "impossible" happened—the next day, on her actual birthday, she got the best birthday present ever . . . a lifesaving liver and kidney transplant! We were all reminded that God is so good—all the time. I was prepared for God's answer to be no since He even had to say no to Jesus' agonized pleas to take the cup of suffering from Him the night before His crucifixion. I truly believe God knows best and can make good out of every bad circumstance. When our patients are unable to receive a cure, it does not mean God does not love them. We live in an evil world, and heaven is to come.

The day I had flown from San Diego to New Orleans, it was a dreary, rainy day, and yet once the plane ascended above the clouds, suddenly the sun and blue skies appeared. They were always there, but I could not see it under the rainy clouds on earth. It is a simple metaphor, but one I try to remember often when I am losing hope or have fears, since even when we are living in the "unknown," we can have confidence that God is in His heaven and is ultimately in control and knows best. Our fears of the "unknown" can be erased with our knowledge of a God that hears our cries and prayers and loves us all more than we can begin to imagine.

Melissa Torrey, LLUSM class of 2001, currently practices medical hematology/oncology in San Diego, California, at Scripps Clinic/MD Anderson. She has a passion for treating breast cancer patients and enjoys clinical research in this capacity as well. In her "free" time she enjoys traveling and exploring new cultures, reading, interior design, playing her harp and piano and making wonderful memories with family and friends. November 11 is her mom's birthday and also the date of her mother's lifesaving liver and kidney transplants. Melissa thanks God daily for these miracles.

November 12

The Gigantic Impact

What wonder! To see
A silver sliver of moon
Hanging in the dawn sky
With delicately poised grace;

A tiny piece of celestial choreography
Where galaxies spin, stars dance,
Worlds pirouette, meteors whirl...
Sometimes they collide.

Scientists postulate
That the moon did not exist
Till earth was pummeled
By a giant meteor half her size.

In the chaos that resulted,
The moon was born.
Earth held on to her new satellite
With the fierce power of gravity.

What must it have been like,
That giant meteor strike?
Powerful beyond any nuclear blast.
Disrupting orbit, surface, core.

And yet, beauty has resulted.
And joy! To see the moon
Twirl 'round the earth,
Reflecting the light of the sun.

I too experienced a gigantic impact:
My beloved's neck was broken.
The shock still reverberates
In my being.

Chaos resulted.
The orbit of my life
Forever altered. The surface
Of how I lived destroyed.

Grief erupted: a volcanic ash plume
Of darkness, obscuring all joy,
Chilling my very existence,
Shaking me to the core.

Quadriplegia. Stark reality.
Dreams shattered; career surrendered.
Immersion in legal and insurance
Matters never anticipated.

Ventilator, Hoyer lift,
Feeding tube and Foley,
Stage III decubiti, neurogenic bowel;
An in-exsufflator (who knew?)!

Adaptation comes slowly
To these disconcerting complexities.
Gradually the ash settles.
A new normal is born.

I discover that through all this,
The ineffable love of God,
More absolute than gravity,
Has indefatigably held on to me

And kept me spinning in orbit—
Albeit a new and wobbly one.
His grace enables me to once again
Reflect the light of the Son.

Debra Stottlemyer, LLUSM class of 1986, is an associate professor in LLUSM's department of medicine. She has been married to Craig for 38 years. Craig became a quadriplegic as the result of an accident that occurred November 12, 2012, while he was riding his bicycle to work at LLUMC. This poem about Craig was written in April 2015.

November 13

"Likewise the Spirit helps us in our weakness. For we do not know what to pray for as we ought, but the Spirit himself intercedes for us with groanings too deep for words. And he who searches hearts knows what is the mind of the Spirit, because the Spirit intercedes for the saints according to the will of God."
Romans 8:26-27, ESV

This story is the unexpected continuation of the November 13 devotional found in the prequel book *Evening Rounds*.

Homelessness is an ever-present problem in San Bernardino County in Southern California. Whenever I see the homeless, I often wonder what story lies behind each person's seemingly hopeless plight and what could, if anything, be done about it.

Seven years ago I was moved to help a homeless man at a gas station, although not entirely out of the goodness of my heart but rather by the impressions placed on my heart by the Holy Spirit. I was curious: What would make an able-bodied man clean windshields, only to be paid spare change? At the time I was employed as a writer for National Public Radio contributing to a blog called *The California Report*—and I was long overdue for an interesting submission.

I set out to speak with this man, to find out how he had arrived at this point and what, if anything, I could do about it. I heard his story, wrote about it, received many accolades for it, and went on my way, not thinking about it thereafter. Because of this story, I did see homeless individuals in a new light, thinking of them more humanly: intentionally stopping to talk to them when I had time. I also called my new friend, Joe, from time to time to check on him. Then one day his number no longer connected me to the familiar voice on the other end of the phone line.

A year and a half passed, and curiously, I received an email. The subject line read one name, "Joe Sheroan," the name of my homeless man. I opened the page-and-a-half-long letter, and I was immediately speechless. The letter was written by Joe's daughter, who had been mentioned in my blog post as being one of the things in Joe's life that brought him joy. The blog continued to say how Joe missed his daughter and how he had longed to spend more time with her.

Yes, Joe had died. And because of the estranged relationship he had with his daughter, she knew little about him. Now tasked with writing his eulogy, she took a chance and entered his name in her computer search engine... and guess what popped up? The story I wrote! She said this brought her to tears, reading about her dad and how he missed her so. She said that it made her so appreciative that someone had taken the time to learn about his life and spend a little time with him. She knew his lifestyle and where it had taken him, but she was forever grateful that at least one person did not dismiss him. And it was only by the grace of God that I had not.

Bobbi Albano is a business owner in San Bernardino, California. She began her MBA at LLUSPH while working for Loma Linda Retail Services and before starting California Curb Appeal in 2018. The vision and mission of her business are ones that elevate service, commitment, and love—much like the values of LLUH.

November 14

"Train up a child in the way he should go, and when he is old he will not depart from it."
Proverbs 22:6, NKJV

Statistics show that children of teenage mothers are more likely to experience abuse and neglect, drop out of high school, fall into poverty, be incarcerated, and become teenage parents themselves. Statistically, that should have been me—yet by God's grace and intervention, that is not my story.

I was born when my mother was still in high school and totally unprepared to be a parent. It was a tumultuous and distressing time for the whole family, but my grandparents were certain of one thing: They did not want their daughter to bear this responsibility alone. They feared how she might struggle as a teenage mother and worried about the future of their grandchild. To help my mother finish her education, my grandparents stepped in to help care for me. As a result, I grew attached and did not want to leave them when my mother moved away, so they became my de facto parents. They tell me that they have never regretted raising me as their own child and that God always provided for their needs.

My (grand)parents had a very formative influence on my life. They encouraged me to read the Bible as soon as I was able and to trust God with all of life's challenges. Their example strengthened my faith as I witnessed how loving and kind they were to family and strangers, and how diligent they were in their daily responsibilities. Impacted by their mindset, I was inspired to choose a profession in which I could serve others, leading me to pursue medicine. Given that my grandfather was a retired mechanic and my grandmother a teacher's assistant, funding higher education would have been challenging. Yet, with their support and more of God's grace, I earned a full scholarship to attend the University of Arizona.

In college I learned that a competitive application to medical school would require many extracurricular experiences. I was completely new to Tucson, with no prior connections, but again God opened doors. I was blessed with opportunities to do research with wonderful mentors who taught me to pursue excellence and aim higher. Additionally, volunteering at a hospital and free clinic provided interactions with patients, families, and dedicated staff that gave me greater perspective on the challenges and joys of working in health care. All these amazing people that God brought into my life confirmed my desire to help others as a physician. The sequence of incidents, relationships, and God's guidance culminated in something that seemed so distant at one point—an acceptance to medical school.

As I near the end of my first year of medical school, I often find myself reflecting on how my life could have turned out drastically different at so many points if it were not for God's care. One of those turning points was when my grandparents "adopted" me. When someone shows us compassion, we often feel indebted to reciprocate that courtesy, but there are some acts of love and service we can never repay no matter how much effort we give. This is how I feel about my grandparents' voluntary role in my life. I'm inspired to pay forward all the kindnesses shown to me by working in the mission field after I graduate. I do not know where that will be or what that will entail, but I trust that God will continue to be faithful, just as He has been all along.

Benjamin Rivera, LLUSM class of 2023, is a deferred mission appointee who looks forward to serving wherever God leads.

November 15

> *"Philanthropy is the secret that unlocks the storehouse of life's blessings."*
> Douglas M. Lawson (1936–2020): American author,
> educator for philanthropic services, and speaker

As a fundraiser, I meet a lot of people over the course of my work. One who stands out is a woman I met at her reunion. She was this ball of energy working the room to make everyone feel welcome, including me. I was there to help troubleshoot—working with the caterer on setup, handing out name badges so people could identify each other 55 years later. She introduced herself and, upon learning that I was just pitching in to help and was not an event planner, she thanked me and reassured me that everything was going to go smoothly.... I think this was actually my job to do for her, but it made me feel better all the same.

When she called me a week after the event to thank me again for my help, she shared how hard my job must be to get people to give. I shared that my job isn't to get people to give, but rather to assist people who want to make a difference find the best place and best way to make their gift. My role was as a philanthropic problem solver and matchmaker. She paused, then shared that she wondered if I could help her.

Her husband, whom she had met at college, had passed away three years earlier after 52 years of marriage and 3 children. She missed him every day, and one of the reasons she volunteered so much as an alumna was because being on campus reminded her of their life together. While she had been a social worker, John had been a lifelong teacher, and she wondered if she could create a scholarship in his name so that he would always be remembered at this place that meant so much to them as a couple. I told her this was definitely something she could do, and invited her to come in so we could talk through some possibilities. At first, hearing how much it took to create a scholarship, she seemed discouraged. But we talked through options she had, including funding the scholarship with a bequest gift, paying it over a few years, and donating the small vacation home they had purchased in the early seventies in the nearby mountains. During the next four months she talked to her accountant and her children about her idea, and they all encouraged her because they saw how excited she was.

When she told me she was going to move forward with starting a scholarship, I thanked her for her generosity and reassured her everything was going to go smoothly. That was six years ago, and she and her family have now met four of "their" scholars at the annual donor appreciation luncheon, and I look forward to seeing her annual photo with them on Facebook.

I have a unique privilege to help people establish a legacy, and while it is not always easy, it is always rewarding, and I thank God for this calling each time I see one of this gracious donor's photos.

Patience Boudreaux, MBA, is a planned giving officer at LLUH and has been a fundraiser in higher education for nearly two decades. Note: National Philanthropy Day is observed on the 15th of November every year as a way to recognize the contributions that philanthropy has made to the world and to encourage people to become more active in charitable acts.

November 16

"One of them, when he saw that he was healed, came back to Jesus, shouting, 'Praise God!' He fell to the ground at Jesus' feet, thanking him for what he had done. This man was a Samaritan. Jesus asked, 'Didn't I heal ten men? Where are the other nine? Has no one returned to give glory to God except this foreigner?'"

Luke 17:15-18, NLT

People are often thankful for our efforts as health care providers, especially when the outcome is positive. I experienced this when I was in solo practice in a small, rural town. Small tokens of appreciation would appear at the front desk for performance of routine duties or on special occasions. I was always fascinated by who was thankful and for what seemingly small acts prompted a thankful response. I was likewise perplexed when extraordinary effort was ignored.

One case that I never understood was a case of a ruptured abdominal aortic aneurysm (AAA). I was called at 2:00 a.m. to the small hospital ER for a patient in acute abdominal distress. Getting out of bed, I hurriedly dressed, shook the cobwebs from my mind, and rushed to the hospital. As I arrived I observed a rotund man in his 60s complaining of abdominal pain. I began my physical exam, ordering IVs and oxygen and a set of abdominal films. He was clearly in distress, but without an obvious diagnosis. A few minutes into the examination the periumbilical discoloration of the Cullen Sign appeared. I made the preliminary diagnosis of a ruptured AAA, inserted additional lines, pushed fluids, and ordered a medivac and called the surgeon 25 miles away. I anxiously waited for what seemed like hours and watched the chopper's arrival through the night's sky. As the bright lights split the darkness and became fixed on the landing zone, I prayed that it was not too late. The man was loaded and whisked away.

Later that morning I received a call from the surgeon telling me that as the patient was placed on the OR table he crashed, his BP becoming undetectable. With no time to prep, they splashed him with betadine, then went in and cross-clamped the aorta. The patient survived with his new vascular graft and retuned to good health. I never saw him at the hospital again, but many years later I ran into my former patient; he muttered a quick thanks. I never quite understood why he made so little effort to say thank you. Perhaps I expected too much. Spanning the years of my private practice, including more than 25 years working in prisons, I came to find that true thankfulness was a rare trait.

This has caused me to ponder the question of my own thankfulness. In football there is the phenomenon of "the twelfth man,"* but in the Scriptures we have an example of a tenth man: the one who was thankful for what Jesus did for him. Do I practice thankfulness? Am I thankful for everything that He has given me, even the seemingly small stuff? Have I thanked the One who has given me eternal life? Am I the tenth man?

What has Jesus done for you? Have you thanked Him? After all, He has freely provided to you the most precious gift of all: life everlasting. Pray with me today as I resolve to walk with Him in thankfulness and give Him the only gift that I have: my heart.

*The twelfth man is the stadium-filled football fans cheering loudly for the home team's 11 players on the field.

Dwight Winslow, LLUSM class of 1982, completed an internal medicine residency at a University of Washington affiliated program. Most of his career has been spent in correctional medicine with the California Department of Corrections and Rehabilitation. He continues to work as a correctional health care consultant and resides in Northern California and Eastern Washington State. He and his wife of 41 years, Janice, have two daughters and five grandchildren.

November 17

> *"This service that you perform is not only supplying the needs of the Lord's people but is also overflowing in many expressions of thanks to God."*
> 2 Corinthians 9:12, NIV

I felt the warmth of the summer sun slip away as it tucked behind vast New Mexican horizon, its light giving way to ubiquitous twinkling stars as the inviting cool of the desert evening emerged. After 11 years of medical training, the entirety of our marriage, we had arrived at Nathan's final graduation. Nathan would now begin his career as an attending perinatalogist. I was a bit overwhelmed thinking of what it took to arrive at this poignant end of an era.

I thought of medical school, hours spent studying in our Loma Linda apartment, the classmates whose company had made it bearable for Nathan and the friends who never let me feel alone. I thought of the treasured gift cards slipped to us by our parents used to buy clothes and sneak date nights when we could barely afford to pay our rent. I thought of the mentors who assured us we would make it through. I thought of how the elation of medical school graduation gave way to the reality of residency.

I remembered becoming a mother to Ansel, how the combination of joy and exhaustion left me feeling so broken. I thought of how my church families made me know that though I often came to church alone, I was never alone once I got there. I thought of Nathan's mentors through residency, how they shared the knowledge and modeled the values necessary for him to learn to care for his patients and discover the kind of physician he wanted to be. I thought of that last year of residency when we became parents of two.

We juggled setting up life in a new state while working a combined 120 hours a week. I remembered our family members driving hours through traffic to our little Pasadena bungalow to hold newborn Autumn while I put 2-year-old Ansel to bed when Nate worked 24-hour shifts every fourth night.

I remembered four grandparents forgoing summer vacations to move us into our New Mexico home, and Nathan's brother driving our car across three states of desert sans air conditioning. I remembered when Autumn started having seizures and developmental concerns and how Nathan's medical school classmate turned pediatric neurologist instructed me to call her anytime even if all I needed was prayer. I remembered those who held me up during those moments of holy unknown. I thought of our children's caregivers whose high-quality care made it possible for me to give to the children of others.

As I considered how the living, breathing love of God transmitted through so many beautiful souls had carried us to that moment, I was overwhelmed with heart-stopping gratitude. When a season comes to an end, it is natural to look forward with excitement for what is to come, but I was reminded of how important it is to look behind and remember how we arrived. When we recognize how love has propelled us, we will move forward with intention to do the same for others.

Cheri Blue is a speech-language pathologist and PhD student at the University of Utah. Both she and her husband, Nathan Blue (LLUSM class of 2011), graduated from LLUH. They have a son and daughter, Ansel and Autumn, who love outdoor adventuring, as do their parents.

November 18

"It is well to preach as I do, with my lips. But you can all preach with your feet and by your lives, and that is the most effective preaching."
Charles Spurgeon (1834–1892): English Baptist preacher, author, and philanthropist

Peace. After finding UCLA to be a chaotic place to work, I left in 1971 to start working at a hospital I knew little about. The first thing I noticed at my new place of employment, Loma Linda University Medical Center, was what happened on Friday evenings. There was a hush that came over the oncology unit as a few medical students gathered and would go from room to room playing guitars, singing hymns to dying patients. This created an atmosphere of such peace and healing. Back then, while I was mixing my own 5FU chemo from a vial behind a four-inch glass plate, I began to wonder, Who were these genteel, educated, and kindhearted people?

Suffering. The suffering on the unit was immense. Trying to find a spot on my patient's hip to give a shot for nausea was a challenge because of the ravages of cancer. Young mothers saying goodbye to their toddlers because of leukemia was heartbreaking. One tall 14-year-old patient named Patrick weighed a mere 45 pounds at the end. I had so many questions, and I starting seeking God.

Questions and Answers. Before long I sought a hospital chaplain for Bible studies. She was loving, as was my new friend Carmen, who shared her yummy vegetarian recipes. Spiritually I had always felt there was something more out there. I would say to the different medical students I met along the way, "You are an intelligent person; how can you buy all this stuff about Mary and Joseph, etc.?" Each would just say, "Keep studying and praying." It was when I studied the prophetic timetable in the Hebrew Bible that I discovered the concrete evidence that sealed my faith. I realized that God has a great plan of salvation and that He is in charge. The Old Testament had dates that pointed to Jesus, who fulfilled the prophecies in the New Testament. This was amazing news that my patients and I could choose everlasting life without any more pain and suffering.

Response. I made the decision to follow God, and it changed my life for good. I have never wavered, nor looked back. I also knew that when I married someday, my children would have a better life because of my decision. And that came to be true because of the church and school villages that helped me raise my four children. Now my grandchild has started at the same Christian academy where his dad, my son, went to school. While I am not perfect, nor are my children, all of us, including spouses and adult children, are in a service type of teaching or medical career in the Adventist system. What a gift my decision from so long ago has been to my entire family and me!

Appreciation. This hospital is where I originally felt the perfect Spirit blowing through me. I felt the love and learned healthy modeling from you, the Christians at Loma Linda University Medical Center with whom I grew up. I have been ever so blessed ... thank you, my newfound (now five decades later) and forever family!

Nancy Carter Zinke, RN, worked at LLUMC on the oncology unit and psychiatry unit. After having four children, she taught private K-12 Christian-based art lessons. She is currently recording a series of art lessons. She is married to Ernest "Ernie" Zinke (LLUSM class of 1976-A), and they live in Redlands, California.

November 19

> *"And tongues that looked like fire appeared to them, distributing themselves, and a tongue rested on each one of them."*
>
> Acts 2:3, NASB

I hesitate to tell this story lest it sound like I am bragging, but miracles have to be shared, and to God be the glory for what He has done in my life. I hope this story encourages you to believe that God can do greater things in your life.

I have been a career missionary physician since finishing my family medicine residency at Florida Hospital. I was bitten by the mission's bug when as a child I read many of the books about missionaries. This was reinforced by serving a year as a student missionary teaching English during college.

My first medical mission posting was Youngberg Memorial Adventist Hospital in Singapore. When that hospital closed, I moved to the Guam Seventh-day Adventist Clinic. I wanted a foreign challenge, so then I moved to Gimbie Adventist Hospital in Ethiopia. In Gimbie I learned to trust in God more fully, because of my own failings.

Finally I had the opportunity to work at Bangkok Adventist Hospital, but would have to take the medical boards in the Thai language. Others had tried and not been successful. However, the challenges of Ethiopia had taught me that God can perform miracles for weak humans. I decided to try, trusting God would somehow work things out.

While studying, I prayed for a second chapter of Acts experience, in which tongues of fire would come down and give me the instant ability to speak Thai, but God did not see fit to allow that to happen. I studied Thai in Bangkok for 18 months and reviewed the basic and clinical sciences. I had forgotten how many molecules of ATP are produced from a molecule of glucose and many other basic science facts.

The Thai boards came sooner than I felt ready. They consisted of two days of basic science multiple choice questions, two days of clinical science multiple choice questions, one day of clinical essays and one day of practicums with real patients and professors. All of this was in the Thai language. It was one of the most humbling, terrifying experiences of my life. I went to see the posted final results two months later and thankfully found my name on the pass list!

God clearly had a plan for me in Thailand. I have been asked if it was worth all the sweat and tears, and my answer is an adamant yes, for many reasons. I know better now what God can do through me if I let Him. I know He sometimes lets us work for our blessings to appreciate them better. I can speak Thai without a translator and can tell my Thai patients in Thai of Jesus' love and how He helped me get my license to practice in Thailand.

This story is all about God and not me. Find out what He can do through you today if you let Him.

Nick Walters, LLUSM class of 1989, is board-certified in family medicine and has a diploma in tropical medicine. He is married to Phosfe, and they have two sons, Christopher (LLUSD class of 2019) and Ian (LLUSM class of 2021). He is a missionary physician and has been one since 1992. He currently serves in Thailand and previously served in Singapore, Guam, and Ethiopia.

November 20

"But when Jesus heard this, He said, 'This sickness is not to end in death, but for the glory of God, so that the Son of God may be glorified by it.'"

John 11:4, NASB1995

The scars on my son's neck, his chest, and his abdomen are a daily reminder of things in life we often take for granted. The first 24 hours after the arrival of my firstborn son was a flood of wonder, amazement, and hope. He was perfect. As he stared at me through his dark piercing eyes, furrowed eyebrows, and full head of black hair, I dreamed of watching him grow up, playing catch together, all the joys of fatherhood. Little did I know that in 24 hours I would be picking up the shattered pieces of my dreams as they all came crashing to the ground.

He never passed meconium, and his progressive abdominal distension led to confirmation of a bowel obstruction. As he was loaded into the ambulance for transport to the nearest children's hospital, I never anticipated that the next time I would see him he would be almost unrecognizable, sedated, intubated, mottled from sepsis, requiring full hemodynamic support in the NICU with invasive lines and monitors. My mind went numb as the pediatric surgeon discussed the informed consent before they rushed him to the operating room for a bowel perforation. I felt completely and utterly helpless. My son had just entered this world and was already fighting for his life. It was not fair.

His postoperative course did not provide any respite. His lungs started to fail, requiring ECMO, in addition to TPN for an enterocutaneous fistula, functional short gut, and an ileostomy. Those eight weeks in the NICU were a blur. But what buoyed us through the storm were the comforting words of the surgeons on rounds each day, the tender loving care provided by the nurses day and night, and the prayers going up to the throne of God from family, friends, and even strangers.

In the moment of my greatest need, I was able to witness a glimpse of God's love manifested through the powerful extent of human compassion. Ten years later my son's scars are a reminder of our valley of death experience, but even more, it reminds me of the power in medicine to show compassion to the suffering, offer hope to the hopeless, and knit relationships that will last for eternity. I will never forget the surgeons and nurses who cared for us. Their lives are forever entwined with ours.

In heaven my son's scars will be no more, as "old things have passed away; behold, all things have become new" (2 Corinthians 5:17, NKJV). However, Christ has chosen to keep His scars as an eternal reminder of His love for us. As He said to Thomas: "Reach your finger here, and look at My hands; and reach your hand here, and put it into My side. Do not be unbelieving, but believing" (John 20:27, NKJV). Thank You, Jesus. To God be the glory.

Jukes Namm, LLUSM class of 2005, is an assistant professor in LLUSM's department of surgery, division of surgical oncology. He serves as the program director for the general surgery residency program. He married his medical school classmate, Aileen. They have three children: Ian, Ella, and Audra.

November 21

> *"For Christ also died for sins once for all, the just for the unjust, so that He might bring us to God, having been put to death in the flesh, but made alive in the spirit."*
>
> 1 Peter 3:18, NASB1995

Yes or no?

"No." This simple word once gave me the power to end someone's life. As a college student I had joined a bone marrow registry called "Be the Match." I soon forgot about this until I received a phone call telling me how I could help a baby girl suffering from acute myelogenous leukemia. Legally I could not be told any more about her. No name, no face. Just "the recipient." She, a complete stranger, now clung to the slim chance at life that my bone marrow offered. Though I had no obligation to proceed, I hoped that if I were in a similar situation, some nameless stranger would also help me. Let the testing begin.

And test they did. After several rounds of testing I met with my physician to discuss the procedure. "For this procedure there is no tangible benefit to you, only risk," the oncologist intoned. "The risk of serious complications is between one in 10,000 and one in 100,000." He moved on to discuss the risks of bleeding, infection, and pain, while my mind stayed on the "serious complications."

"The risk is low, but not zero." I have used these same words with my own patients when discussing informed consent, but now that I'm on the receiving end, the words somehow sound different. And though my participation is voluntary, there is a catch.

About a week before my own donation, the recipient would begin chemotherapy, targeting her cancer at the expense of destroying her bone marrow. Once begun, she was totally dependent on my continued consent. I had no such limitation. With one no, I could walk away from the proceedings, causing a family to lose their little girl. Never before did one word carry such power. This experience has taught me a new connection between me and my Savior, Jesus Christ.

Before His crucifixion, Jesus could also have walked away. In the Garden of Gethsemane, after one of His disciples violently tried to thwart Judas' betrayal, Jesus interrupted the fighting saying, "Thinkest thou that I cannot now pray to my Father, and he shall presently give me more than twelve legions of angels?" (Matthew 26:53, KJV). Expecting His death the following morning, Jesus reminded His disciples that not only was this betrayal expected, but also that His coming sacrifice was voluntary. After all, Judas' betrayal was foretold in Psalm 41:9 and 55:12-14. Jesus already knew of the suffering that He was to experience, with no tangible physical benefit to Himself (Isaiah 53). The path to the cross led to only risk, only pain, only death.

To my eternal gratitude, Jesus did not turn away from His chosen course. He endured indignities and pain beyond my imagining. He gave of Himself so that I could live. My own small sacrifice pales in significance next to what He has done for me. I cannot—will not—say no because my Savior did not say no. I must go on. And as the anesthetic takes hold, I decide, yes.

Ken Mindoro, LLUSM class of 2003, works for the California Department of Corrections and Rehabilitation in medical informatics helping physicians to get home in time for dinner. He and his wife, Audrey, live in Camino, California, and have a passion for evangelism and international medical mission work.

November 22

*"The L*ORD *is my light and my salvation; whom shall I fear? The L*ORD *is the strength of my life; of whom shall I be afraid?"*
Psalm 27:1, NKJV

Driving my daughter and her friend to school, I knew I was in trouble. The sensation had returned with a vengeance. Two days prior I was relaxing at home when I felt a tense uneasiness in my chest. Running through the cardiac risk factors, I counted zero. Thinking, *I'm 47, I walk or run three to six miles every day, and this isn't pain anyway*, I convinced myself that I was just stressed. Now I knew something was wrong. Barely making it to work, my colleague Duncan Leung (LLUSM class of 1982) saw the EKG changes and acted quickly, whisking me off to the ER, where I ruled in for MI. Lying on the cold cath table, I listened dazedly as my cardiologist told me the extent of my disease: quadruple vessel occlusion. I underwent heart surgery the following day.

I'm comfortable in the hospital as a physician, but as a patient I was a nervous wreck. The flip side of medicine is scary: You go from being in control of almost everything to having no control over anything. It was an unnatural environment for me. But I was the recipient of genuine kindness from so many strangers. The skill and encouragement of fellow physicians, the caring touch of nurses and therapists, and the gentleness of radiation techs and orderlies calmed my trepidation.

Through my experience as a patient, I see we as physicians are uniquely positioned to serve as the hands and feet of Jesus. From the technical expertise needed to perform intricate operations and procedures, to the power of our words and the manner in which we say them, we have a wonderful opportunity to impact people for the Lord that few professions do.

My road to recovery hit major difficulties, yet what I lost physically pales in comparison to what I have gained spiritually. I've been blessed to have my daughters, Taryn and Bryn, and wife, Lacy, by my side every step of the way. After surgery Lacy dressed me, fed me, walked me, and gave me a bath . . . I sound like a dog, don't I? She did for me what I couldn't, with a loving heart. She's truly my best friend and soulmate.

I've been blessed to experience the power of prayer. The Word of God says that the effective, fervent prayer of a righteous person avails much. I know the Lord heard the prayers of those praying for me. My chronic anxiety has been replaced by His peace that passes all understanding. He is my light and salvation. I have nothing to fear.

I'm truly thankful for God's presence in my life. I am thankful for His sustaining love and grace, even when things didn't turn out the way I had hoped they would. And I am privileged to learn what it really means to trust and wait upon the Lord.

H. Roger Batin, LLUSM class of 1993, currently limits his practice to telemedicine at Redlands Kaiser Clinic in Redlands, California. He has been married to Lacy (LLUSAHP class of 1994) for 26 years and has two daughters, Taryn and Bryn.

November 23

> *"With God all things are possible."*
> Matthew 19:26, ESV

"Will I have to go home without installing the equipment?" I wondered. Getting the unit ready, crating and shipping it, preparing the room, and all the travel expenses would sadly be wasted.

It was November of 1998, and I'd traveled to Madagascar to install an X-ray machine for the Andapa Adventist Hospital. Andapa was a several-hour trip north of Madagascar's capital city of Antananarivo. It looked like a small old Western town with tin roofs and dirt streets, with the hospital set on a rise above the lush jungle valley.

I always sent full instructions ahead on preparing the room for the equipment. An X-ray unit requires a good-sized wire for the power supply. I went to the room where the unit was to be installed and asked the technician where the electrical power was. He pointed to a small wire hanging from the ceiling. It was questionable if it would even run a toaster! Two days earlier he had gone to the local power company to look for the wire needed, but they didn't have it. So the local doctor, his friend and I went back to town to talk to the supervisor of the power company. He took us out behind the building where there was a bunch of different wires all around a large tree. Nothing there would work. The wire needed to be about ¾-inch thick, and we needed 450 feet of it!

While the others were still looking by the tree, I wandered off around the building and came to the loading dock. There on the dock lay two large rolls of wire. It was exactly what we needed! The doctor and his friend were in tears. Everyone there, and back in the capital city down south, said it was impossible. There was no reason for large wire like that to be there in that remote place. They had no use for it. We truly believe that wire was put there by unseen hands!

We had our large wire. Now for the second half of the story!

The seven-way conductor cables that I'd made for connecting the components of the machine together were missing. They had probably been stolen in customs. What to do? Would our efforts be wasted?

There was a small store in Andapa that sold pots and pans, dresses, umbrellas, and such. The doctor and I went there, and he told the owner what we were looking for. The man went to the back of the store and, after a while, came out with a coil of wire. Unbelievably, it was a seven-way conductor wire, the exact thing we needed, and exact amount we needed! This wire is usually used only on equipment requiring multiple connections. *There was no reason for it to be there!*

I had carried my tools, schematics, and extra connectors from California just in case, and was able to make new cables. So, with unseen help again, I was able to install a fully functioning X-ray machine. Why was it out there in the jungle? God only knows!

Donovan C. Nelson, RT, worked at LLUMC for 48 years, first as chief radiologic technologist and then as senior service engineer for radiology. On his own time he acquired and refurbished approximately 35 X-ray machines and installed them for SDA mission hospitals all around the world. He and his wife, Carroll, were married for 64 years. He is most proud of his 4 children and delights in his 10 grandchildren and 2 great-grandchildren.

November 24

Thanksgiving Day, 2022

> *"There is nobody you couldn't learn to love once you've heard their story."*
> Fred Rogers (1928–2003): American host of television's Mr. Rogers'
> Neighborhood (1968–2001) and Presbyterian minister

When I was in high school, I was hired to clean up some yard waste. I borrowed my dad's trailer and loaded broken cement, branches, and dirt for hours.

I worked quickly so I could get to the landfill before they closed Friday night. I was just in time! I joined the line of cars waiting to pay just 10 minutes before closing.

As I got to the window, the aging cashier said, "That'll be $30, please." That wasn't good—it was almost always $20. I guess the cement was heavier than I thought, but I had only $20 in cash.

I told him, "I'm sorry. I was expecting it to be $20; that's all I have in cash. Can I pay with my debit card?"

"Nope. Machine's broke."

"Well, I don't have time to go to the bank and get back before you close. Can I pay with a check?"

"Nope."

I took a deep breath. My dad wanted his trailer back tonight so that he could use it over the weekend. I was not looking forward to unloading the trailer, then reloading it again next week.

I took a deep breath. I said, "Well, I guess I'll have to come back, then." I tried to smile and added, "I appreciate you being here; I'm sure it's hard to tell people no. I'll see you Monday—have a good weekend."

As I was getting into my car, he called me back to the window. He had tears streaming down his cheeks. He said, "I have worked here for 22 years. I've had to turn away a lot of people; you are the first person ever to thank me anyway. Give me your $20, and you can go on in."

So I did.

One lesson might be "Be nice to people so you can get what you want." But the tears on his face bothered me more than reloading the trailer would have.

Many people are suffering in ways we don't recognize.

Being kind can make a difference. If he hadn't called me back, I could easily have missed the impact of my words.

I want to live in a world in which people are kind. Even though I may be frustrated, I want to be kind to the patient who needs something explained, again. I want to be kind when everyone is frustrated. I want to be kind to the cashier working the night shift on a holiday.

I want to be kind as others have been kind to me.

If we can remember Jesus' ultimate kindness, we can stay on track. Kindness and love are not weaknesses.

W. Tait Stevens, LLUSM class of 2000, is an assistant professor in LLUSM's department of pathology and human anatomy, division of pathology. He enjoys photography and exploring the local deserts and mountains with his family.

November 25

"But let all who take refuge in you be glad; let them ever sing for joy. Spread your protection over them, that those who love your name may rejoice in you."

Psalm 5:11, NIV

Every medical student needs an escape from the books. For my group of five friends our getaway was the ocean, and on Black Friday we chose to forgo the chaos of sales and shopping in exchange for sand, sun, and surf. What differed this Friday from our other surfing expeditions was that the surfboards would be strapped to the roof instead of placing them inside the SUV. I was a little apprehensive about the strap setup, as a quick Google search for instructions produced online tutorials with such ominous warnings as "Flying surfboards can kill people!" Making sure we triple-checked the strap security, we started the journey. The car was filled with the usual chatter, discussing how many slices of pies had been eaten the day before, etc., when abruptly one of the girls said, "Wait! We didn't pray!" Right at the red light heads bowed, and we asked for God's hand of protection over our day.

Less than one minute later we were on the highway when I started hearing bumps and rattling from the top of the car. Suddenly I watched my worst nightmare unfold in my side-view mirror. In the blink of an eye four surfboards went flying across all four lanes of the interstate, hitting the pavement and careening toward the incoming, unsuspecting traffic. As I pulled to the shoulder, I envisioned everything that could go wrong—a 10-car pileup, crushed surfboards, and potentially much worse.

But by the grace of God, two semitrucks behind us stopped on a dime, blocking all traffic. One truck driver leaped out, grabbing one surfboard and bringing it to the side of the SUV while we sprinted down the highway to retrieve the others. He hopped back into his semi as we shouted thanks, and within seconds traffic resumed as normal; no one even honked their horn. There was not one collision; not one car was scratched; and the surfboards were just fine despite flipping across four lanes of traffic. Lying on the side of the road was the culprit responsible for this harrowing experience—the attached metal roof rack had ripped off our vehicle, taking all the strapped surfboards with it. Huddled together on the side of the highway, we were struck by how differently this situation could have played out: The heavy metal rods hurtling through the air at 60 miles per hour could have easily pierced through a windshield.

Literally seconds beforehand we had prayed for God to protect us. In a situation we never even dreamed would unfold, He had done just that—shielding us and every person on the busy highway by sending two semitrucks to be behind us at the perfect moment. Our next words to God were of deep gratitude.

Prayer is profoundly powerful. Surfboards, semis, and Interstate 10 reminded me of this in a way I will never forget.

Briana Greene, LLUSM class of 2023, spends her free time surfing and is dedicated to her nonprofit From Hearts 2 Hands, Inc., which works to help needy children in Tanzania. God willing, she hopes to serve as a mission doctor in Tanzania.

November 26

> *"Now faith is the assurance of things hoped for,*
> *the conviction of things not seen."*
> Hebrews 11:1, ESV

In 2004 my parents sat my sister and me down for a talk that would change our lives. "*Hijitos* [children], I want you to know that what we are doing is to better your future," my dad said as I tried to make sense of the recent sale of our house, furniture, and everything in between. It hit me so fast I had trouble grasping what was really going on. "We love you both so much, and we hope one day you will understand," my mom said in tears. As they wrapped up the conversation, he told me that I had two suitcases to pack all my valuables and belongings. One week later I put on my lucky, multilayered green-and-gray shirt, said farewell to our grandma in Lima, and set off to the land of opportunity.

Six months after our arrival in the U.S., our lives were dramatically altered. My dad exchanged his white coat for factory gloves and my mom's stethoscope for a student account. Our family traded in the comfort of yearlong sun in the tropical jungle of Peru for the frigid temperatures of Massachusetts. We left behind our friends and family for the uncertainty ahead.

Yet somehow it all seemed to work out. God's loving and caring nature created so many miracles and opportunities for us. Our short supply of food lasted beyond a week's notice. Random strangers gave away their clothes to us when we needed them most. Others allowed us to hitch a ride to church or school in the cold winters and scorching summers. Some shared how we could check in at a clinic for the underserved at no cost.

God never left us. My parents had unwavering faith in Him even when our bank account had only two digits. A language barrier was not strong enough to tumble us. If anything, struggles became the solid foundation to rely on Him more—to trust His timing and plan that He so delicately designed for us.

Daily we remind ourselves of blessings that have been placed along and poured on our path. Had it not been for the random acts of kindness from people, the unexpected hours given for my dad to work, or the food bank willing to provide us with meals for our table, our life story would have a different ending. But God had something special in store for us.

As the plane took off on that misty spring day, my parents prayed this new beginning would be His will. We had no clue what was going to happen to us or where we would end up. What we didn't realize is that He had already crafted an amazing, unparalleled plan for us—one that brought forth experiences we learned from and later would become the boxing gloves to fight hardships that would come our way.

Trust in Him, and you will realize that He, too, has a plan for you.

Ricardo Chujutalli, LLUSM class of 2021, received his MBA from La Sierra University in Riverside, California. He enjoys reading, traveling, and exercising in his free time.

November 27

> *"He will wipe away every tear from their eyes, and death shall be no more, neither shall there be mourning, nor crying, nor pain anymore, for the former things have passed away."*
> Revelation 21:4, ESV

I held you in my arms. The weight of your shoulder and torso felt heavy, as if the whole world collapsed beneath your feet, and there was nothing left to slump on besides me. My MRSA-ridden, pen-stained coat soaked in your tears. From the tip of my shoulder, the salt spread like vines and tree buds of a newborn spud. The trail of sea water left dark, black stains of mascara and eyeliner, veiled in foundation and blush. I stood unmoving. You stood unmoving, and the room was dark, somber from the evening light. All inanimate life was shadowed by the dense, gray blinds. and it made everything feel worse. Your husband lay in bed unmoving. His eyes fell shut from fatigue. His mouth cracked with blood from plastic tubing. His hands frail. His body frail. His skin like paste, dull and doughy.

I hope he heard us. I hope he could hear. Our quiet prayers for him, for God to spare, the suffering, the pain, the gasps for air, the wear and tear, and most of all, the trepidation and wreckage of mind and spirit. My Spanish was poor. I hoped it was good enough. Maybe God could hear our calls for *Dios*, our calls for help, our calls for translation, unspoken and urgent.

And can I tell you the truth? My heart ached. It ached so bad. Your weight felt whole, yet so severe. Like an entire whale, it floated, yet crushed my entire core. The weight presented in my chest—deep, down within, not on my drenched shoulder; sturdy, yet thin. I wished it would dissipate. Still I held you close. And told my nasolacrimal ducts to start working. Hurry, hurry, hurry! Absorb back those lousy tears. This was not the time. Please, not now. Ugh, you flimsy, little specks of salt and despair.

Here you are. And here he is. Your loved one unrecognizable against a stark, pallid room. Filled with machines and monitors, lines and chimes, drips and stale day-old bread. The atmosphere clouded in dread. You step back away and hold my hand. Your wrinkled little palm sat still in my hand. The palm of an 80-year-old woman, whom I barely knew, but felt the greatest sentiment with, the suffering and hurt intense. I am overcome with emotion and quickly step outside. Can I tell you I ran to the bathroom to cry my own cry?

And at the end of the day I lie in bed. And I cry a long cry without clarity of why. I wake up anew as the dawn shines through my red emblazoned curtains, giving the room a tiring hue. The puffy eyes are covered with eyeliner and dust. The pouched bags are covered with foundation and blush. The coat is cleaned in the washer with chemical bleach. The coat turns white, but thoughts of you and your husband continue to saturate the fibers of my heart. You are stained within me with permanent ink. And I carry his death with the deaths of the past, and I think he and the others forever changed me. How long will we last?

Thi Khuc completed her internal medicine residency at LLUH in 2020. She is currently a gastroenterology fellow at the University of Maryland. She has a passion for indulging in ice cream, hiking outdoors, and serving others.

November 28

Early on the morning of November 28, 1967, two Army officers in full dress uniform knocked on our door, and my world fell apart. My husband, James Brannon Meek, had been serving as a conscientious objector combat medic in the jungles of Vietnam, but he would not be coming home. At 19 I became a Gold Star wife and a "hero's widow." Jimmy and I were both raised in Adventist homes, and he had attended Adventist schools since the first grade. We were grounded in our faith, believing that angels would be there to protect us. My first thought was *How could this be?* I had never let myself think that God wouldn't bring him home.

The ceremonies and honors that followed praised Jimmy's short life, awarding him the Bronze Star, the Purple Heart, and other citations and medals. From the first moments of shock through the heart-wrenching days of despair that followed, my journey through grief was supported by our family, friends, and the letters that I received from the guys in Jimmy's company still in Vietnam. Jimmy's caring Christian example had impressed those young men so profoundly that for years afterward they kept in touch with me, though most knew me only through the letters and care packages that I had sent and Jimmy had shared. Many of the wounded that Jimmy had cared for in the field and whom he had carried to safety made it home. They told me stories about how he would pray and share his faith in the precious peaceful moments they had in the midst of the hell of war.

Soon after the funeral, the president of our local chamber of commerce received a letter from Jimmy's commanding officer with a check—money collected from the men in his unit, asking for a monument to be erected in remembrance of "Doc," the medic they had all learned to love. The monument at the base of the flagpole on the campus of Forest Lake Academy in Florida is a permanent reminder to future generations of the courage, faithful service, and sacrifice made by those in uniform and especially by my young husband.

After the war Leon, the unit's radioman from Michigan, made good on a promise that he had made to Jimmy, and sang at the Forest Lake church. John, the front man from Hawaii, who was with Jimmy when he died but whom he knew only as "Doc," searched for Jimmy's family for years before we reconnected so that he could tell me about how my husband had made a difference in his life. Fifty-two years later we still keep in touch and I can count on a package of macadamia candies from Hawaii in the mail every Thanksgiving.

God did not bring my husband home safely, but in the years that followed He showed me time and time again that He was keeping the promise of Jeremiah 29:11. Though His plans had not been my own, He had prospered Jimmy's short time on earth, and He was prospering mine. Four years after that horrible morning, His plans for me included learning to love again, and I married Tom. For 47 years Tom has loved me for who I am and for who I was, and has allowed me the freedom to do the one thing most important to Gold Star families: to never forget. Every day Gold Star families honor the memories of those who did not come home, and our hearts look forward to the heavenly reunion when we can claim the promise of Isaiah 25:8, which says that Jesus will swallow up death in victory and wipe away all tears.

Suzonne Weeks Meek Murrell and James B. Meek met at Forest Lake Academy and were married in July 1967. Jimmy lost his life on November 28, 1967. Sue married Tom Murrell (LLUSAHP class of 1972) in 1973. They have two daughters, including Monica Wernick (LLUSM class of 2006), and four wonderful grandchildren. She and Tom are involved in outreach by the U.S. Department of Defense to honor Vietnam veterans and Gold Star families who were not properly acknowledged or thanked for their sacrifice following the action in Vietnam. They, along with Jimmy's family (Bill Meek [LLUSM class of 1971] and Neva Mason Meek [LLUSM class of 1970]), strive to keep Jimmy's memory alive and honor his sacrifice.

November 29

"When you pass through the waters, I will be with you; and when you pass through the rivers, they will not sweep over you. When you walk through the fire, you will not be burned; the flames will not set you ablaze."

Isaiah 43:2, NIV

It was almost two decades ago when I was a first-year medical student at Loma Linda School of Medicine, yet I will never forget that summer. It was a dream come true to be accepted to medical school and pursue my calling of studying medicine. Within the first couple of months into my studies I found myself deep in the waters and the blazes of trouble. I was afflicted with a serious medical condition that was slowly weakening my body, mind, and spirit. My learning was impaired; my concentration, broken. I felt lost, alone, and terrified. Everything that I had worked so hard to achieve was quickly slipping away from me. I remember walking into the anatomy lab, surrounded by the cadavers, their bodies dissected for our studies, their mouths open and distorted facial expressions. For a brief moment, I felt like I was in the throes of hell itself, surrounded by death and hopelessness.

One morning, as I was walking aimlessly on campus, carrying my heavy backpack full of notes and books that had ceased to make sense to me any longer, I happened to run into the dean of students. The despair and fear on my face was unmistakable and obvious. Dr. Henry Lamberton walked me to his office, and we talked. We talked for a long time, and I shared my struggles, fears and failures. He simply listened. He listened and then offered to pray with me and for me. We sat in his office and for the first time in my life, I heard a person utter the most genuine and powerful prayer that touched my heart and awakened my hope that God was with me, in that very instant. I was able to take medical leave, and although my journey through medical school was marked with deep valleys and peaks, I was able to graduate and earn my degree.

I have always said, I met God at Loma Linda, and it's true. I grew up in the former Soviet Armenia where Communism had stripped its people of their spirituality and religion. Ancient churches had been converted to warehouses for storing potatoes and discarded furniture. Many parades and Communist marches had become religion itself. At the time, when I was going through my struggles as a medical student, I did not know that the cross I had come to bear was a gift bestowed upon me to grow me in wisdom, strength, courage, resiliency, and love. It was the same cross that Jesus had given me to liberate me and show me who He truly was. I met God in the prayers of the chapel we had every week at Loma Linda. I met Him in the friendships and kindness of its faculty, teachers, and attending physicians. I met Him in the eyes of the patients I cared for and in the newborn babies I helped deliver. I met God at Loma Linda and will be eternally grateful to have been given the opportunity and privilege to spend those few critical years of my medical education at this very special place—a place that valued spirituality and spiritual growth; a place that understood the bigger picture and the larger purpose for us as individuals, students, and budding physicians. It was this kind of education that taught me to sit down with a dying patient in silence and simply pray; to hold their hand and connect with my heart. This was the type of education that enriched me as a physician and has allowed me to wholly take care of my patients today, decades later. I will forever be indebted to this wonderful organization and am proud to be its alumna.

Kristine Tatosyan-Jones, LLUSM class of 2007, is a faculty physician at Vanderbilt University Medical Center in Nashville, Tennessee, department of family medicine.

November 30

> *"They will have no fear of bad news; their hearts are steadfast, trusting in the Lord."*
> Psalm 112:7, NIV

More than 18 years ago, when she was 19, my daughter nearly died. Every day, I am grateful that she is alive. Unfortunately, my experience is not everyone's—I know many people whose children have not survived. I do not believe that God chose to save my child that day, because if I believe that, then must I also believe that He chose not to save someone else's child? I do not believe that God performed a miracle to save my daughter, because if I do, how can I explain why God would grant us a miracle and not give one to my closest friends? I hope that you never experience either of these tragedies, but if you have or know someone who has, I'd like to share some of what I learned from my experience.

I do not believe that because my daughter survived, God has a special plan for her life. I found that this belief, rather than comforting, put a great burden on the person who survived. I do believe that God can help all of us become more understanding and empathetic because of our experiences, and if we do, we can show a more complete picture of God to those around us.

I have learned that life itself is a miracle.

I have learned that the guilt of surviving while someone else didn't is very hard to live with.

I do not believe that God blessed me or my child—because if I do, why didn't He bless someone else the same way? How can I possibly say "I am blessed" when my child survived but yours did not?

I have also learned that God provides for us in ways we can never imagine. He provides people with the ability to learn, to develop new techniques, to perfect their skills in diagnosis, surgery, and caring for others. In my daughter's recovery, from the surgeons who operated on her back, hips, and leg, to the physical and occupational therapists, the nurses, X-ray technicians, people who brought the food trays, blood donors, and a myriad of others involved in her care—God gave these people the ability to care for and treat others. God also provided us with family, friends, and strangers who supported us physically, emotionally, and spiritually on a daily basis. Perhaps, these are the miracles we prayed for.

Last, I have learned to be grateful for life every day and treasure it while I am able because I know that life can change in a split second.

Even though I cannot explain the good and bad of life, I believe that God is with us through it all and that He will give us strength and courage in whatever we face. And I believe that ultimately God will make all things right. That He will bring back those who have left us too soon and heal the hearts and bodies of those left behind. Until that time, my prayer is that I trust Him and that I can be a support to those in need.

Merrilee Scofield, LLUSPH MPH class of 1981 (nutrition and health education) and LLUSPH MS class of 1982 (nutrition), spent most of her career as a pediatric dietician and certified diabetes educator. For the past 26 years she has worked for the pediatric outpatient diabetes specialty team clinic at LLUCH until her retirement in June 2021. She enjoys gardening, hiking, spending time with her two daughters and their husbands, going to the beach with her husband, Ken, and most of all, playing with her four adorable grandchildren.

DECEMBER

⋅ HUMANITY ⋅

"Humanity should be our race.
Love should be our religion."

Anonymous

December 1

> *"Beloved, let us love one another, for love is from God,*
> *and whoever loves has been born of God and knows God."*
> 1 John 4:7, ESV

It was about 1:30 a.m. on a cold December night at the former Riverside General Hospital in Riverside, California. Our internal medicine team was on call and, as usual, we were at the limits of being overwhelmed with really sick patients. As the senior resident I made frequent visits to the ER, and Dr. Naftel made sure I was always within reach. Our two interns, Claudia Foster and Larry Loo, worked like three and incorporated the medical students into all of our activities. We were already 15 admissions deep when I was called to the ER. With two medical student escorts, I hurried to the ER to see a doctor and two nurses busily attending to a obtunded man who shouted incoherently at times. He was gaunt, had long matted hair resembling dreadlocks and an unkempt graying beard with remnants of prior meals, chips of autumn foliage, and dried spittle. His skin was dry and wrinkled, and he had what appeared to be a well-weathered tan on the exposed areas of his face, upper chest, and arms. He had the odor of stale alcohol mixed with smoke and "street" . . . an odor not unfamiliar to ER personnel.

The ER doctor reported "bloods cooking" and a "portable chest," then added, "He's a sick puppy . . . a keeper, no wiggling out of this one," his last comment alluding to the common practice of senior residents to look for every way possible not to have to admit yet another patient over the often vehement objection of the ER docs. I approached my new patient, introduced myself and the student, and said we were there to help him. "What is your name, sir?"

He opened his eyes with much effort and whispered, "Filthy McNasty." His eyes were a dirty blue but kindly; it was agonizing for him to speak—the poorly placed nasal cannula didn't seem to bother him. One student dutifully wrote his name without catching its obvious meaning. It would take several hours of working with him that night and into the following day: trans-tracheal sputum collection, blood cultures, IV antibiotics, bath, clean hospital clothes—a virtual makeover. His "skin tan" disappeared into the bath to expose his pallor, and his wrinkles smoothened out as he received IV fluids. He had a lung abscess and multiple abnormalities on his blood chemistries and his CBC.

Our students tenderly cared for him—a pedicure, manicure, and lip balm. The social worker managed to contact his niece in Fresno. She came to see him and make arrangements to take him home. Our nurses and students showered him with attention and acknowledgment as a valued and valuable human being. During the ensuing days he replaced his self-deprecating moniker with his real name. Transformed, he was no longer Filthy McNasty! He was somebody, he belonged—a child of God!

Amazing what antibiotics, fluids, folate, and multiple vitamin injections can do. Ahh . . . but kindness, compassion, love, and caring are potent therapeutic agents: a soothing balm even for deep wounds and lung abscesses. We are privileged to dispense these freely in unmeasured doses.

Zeno L. Charles-Marcel is an adjunct associate professor in LLUSM's department of medicine. In 1980 he graduated from Howard University College of Medicine in Washington, D.C. Currently he is vice president of medical affairs at Wildwood Health Institute in Georgia, and associate director for health ministries for the General Conference of Seventh-day Adventists.

December 2

"A Christian reveals true humility by showing the gentleness of Christ, by being always ready to help others, by speaking kind words and performing unselfish acts, which elevate and ennoble the most sacred message that has come to our world."

Ellen G. White (1827–1915): instrumental in the founding of Loma Linda University, one of the founders of the Seventh-day Adventist Church, and American author; in Life Sketches, p. 86

The call from the nursing home relayed that an 85-year-old male was coming in by ambulance complaining of increased shortness of breath. Once the patient arrived, it was clear that he was in the process of dying. While I was preparing for aggressive resuscitative efforts, my attending physician was shuffling through some paperwork that had come with the patient and discovered a "do not resuscitate" order, signed by the patient. The paperwork also stated that he had advanced cancer. It was clear why the patient had decided he did not want any procedures to be done. With this added information, we put a stop to our efforts, followed the wishes of the patient, and made him as comfortable as possible in his final moments.

My attending asked the paramedics about the patient's family, and they said they would be arriving in 5 to 10 minutes. At the time I was the senior resident in charge, and I was feeling the increased pressure of wanting to see more patients and to get some charting done. A 5-to-10-minute wait may not seem like much, but in the shift of an emergency physician it can feel like an eternity. However, my attending didn't leave the patient's side, and he held his hand the whole time.

After several long minutes our patient's family arrived in the emergency department. We talked over the care of the patient, and the family quickly understood the entire situation. With tears in their eyes they still had one request from us: They asked that my attending and I participate with their family in prayer. Of course, we could not refuse. As we gathered around the bedside, all holding hands, we instantly felt for that brief moment as members of the family. The more we listened to the prayer, something incredible happened. The patient, whom we had no previous connection to and knew nothing about, quickly became very real to us. During the prayer the family described our patient as not only a wonderful and loving person, but also the rock and foundation of this entire family, and that this dying patriarch would be missed beyond measure. What an unforgettable moment that was, to instantly connect to our patient and his family during his last moments on earth.

Then I had an epiphany—what would it have looked like if the family had arrived and no one was at the bedside? It would have looked like their loved one was being abandoned in his final hour. But his family arrived to see my attending holding the hand of their loved one, and he was able to explain the entire situation the moment they arrived. In emergency medicine we train to save lives. We live for chest tubes, charged paddles, and difficult airways. In reality, the most important and meaningful thing we can do sometimes is as simple as staying in the room a few more minutes.

Jesse Kellar, LLUSM class of 2010, LLUH emergency medicine residency class of 2013, is the founding program director for a new emergency medicine residency in Fresno, California. He and his wife, Louisa, homeschool their three sons on a small farm in the foothills of the Sierras, where the guys all forge knives and ride motorcycles.

December 3

At Reagan International Airport my wife, Eileen, and I had an hour's wait for our flight to California via Chicago. After settling in with our carry-ons, Eileen went for a walk.

Shortly an elderly Black woman walked up, pushed Eileen's bags aside, and sat down next to me. Well! So many empty seats, and this woman chooses my wife's seat? I felt this was an intrusion into my personal space. With a quick glance I noticed her snug black knit cap and thick glasses, so thick that her gaze seemed unfocused. I like people and a good conversation. But this woman?

"Pardon me, sir," she said. " Could you tell me the time?"

I glanced at my watch: "Eleven," I said. She nodded a thank-you smile. "Where are you going?" I asked.

"Chicago," she said. "My plane leaves at 1:00."

"Have you lived long in Chicago?" I asked.

"Yes, many years."

"What brought you to Washington? Were you visiting family?"

"No," she said. "I came here to receive an award."

"An award!" I said, intrigued. "Tell me more, please."

"Have you seen the morning paper?" She handed me a copy, pointing to the headline: "FIRST LADIES." "Oh! I have a copy of the program, too."

"I'd love to see it," I said, noting the program's title, "First Ladies Salute First Women."

I recognized many names: Barbara Walters, Mistress of Ceremonies; Hillary Rodham Clinton; The Honorable Madeleine Albright; The Honorable Dianne Feinstein; The Honorable Shirley Chisholm; The Honorable Sandra Day O'Connor.

Then names of five women receiving the National First Ladies Library Award. First was "The Honorable Madeleine K. Albright." Second was "Gwendolyn Brooks."

"That's me! What an honor, and a lot of fun!"

I read her biographical sketch: "Gwendolyn Brooks, first African American female Pulitzer Prize winner for poetry; the second poet laureate of Illinois, succeeding Carl Sandburg; 1997 recipient of the Lincoln Laureate medal; current writer-in-residence at Chicago State University, where the Gwendolyn Brooks Center for Black Culture and a chair have been named in her honor."

There was much more. "Miss Brooks, the recipient of more than 75 honorary doctorates . . . and in 1995, awarded the prestigious National Medal of the Arts. Gwendolyn Brooks, author of more than 26 books."

Eileen returned, and I introduced her to my new friend. Miss Brooks took us on a fascinating tour of her life.

Near our departure time she apologized. "Oh, I'm sorry. What do you do, sir?"

Humbly I said I was mayor of a small California town and a university professor.

"Wow! I'm so impressed to be sitting next to the mayor!"

What? Gwendolyn Brooks, a Pulitzer Prize winner with over 75 doctorates, glad to be sitting next to me?

"Please keep that program. Here, I'll sign it for you, and if you write to me, I will send you an autographed copy of my latest poetry book."

On the way to our gate I turned back for a last look. None of my first impressions mattered—not the funny knit cap, thick glasses, age. I had just spent an hour in the presence of royalty.

Thank you, Gwendolyn Brooks. Thank you for talking to a small-town mayor and his wife. Thank you for showing me that a caring life transcends age, color, appearance—everything else. Thank you for sending me your autographed book of poems as you promised. And thank you for intruding, and kindly teaching me never to judge another.

Floyd Petersen, MPH, taught biostatistics at LLUSPH, LLUSN, and LLUSM for 22 years. He also served on the Loma Linda City Council, including 10 years as mayor. Before LLUH he had taught seven years in Zambia and eight years in Canada. Note: Gwendolyn Brooks died in December 2000.

December 4

"The Spirit of the Lord God is upon me, because the LORD has anointed me to bring good news to the humble; He has sent me to bind up the brokenhearted, to proclaim release to captives and freedom to prisoners."
Isaiah 61:1, NASB

When I attended medical school at LLUH, I expected to someday go overseas and work in a mission hospital. My husband, John (LLUSM class of 1981), and I took an elective quarter our last year and went to Phuket, Thailand. It was a wonderful experience working in the hospital and clinic there, and it opened my eyes to other cultures and the many needs in the mission field.

I chose a career in family medicine. My experiences included private practice, pain management, medical director of a community health center, addiction medicine, and lead physician in an Indian health center.

Two years ago my career ended because of medical issues. These past two years in retirement I did a lot of soul-searching, looking for purpose in my life. I felt as though my identity as a physician was such a part of me that there was a big void in my life. I looked back at my career, questioning why John and I hadn't returned to the mission field.

Then God brought to my mind the faces of patients I had helped in my career who had lived a life of brokenness, suffering from PTSD, addiction, childhood trauma, domestic violence, mental illness, and spiritual emptiness. I realized I didn't need to go to a developing country to reach God's needy and broken people. They are everywhere.

The face of a female patient comes to mind. She had been released from prison, having served time for killing her children. Several years after her release she took her own life. I remembered a Vietnam veteran who always visited the office with a soda can in his hand, never parting with it, terrified of ever going through extreme thirst again as he did during the war. I see a patient who sat with me in a psychiatrist's office, revealing her multiple personalities to him. I had been the first professional she had opened up to regarding her mental illness. I see the Native American physician assistant I worked with whose life changed at the age of 8 when she was removed from her family home and put in a dormitory school, not allowed to speak her language or see her siblings or identify with her culture.

I was able to recognize human brokenness in my patients. The Holy Spirit showed me the needs of people around me—in my patients, staff, and colleagues. Practicing medicine for me meant listening, crying, laughing, and praying with my patients. The healing came just as much from these moments as from the diagnostic and therapeutic medicine I practiced.

May I recognize opportunities in this new season in my life to help the brokenhearted, and that in doing so, they will see Jesus in me.

Sandra Ritland, LLUSM class of 1981, served as a family physician for the U.S. Department of Public Health, followed by private practice. Later she was the medical director of a community health center, finishing her career as lead clinician at Muckleshoot Indian Health Center in Auburn, Washington. She is retired in Olympia, Washington, with her husband, John. They have three adult children and four grandchildren. She sees her mission now as nurturing her family and friends, as well as spreading God's health message, compassion, and love to the community around her.

December 5

"Therefore, since we are surrounded by such a great cloud of witnesses, let us throw off everything that hinders and the sin that so easily entangles. And let us run with perseverance the race marked out for us, fixing our eyes on Jesus, the pioneer and perfecter of faith. For the joy set before him he endured the cross, scorning its shame, and sat down at the right hand of the throne of God. Consider him who endured such opposition from sinners, so that you will not grow weary and lose heart."

Hebrews 12:1-3, NIV

On a cold Monday evening, after dinner, I returned to Centennial Complex and walked to the library, where I would try to study the biochemistry, PDX, anatomy, or whatever classes and Anki Decks (a flash card app) I had to review. I frantically whispered presentations of different murmurs to myself in a turbulent flow of words without any easy mathematical formula to break down exactly what was going on. The first test of Test Cycle 3 was tomorrow. My heart pounded terribly like waves crashing a boat as I walked with my iPad in one hand and some coffee and burritos in another. Suddenly a pregnant woman waved at me and asked for some help.

She was sitting on a bench near the walkway with a large bag and a small pink rose she had picked from nearby rosebushes. She looked like a six on the pain scale, her hands were clammy, and she was taking short, quick breaths. Her boyfriend was angry with her, and she was looking for a bus to take her to the underpass she called home. She cried in pain and asked if we could find a restroom. I led her to the library restroom, but she didn't want to go inside, because she was afraid of buildings. We walked toward the bus stop and spent the time talking about her life as a pregnant, homeless woman. She wanted prenatal care, but it was difficult to find a nearby clinic. Even if she was able to find one, she did not know how she was going to support her future child. Before I left, I gave her my extra burrito and had a prayer with her. She said that most people ignored her and walked on by, but she was glad that I took the time to help her, talk with her, and listen to her.

As we waved goodbye and her figure disappeared into the dark sea of night, the last thing I saw was her small pink rose. I remembered Christ's words: "Whatever you did for one of the least of these brothers and sisters of mine, you did for me" (Matthew 25:40, NIV). She helped me remember why I was studying all this material and why God brought me here. It is too easy to get caught up in the details of which nerve innervates which muscle or which murmur occurs in systole or which symptoms indicate which disease. It is too easy to walk past those who are suffering and those who we claim to help and heal. She helped me stop and remember the mission of my calling to medicine.

I heard the clattering and creaking of a train in the distance. When I left from the long day of studying, I felt as though I was creaking slowly along the track, and yet, like the train, I was still moving forward with the fuel of a renewed passion from the pregnant, homeless woman. Sometimes it takes little reminders to snatch our attention away from ourselves and toward Christ and those who are His children. Sometimes it takes a single moment to look up and see the broken people around us like a reflection of our own brokenness. Sometimes it takes a small pink rose shining like a beacon in the night.

Matthew Moran, LLUSM class of 2022, enjoys playing piano for church, traveling, and all things Disney. He looks forward to integrating his passion for mental health and wholistic well-being in his future practice.

December 6

"But if I were you, I would appeal to God; I would lay my cause before him. He performs wonders that cannot be fathomed, miracles that cannot be counted."
Job 5:8-9, NIV

There he was again, this little kid, perhaps 3 years of age, riding a tricycle down the hill—pedals rotating in sync with a wobbly front wheel. A few days later he was observed down the road kicking a ball with gusto. Who was this tyke? One day he just appeared in the neighborhood. Where did he live?

Soon it was learned that he was the grandson of an older couple who lived several houses down the block. Word began to circulate that the little guy had been placed in foster custody of his grandparents.

A few weeks later a neighbor woman met the grandmother in the local market. The neighbor greeted the grandmother and acknowledged the little boy. Nodding toward him, the grandmother stoically remarked, "He is our grandson," and without a pause continued: "Do you know of anyone who may want to adopt him? We are too old to take him, and he needs a good home."

The young woman went home, and as she put away the groceries the incident at the market tugged at her heartstrings. When her husband arrived home from work, the wife recounted the experience. The husband, without hesitating, avowed: "We will adopt him." The wife reminded her husband that that would be all but impossible: The grandparents had adult children; we were not in the Fost-adopt system; and the big obstacle: There were families already in the system who had been waiting to adopt a child.

The couple, however, appealed to God. They made arrangements to enroll in the Fost-adopt program. In time they were assigned a social worker. The rigors of background and lifestyle checks that required licensing became routine. To say the least, a little nerve-wracking for this childless couple, who knew their hopes could be derailed at any step during the process.

One day the social worker called and excitedly exclaimed: "Congratulations! I don't know how to explain this; when I left my office on Friday, there were no files on my desk. When I returned today, there was this thick file on the desk, along with a note that stated: 'To the Parks.'" After the wife caught her breath, the social worker briefly explained what to expect going forward, and then closed the conversation by reiterating: "I just can't explain it. I have never experienced something like this before."

The transition process began, and after several months the Fost-adopt program transitioned into a full-fledged adoption plan. Approximately a year later the little fellow and his legal parents left the courtroom clutching the adoption papers in hand. That was 32 years ago, on December 6, 1988. Today that little kid is a strapping six-footer, college-educated, working in the computer field. Needless to say, he is the pride and joy of his mom and dad.

By now you may have guessed that the couple in this story is the author and his wife, Pauline. Incidentally, we know how that file made it to our social worker's desk—divine intervention: because they laid their cause before Him.

Dennis Park, MA, writer, editor, campus historian, and a retired executive director of the Alumni Association, School of Medicine of Loma Linda University. In 2006 he was given the Outstanding Citizen Award by the San Bernardino Medical Society. He was named an honorary member of the Alumni Association, SMLLU in 2007. He received the Alumni Association's Iner Sheld-Ritchie Presidential Award in 2011. For the past six years he has had the privilege of documenting the Loma Linda University Campus Transformation project. Dennis enjoys photography, astronomy, traveling, and woodworking.

December 7

"Father, give us courage to change what must be altered, serenity to accept what cannot be helped, and the insight to know the one from the other."
Reinhold Niebuhr (1892–1971): American theologian and ethicist

It was my second month in residency, rotating at the emergency department. Mr. B was a Caucasian male who had been involved in a motor vehicle collision. He had lower extremity pain and bruises, but otherwise no apparent injuries. I signed up to be his physician. I walked up to him, introduced myself, and began asking questions typically contained in a complete history. He seemed uncomfortable and distracted. Midway through my interview he asked me a few unexpected questions. "Where did you attend medical school? How long have you been a physician? Are you authorized to treat patients, or am I an experiment?" I answered to the best of my ability. "I am about two months into residency. No, you are not an experiment; this is a teaching hospital, with other residents like me." After completing my history, I moved on to doing a physical exam. As I touched his leg to examine his bruises, he withdrew his leg. "I am sorry; I just can't. I cannot be touched by people like you, Black people." He followed this with more apologies. I attempted to be empathetic and provide reassurances, but he still maintained he could not be seen by a Black physician. He asked to be seen by either of the two Caucasian interns that he could see sitting in the office space right across from his room. With embarrassment I told the attending physician on call that night what had happened. Without hesitation or much contemplation, the attending walked up to the patient and said, "Good evening. Dr. Afolayan is your physician tonight. If you do not want him to be your physician because he is Black, you can leave this emergency department." Mr. B got up and limped out of the emergency department.

I have had a handful of racially charged interactions during training. I used to simply keep quiet and move on, having developed a resistance to emotional responses that can sometimes ensue. However, after a very recent experience during which a patient called me the derogatory N word, I realized the detrimental effect of my silence. Incoming residents would undoubtedly soon face a similar experience in their training. Furthermore, my silence ensured there were no consequences for those actions and a strong support for racism in its own way. By reporting my recent experience, an institutional policy development regarding the management of bias incidents involving patients and their family members, which had been stalled, was completed, and is being instituted.

Bias and microaggressions should not have a role in medical training regardless of its source. Every experience with racial bias was an opportunity to effect change. Policy changes, education, and widespread institutional awareness represent examples of a starting point to bring about such change. Trainees should have an avenue (possibly with anonymity) to share such experiences, which would provide an opportunity to evaluate newly implemented changes. Though I regret my hesitance to be more vocal over the years, it's not too late for change.

Oluwatobi Afolayan, LLUSM class of 2016, started a fellowship in cardiothoracic surgery at Baylor Medical Center in Dallas, Texas in July, 2021. Prior to this, he completed a general surgery residency at the University of Washington.

December 8

> *"Don't forget to show hospitality to strangers, for some who have done this have entertained angels without realizing it!"*
> Hebrews 13:2, NLT

Coleman Pavilion is one of the main buildings of our medical school; it has three large sets of heavy glass doors. On a breezy afternoon I used my shoulder to push one open, my arms full with a computer in one and a bag in the other. As a second-year medical student I had just finished a meeting and was rushing to nowhere in particular.

As I stepped out, I caught something moving out of the corner of my eye: an elderly woman in colorful layered garb from a culture I couldn't identify, shuffling my way. She could not have been even five feet tall and was hunched over. She came from a distance at which I wondered whether holding the door for her would be helpful or only rush her. Something told me to wait with it open anyway.

As she reached the door, she turned her yellow-scarfed head and peered up at me.

"Are you a doctor here?" she said with an accent I couldn't place, no doubt noticing my short white coat.

"Um, student. I'm a medical school student."

"Ah, yes. You see, I could tell because of the way that you hold yourself. . . . And let me tell you this: You will make it. Not just 'can' make it—you will," she said, grabbing my hand in hers with a conviction that startled me.

Stunned, I struggled for a reply. Where had this mystical sage come from? Why was she telling me this? Just because I opened the door for her?

As almost a reply to my thought, she continued: "You are tall and beautiful, and you are not Miss America or this or that, but you have it inside you," she said, pointing to my chest. "You have a pure heart, and you will be OK."

"Why, thank you. That's . . . really inspiring."

"Oh no, you don't need me for inspiration; you already have it," she rebutted.

She was forceful and insistent, and proceeded to talk to me for the next five or six minutes about confidence. About tenacity. About true beauty and listening to your gut. My arms burned under the weight of my disorganized rushing.

As I listened to her, I looked in her eyes and saw the misty lipid deposits circling her iris, the glistening opalesque cataract just past her pupil, things my clinical training had conditioned me to notice. But it was my upbringing that taught me to wait and spend this moment with her, to keep her hand in mine and be fully, completely present.

"Don't wait for anything to come. You have decided you will do this. Not you want, but you will. Remember that. You have it inside you. Just listen."

"I will," I said, and I meant it. "Now go and do, Doctor," she said with a smile, and we parted ways.

Of all my encounters with strangers, none have been as beautiful and bizarre as that. But how thankful I am to this woman who did me a much greater favor than I did for her!

Lauren Ivey Yorozuya, LLUSM class of 2020, matched to an internal medicine-dermatology combined program at the University of Minnesota. She majored in Asian studies in college. She enjoys spending time with her husband and baby girl, painting, and writing.

December 9

> *"Greater love has no one than this: to lay down one's life for one's friends."*
> *John 15:13, NIV*

The radio call broke up the usual noise of the emergency department. On the other end I could hear the familiar wail of the ambulance siren cutting through the calm of the evening air. The paramedic was speaking rapidly. He was short of breath. I could tell from his voice that this call would be bad.

"We have a 20-something-year-old female. Pedestrian versus motor vehicle. Multiple injuries. Unconscious at the scene. She is tachycardic with a thready pulse. Having difficulty getting a blood pressure on her. Starting IVs. We'll be there within five minutes."

Our team started preparing trauma bay 1 for her arrival. In a few minutes we heard the wail of the ambulance as it pulled quickly into the ambulance bay. The paramedics almost ran with her on the stretcher into the emergency department, and immediately we jumped into action.

The paramedics gave us an update as we quickly moved her from the stretcher to the bed. One nurse grabbed the left arm as the other grabbed the right, both starting large-bore IVs. We quickly ran down our trauma protocol, doing what we could to assess her injuries and respond in whatever way possible to keep her alive.

But it quickly became apparent that we were losing the battle against death. Even as we worked on her, we lost her blood pressure. She stopped breathing. We kept working hard . . . but we lost. We lost the fight with death . . . again.

Some of the local roads run directly east and west, and an older gentleman was driving his car westward into the setting sun. As he came up over a small hill, the sun was setting directly over the road in front of him, obstructing his view. He didn't see the child playing in the road in front of him.

The woman—the one who had died in my hands—saw what was going to happen and dashed into the road, pushing the child out of the path of the vehicle and saving his life. In doing so, she took the place of that child and was hit by the car. The child that she saved was the neighbor's child. In her own yard stood her husband and two small children, witnesses of her saving act.

Just like God, she stepped into harm's way and took death so another could live. That day I met a hero, and she died in my hands. I will never forget her and the sacrifice that she made.

There is another Hero, though, and He died in my hands as well. But this time my sin killed Him. My hands nailed Him to the cross. He took death for me, and for her, and for you. It was nothing less than infinite love that motivated the Father to give His Son so that you and I can live—eternally. With such a sacrifice made for you, is it too much to ask for your heart in return?

Mark Sandoval, LLUSM class of 2005, practices emergency medicine and lifestyle medicine. He is the health ministries director for the Gulf States Conference and medical director at Uchee Pines Institute in Seale, Alabama. He and his wife, LeEtta, have seven children.

December 10

"Therefore, if anyone is in Christ, the new creation has come:
The old has gone, the new is here!"
2 Corinthians 5:17, NIV

"We just don't think that he is going to be able to come off the ventilator. It's time to make some hard decisions." The face of the young mother became pained, but the PICU attending barreled on.

"You know he was a premature infant, and he has a chromosomal abnormality. He is not going to have a quality life." The mother started to speak, but the physician wasn't really looking at the mother, so she continued in her well-thought-out presentation: "The first thing we need to do is a tracheostomy."

"But, but ...," started the mother, tears beginning to flow down her smooth skin.

At that point, as the child's primary pediatrician, I had to intercede. "We need to hear what Ms. Smith has to say." Reluctantly the PICU attending yielded. "But Caleb came into the hospital breathing just fine. He had RSV, you told me. He was getting better and started breathing off the machine. But then he got sick again, and you told me he caught influenza and it has turned into pneumonia. His last chest X-ray still showed pneumonia. I think the reason he can't come off the machine is that he is still infected. Can't we wait and see if he will breathe on his own once the infection is gone?"

The PICU attending was not to be deterred from her management plan. "Well, you know he is never going to be a normal child and you have two more children at home." The mother quietly said, "That may be true, but I love him."

The advantage of being an attending pediatrician is my role to advocate for this young mother and her son—we waited a few more days, and he was extubated sucessfully. No, he is not a "normal" child, but he is a loved child making slow but definite progress.

The enemy, Satan, argues truthfully, we are "messed up." "They will never be perfect. Just look at them—can't stop lying, can't stop cheating, can't stop doubting You!" he accuses. But Jesus, the ultimate Advocate, says: "True, but—I love them. I will infuse the transforming power of My blood—the greatest antibiotic, the only true gene modulator for the inherited condition of sin. And slowly but surely, as long as they keep the IV of My love connected, they will become new!"

Dear Father, may I accept the transfusion of Jesus' love; may I allow His transforming power to make me into the new image of Your dear Son—the Great Physician.

Denise Roberts Johnson, LLUSM class of 1984, served as the medical director for a multispecialty community health center in St. Louis, Missouri, for many years. She has been a solo pediatrician for more than 20 years and is an associate professor at Washington University in St. Louis.

December 11

"The righteous shall live by his faith."
Habakkuk 2:4, ESV

I had just entered the chaplain's office when there was a knock at the door. A young couple introduced themselves to me, and we sat in the chairs near the secretary's desk.

"We have just come to speak with you and get a final opinion," the husband said. "We want to make sure we are not doing anything wrong," continued his wife. She had recently given birth, but their baby was in serious trouble. The final tests had come back indicating that he had no brain function, and they were going to turn the life support off that afternoon. After talking it over for a few minutes, they declined any further help other than requesting to use the chapel for one final prayer. Then they would go upstairs to say goodbye to their baby—their dream.

This couple had hardly left when there was another knock at the chaplain's office door. Composing myself, I opened the door to find another young couple standing there with a baby.

They were as radiant as any proud parents I have seen. "We are so thankful that God has given us a beautiful healthy baby," he said. "We want to dedicate her to God and were wondering if you would pray with us in the chapel," she concluded. After checking that the chapel was empty, we filed in for a prayer of dedication and thanks.

This second couple had no idea of how difficult it was for me to concentrate, knowing that probably at the very moment we were offering prayers of thanks and dedication to God for this child, there was another young couple upstairs turning off the machines that maintained the last vestiges of life for their child.

Again, I was reminded that much of the sense of futility that we experience comes because we hang on to the questions raised, rather than recalling the insight gained in utilizing our faith so that we can face that which we do not want to be true.

The prophet Habakkuk, who was very forthright with his questions to God, chimes in with ". . . but the righteous will live by his faith." At first glance we might dismiss his statement as a tired cliché. However, when I survey the passage through time and experience, I recognize that faith permeates almost every aspect of life. The prophet goes on to conclude his oracle by stating: "Though the fig tree should not blossom, nor fruit be on the vines, the produce of the olive fail and the fields yield no food, . . . yet I will rejoice in the LORD; I will take joy in the God of my salvation" (Habakkuk 3:17-18, ESV).

My experience with the two young couples ultimately affirmed that while we have little or no control over life events, faith gives us the ability to scramble over the battle-strewn landscape of life. We will still experience peace, while continuing our unique mission of providing help and support to whomever we meet, in all circumstances.

Lance Tyler, DMin, moved to the United States more than 30 years ago from Australia to pursue chaplaincy as his calling in ministry. This life choice has been confirmed through service in three health care environments: the veterans' hospital, hospice, and inpatient level 1 trauma care. While the care of people in the times of their greatest need challenges him every day, it has been the most rewarding time of his life. He is eternally thankful for God's confidence in using him.

December 12

*"The second is this: 'Love your neighbor as yourself.' There is
no commandment greater than these."*
Mark 12:31, NIV

When I can't sleep . . . I pray. Sometimes from bed, and sometimes I get up and go into the living room. I tell God whatever concerns are on my mind. I tell Him how thankful I am for my family, for our friends and acquaintances, and for their families. I pray for those in need, or those in pain; for those unhappy or sad; for those with anxiety or depression, illness or sorrow; for those with loneliness, or perhaps the agony of a bad relationship, whether past or present. And I pray for those in joy! For answers given and received; for those who are awaiting the answers prayed for . . . hoping God answers the desires of their hearts; or I pray for them (and me) to trust the Lord to open or close doors as He sees best. "Thy will be done" is one of the hardest prayers to pray sincerely, but so important to help "growth" in trusting God through all things. I also pray for those who are in the midst of medical treatment (whether from illness, accident, or whatever reason) that God will reach down with His healing arms of love, hear them, and heal them—soul, mind, and body.

Sometimes we can become so self-involved with the challenges in our own lives that we lose track of those we wanted to pray for. Or we can become so concerned for others that we forget to take care of ourselves. Balance is so important. Our verse today reminds us to "love your neighbor as yourself." And if we love ourselves, we should take care of ourselves, eat healthy, drink water, exercise, take time for prayer and devotions. It's important to keep our own bodies and souls refreshed and at peace; thus we have the energy to reach out and not only pray for others but share ourselves with them, as we feel led by God's touching of our heart.

What happens to our sincere prayers? I believe that the best measure for answered prayers is by God's touching of their (and our) hearts, not by the number of yeses to our requests. Prayer is the soothing of a soul's heart. It's God reaching down from heaven to say, *There is a reason I woke you tonight, or brought someone to you today, My child. Pray for My other children—pray for your own children. Pray for those who love Me, and for those who don't even know Me. For I am meek and lowly of spirit. I will give them rest.* And in so doing, He touches our hearts as well.

Many times through the years I have been touched to have someone who comes up to me and says, "Do you remember when you prayed with me for such and such? I felt so much better, and God has become *so* important in my life." God's sweet peace that "passes all understanding" (Philippians 4:7, RSV) is a gift we could all use. Share, and ye shall receive!

Judi (Lacy) Hewes, LLU La Sierra campus BSW class of 1975, MSW, LCSW, has been married 46 years to Robert "Bob" Hewes (LLUSM class of 1976-B). She is the author of You Are His Masterpiece: Hope When Life Throws You a Curve, *published in 2018.*

December 13

"So we do not lose heart. Though our outer self is wasting away,
our inner self is being renewed day by day."
2 Corinthians 4:16, ESV

The day I met "the enemy" was December 13, 2016. The enemy was PSC, primary sclerosing cholangitis. Of unknown etiology, this disease of small bile ducts causes cirrhosis of the liver, with associated complications, liver failure, and death. It may go undetected for 10 years or more. There is no truly effective treatment save liver transplantation. Earlier I had consulted my gastroenterologist, who treated me for a year with ursodiol (bile salts) because of a long history of elevated LFTs (liver function tests). For a week or two I had noted dark urine; this I attributed to inadequate hydration, but noted no response to greater water consumption

On this day I decided to consult my urologist and friend, Dr. James Wooley (LLUSM class of 1980-A). He took one look and announced, "Hey, you have jaundice!" Then things began to happen. Lab studies confirmed a markedly elevated bilirubin of 10.5. I was referred to California Pacific Medical Center, where liver biopsy December 20 confirmed the diagnosis of PSC. Next I was evaluated for liver transplantation at Stanford's excellent liver transplantation program, led by Dr. Waldo Concepcion, former LLU faculty. By the time the committee met, I was judged too well to transplant. In March 2017 I felt fine, with a bilirubin of 1.8. We attributed the improvement mainly to the prayers of dear friends and family, including an anointing led by our son John C. Anderson (LLUSM class of 2000).

Within a year the disease reasserted itself. I developed ascites, weakness, and progressive muscle atrophy. This time the committee concluded that, at 79, I was too old for transplant. After several other programs concurred, I was referred to Indiana University Medical Center, a leading transplant center. After extensive studies, placement of two cardiac stents, and repeated banding of esophageal varices, I was listed for transplantation August 24, 2018. We expected to wait up to six months.

After I experienced progressive weakness and weight loss, with no certainty of transplantation, and the real possibility of delisting because of "improved" chemistries, my hopes faded. I was sustained by the text above, which Paul seemed to have written for me. Friends were deeply concerned, and my classmates, Frances Gutierrez (LLUSM class of 1964) and George Chen (LLUSM class of 1964), organized a prayer event. The evening of October 9, 2018, friends and classmates from LLU, Pacific Union College in Angwin, California, and even Lynwood Academy in Southern California, prayed fervently for either miraculous healing or early transplantation.

Within three days "the call" came. It was late Friday night, October 12. Early Sabbath morning I received what my surgeon described as a pristine liver. My recovery has been essentially uneventful. Indiana University discharged me December 13, 2018, to return to California and outpatient care.

I believe prayer opened heaven's doors, giving me perhaps many years of life rather than further decline, inevitable liver failure, and death within a year or two. This is a miracle for which the only appropriate response is profound gratitude. I have been blessed and, although undeserving, have received what a friend calls "the mother of all Christmas presents."

Bruce N. Anderson, LLUSM class of 1964, practices psychiatry in Northern California and is president of Adventist Health California Medical Group. He is a board member of LLUH's Behavorial Medical Center. He has been married to Audrey Anderson (LLUSN class of 1963) for 58 years. They have three children: Steven, Elizabeth, and John C. (LLUSM class of 2000).

December 14

"For the Lord himself shall descend from heaven with a shout, with the voice of an archangel, and with the trump of God: and the dead in Christ will rise first. Then we who are alive and remain shall be caught up together with them in the clouds, to meet the Lord in the air: and so shall we ever be with the Lord."
1 Thessalonians 4:16-17, KJV

It's too bad that I may not be able to see you graduate," my mom said softly as I sat at the edge of her bed. The fall of my fourth-year of medical school was supposed to be a time of exciting apprehension, traveling and interviews, and preparing for residency. For me, this had been augmented by the joy of the birth of my son. However, what should have been an excitingly terrifying time in my life quickly turned into a gut-wrenching nightmare.

My mom had flown over from Hawaii to help care for my son while I was busy finishing school. He was her first grandchild, and she was more than elated to help around our home; and I relished her company. We even talked about how she could live with us during my residency training. My plan was set, and it was going to be great—that is, until she was diagnosed with pancreatic cancer. We were told that she might survive six months at best.

My parents were my biggest cheerleaders. To them, my medical school graduation was a milestone for the years of endless studying and sleepless nights. It meant so much more to them, especially after my brother's unexpected and tragic death seven years prior, just seven months shy of graduating from college. I had never understood the expanse of love and delight in a child's accomplishments that parents felt until I became a mother. Rather than the fear of dying, Mom was more distressed over the possibility that she would not live to see me graduate. Word of her wish to be present for my graduation reached the ears of the school's administration, and they quickly moved into action.

On a cold December night the dean of the School of Medicine and associates, along with our close friends and family, squeezed into my mom's room. Someone played "Pomp and Circumstance" on the keyboard while I marched in full regalia. My letter of thanks was read to my parents. I poured my heart out in that letter, wanting my mom to know a lifetime's worth of how much she meant to me, though she probably already knew how deeply I loved her. I mentally captured the feel of Mom's frail embrace, and I tucked it away safely in my heart. I didn't ever want to forget the fleeting time while she was still with us. Mom was so overjoyed that she got to see me graduate. Three days later she passed away peacefully, surrounded by family.

This intimate graduation was an indescribably special gift for my dad and me. I am eternally grateful to the Loma Linda University School of Medicine and my mentors for making my mom's dream a possibility, and for giving my family an invaluable treasure. What a glorious day it will be when Christ comes to take us home, and we will be reunited with our loved ones forevermore.

Christal Nishikawa, LLUSM class of 2016, completed a geriatric medicine fellowship in June, 2021, following a residency in internal medicine in Hawaii. She enjoys spending her free time with her husband, Bradley Ching (LLUSD class of 2014), and their son, Luke Brent, and catching up with their family and friends.

December 15

> *"Then the* LORD *God formed the man of dust from the ground, and breathed into his nostrils the breath of life; and the man became a living person."*
> Genesis 2:7, NASB

Chaos ripped through the small crowd circled around one of the emergency department trauma beds. It was after midnight, and we were headed upstairs to the call room to wait for the next shriek from our resident's pager. Turning back, my classmate and I recognized at once this new yet strangely familiar routine.

"Asystole on the monitor!"
"No cardiac activity!"
"No femoral pulses!"

The attending physician drilled an intraosseous catheter through skin and bone into the man's left shin while the nurses shoved IVs into his arms. The resident slid the ultrasound probe down his belly, and emergency responders stood line to compress his heart back into motion. "Any medical students want to come do chest compressions?" the attending yelled out the door into the hallway where we were standing. My classmate jogged up to the bed to swap places with a woman sweating through her gray, embroidered scrubs.

"Good chest rise and fall!"
"When is our next pulse check?"
"This is our third round of epi!"

I stood still in the corner, eyes glued to the elaborate rhythm. There on the gurney was the nameless, faceless man—found unconscious, alone. I'd watched basic life support video reenactments of what to do at a time like this, where the actor falls on the floor of the cafeteria and, conveniently, one or two (depending on the lesson we were reviewing) responders would drop to the ground and begin chest compressions while the other called for help and an AED. At the time I'd been fascinated, not, as I should have been, by the correct number of cycles and compression-to-breath ratios for each situation, but by the moment the camera abruptly snaps from the actor to a chiseled, peach-colored mannequin lying in his place. Somehow in the middle of the dramatized hubbub, the other actors fail to notice that their patient has turned into a lifeless mound of plastic and, unfazed, they promptly begin compressions on the silicone chest of the unfortunate victim with flawless technique and perfect timing while the bystanders wail in agony.

"This is our last round of epi!"
"Asystole on the monitor!"
"No cardiac activity!"
"No femoral pulses!"
"Calling time at 12:44 am."
"Let's have a 30-second moment of silence."

The room drew quiet except for the chatter outside the door.

Who are you? I wanted to ask his body. *And when did you switch, in a heartbeat, from a person to a rubber corpse?*

We shifted our gaze from the clock to the blue paint on the wall.

Your life is precious, I wanted to tell you before you could no longer hear me.

The pause over, we packed up the blankets and tossed out the plastic tubing.

Did you know what your days were meant for?

WayAnne Watson, LLUSM class of 2020, is a second-year otolaryngology (ENT) resident at LLUH. She is proud to be a third-generation LLUSM physician. She is the daughter of Marilene Wang (LLUSM class of 1986) and James Watson (LLUSM class of 1986), and granddaughter of John Wang (CME class of 1960). December 15 is the anniversary of her sister, Whitney's, death.

December 16

> *"And she gave birth to her firstborn son and wrapped him in bands of cloth, and laid him in a manger, because there was no place for them in the inn."*
> Luke 2:7, NRSV

We are in the valley of the shadow of death with this most recent surge in COVID. Loma Linda has run out of ICU beds and has been diverting "not as critically ill" patients to the regular floor—such as diabetic ketoacidosis, which requires an insulin drip but is now being managed by subcutaneous insulin pushes every few hours. The Children's Hospital is now taking patients up to age 30. (I wonder how my peds coresidents are doing?) The morgue is full, and they can't move the deceased patients out fast enough. My coresident told me casually that she had to code six patients on her short call day on CCU—all COVID patients. Some of the codes happened simultaneously. Pulmonology, which is where I've been this month, is getting a constant stream of BiPAP consult requests. BiPAPs are typically managed in the ICU, but not anymore—there's no more room in the ICU.

The COVID hospitalists are overwhelmed. They're now asking for internal medicine resident volunteers to work with the hospitalists to help offset some of the burden and see more patients at the same time. My coresidents and I are volunteering as we can, but many of us just came from inpatient, on-call rotations. The ICU staff are tired, so tired. They've been battling this for months.

It's Christmas, and there's no room in the ICU. No room in this ICU, no room in the next ICU, or even in the next ICU. In this entire Bethlehem of hospitals, there is no more room. There's nothing but the rude stable, the best we can do in a crisis situation, while nonbelievers carry on with their merry lives. Our labor is painful, but unlike the first Christmas, our labor is mostly fruitful of death. But still we press on because we hope we can save at least one person while doing this.

As Christmas comes nearer, please remember, there is no more room in the ICU. If you can pity the Baby Jesus, please pity us and our patients and stay at home.

Eunice Park, LLUSM class of 2019, was a second-year internal medicine resident at the time of this writing (December 16, 2020). She and her coresidents helped with the post-Thanksgiving/Christmas COVID surge, which saw the highest number of COVID patients admitted to LLUMC during 2020. She and other residents were part of the expanded COVID hospitalist/resident teams, COVID MICU, CCU, and expanded backup pools as COVID patients overwhelmed the hospital. In addition to the daily stress of caring for COVID patients, she also had to ensure that she would not bring COVID home to her husband and their 3-year-old daughter.

December 17

"And call the Sabbath a delight, the holy day of the L<small>ORD</small> honorable, and shall honor Him, . . . then you shall delight yourself in the L<small>ORD</small>."
Isaiah 58:13-14, NKJV

The week before Thanksgiving, we joyfully celebrated the news of Aunt Danielle's remission of colon cancer following a year of chemotherapy. After a grateful Thanksgiving meal, she started vomiting that very night ("perhaps she just ate too much?"). No matter what she tried, she could not stop the urge to vomit. Late-night concerned phone call . . . A few days later the oncologist and multiple specialists said they found no other cause ("well, maybe it's a virus"). Then . . . the unthinkable. The chemotherapy had not prevented the spread of metastases to her brain, and three seven-centimeter brain masses were found. The only option was hospice or whole brain radiation to stop the growth of the tumors.

After days of vomiting trauma to her vocal cords, she could not speak well and had trouble seeing because of pressure on her optic nerves. We sat around her hospital bed, simply numb from the hard reality. It would be Christmas in two weeks, but no one had the energy to think ahead. After that traumatic reversal of our "remission celebration" at Thanksgiving, Aunt Danielle asked me to return to her hospital room again for her second week in the hospital, so I drove one and a half hours after my Friday clinic ended to her bedside and slept on the cot in her room while her family took a break.

Every weekend, when I headed home on Sunday night, Aunt Danielle asked if I was coming back the next weekend "to spend Sabbath with me." Christmas Eve landed on Sabbath that year. I spent the day reading her the Christmas narrative in Luke, singing carols, and reminding her that God's love surrounded her. Family gathered around and then left to open presents at their nearby house, but I asked to stay quietly beside my aunt, assuring her with touch and smiles and praying a blessing over her. It was my best Christmas memory ever.

Hopes were dashed when radiation did nothing to shrink the growing brain metastases, and she moved to rehab and then hospice. Still every Sabbath I drove back and re-created her childhood memories of her Sabbath-keeping family, TV turned off, quiet spiritual music, prayer, and Bible stories of hope. We talked about the reality of heaven between ministering to her needs.

The pain grew worse; Aunt Danielle no longer could see well or swallow. On my last day with her, we held our hands high in the air, making the sign language hand symbol of "I love you," and she smiled bravely. She and I knew that God had accepted her repentant heart and that she would see Jesus come in the clouds. Her years of denial of her need of God had been washed away by grace and love on those nine Sabbaths, symbolizing her acceptance of God's rule at the end of her life. My greatest joy was creating nine gift boxes of sacred Sabbath hours packed with love to assure my aunt of resurrection morning and unending Sabbaths together in heaven.

Linda Hyder Ferry, LLUSM class of 1979-B, lives in Yucaipa, California, and practices family and preventive medicine. She has been the chief of preventive medicine at Jerry L. Pettis Memorial Veterans Medical Center in Loma Linda, California, since 1985. She believes that preventing illness is more rewarding than searching for treatable diseases and that preventing the "loss of eternal life" in this end-of-life, spiritual battle beside her aunt was thrilling to witness . . . forever.

December 18

"Education is the knowledge of how to use the whole of oneself."
Henry Ward Beecher (1813–1887): American Congregationalist clergyman and abolitionist

It was my mother's early influence that first sparked my desire to go to medical school. As a nurse and community health educator, she had a passion for health promotion and ministering to others that was infectious to anyone she came in contact with. Inspired by the work my mother did, I began volunteering in the health care field in college. When I experienced firsthand what a meaningful impact a person's influence can have on the health and well-being of another, I knew I wanted to make this my full-time career—and there my dream of becoming a physician first began.

When my mother was diagnosed with a terminal illness, I became more intimately acquainted with another side of medicine: end-of-life care. As I took care of her in the last eight months of her life, I saw firsthand how important and meaningful whole person care can be. My mother's primary physician was a Christian, and when every medical option had been exhausted, he was still able to minister to her by reminding her of the hope she had in the return of her Savior and the complete restoration of health she would receive one day. It gave her peace and helped set her mind at ease when no pill or procedure could.

My mother passed away two years before I started medical school, so she was never able to see my dream become a reality. Although it was challenging to move to another country and secure funding for my education, I have been blessed in being able to attend a medical school where whole person care has been taught and practiced. My education here has been possible only with the dedicated support of my father, a barber who was able to make it only halfway through high school before he had to take over the family business. As a Canadian with no relatives or connections in the United States I was not eligible for any U.S. student loans, and the maximum amount given by the government of Canada covers just under 25 percent of my yearly tuition. At the age of 74 my father continues to work to help fund my education and has had to take a line of credit out against our home to help make my dream a reality.

When I graduate, I will be the first physician in my extended family on both sides and also the first to have obtained education beyond a bachelor's degree. Though it has been challenging at times, I also recognize that I am very blessed to have the opportunity to pursue such a meaningful field.

Chanel Wood, LLUSM class of 2020, is currently a family medicine resident at Providence St. Peter Hospital in Olympia, Washington. She couples-matched with her husband, former classmate and now fellow coresident, Joshua Wixwat. After residency they plan to return home to British Columbia, Canada, to practice full spectrum family medicine.

December 19

> *"They'll know we are Christians by our love."*
> Peter Raymond Scholtes (1938–2009): American Catholic priest and songwriter

Medicine has allowed me to experience humanity in such a special way. I have the privilege of interacting with people at their highest "highs" and lowest "lows" on a daily basis. I have the opportunity to feel the pain of the affluent, to touch the struggles of the indigent, and to be present for everything in between. You never know what you might experience each day, and that's the exciting part. While there are truly no two people alike, we all have some similarities. We all fear, we all love, we all need to be listened to, we all care about something. My journey through medicine as I have transitioned from student to medical resident to now an attending has taught me many things. Most important is that I need to trust in the Lord with all my heart and lean not on my own understanding.

One recent experience comes to mind. An elderly gentleman came into my clinic with mild flank pain. He appeared well and had normal vital signs, but just couldn't seem to get comfortable. Upon evaluation, the possible diagnoses ran through my mind, and the thought that his aorta was the culprit took center stage. While less-serious causes like a kidney stone or muscle strain seemed to be much more likely, my initial impression held firm. After examining him, I sent him emergently to the ER for imaging and, sure enough, he had a large symptomatic abdominal aortic aneurysm on the verge of rupturing. I am thankful for experiences like these, because while my medical education is stellar, I know that there is a God in heaven that gives wisdom.

I am thankful for this wisdom, especially in this turbulent year (2020). As an African American physician, I've had to grapple with medical disaster as well as find my footing in the mix of renewed long-standing racial tensions. This has given me the "opportunity," among other things, to reflect upon moments when I was told such things as "my family won't see you because they don't like Blacks" and "you're good for a colored doctor" in addition to absorbing the occasional slur. I don't write these things to stoke flames of passion, anger, or pity. I write them only to share my experience. I'm not discouraged by these things; rather, I use them as opportunities for open, honest conversation and growth. I'm always amazed by the way God provides the right words at the right time. With God's help, my desire is to be a positive force in my community through excellent, compassionate care for all my patients.

Christ offers us the opportunity to be born anew. He offers us the ability to be one family in Him. That prospect is wondrous to me; it makes every patient encounter memorable because I get to extend my family lines, learn new things, and gain precious experience. I pray the same for everyone. I pray your walk with God is transformative and full of love.

Christopher Holloway, LLUSM class of 2017, is a family medicine physician practicing in Springfield, Ohio, with the Kettering Health Network.

December 20

"You shall know the truth, and the truth shall make you free."
John 8:32, NKJV

At 2:00 a.m. a 68-year-old woman arrived at our emergency department complaining of chest pain. She forced a smile as I introduced myself. Constant pain for four days, which she had never experienced before, pushed her out of bed and drove her to the ED.

I ordered medications along with the usual tests for chest pain, lung disease, and upper abdominal pain.

When the tests came back, I talked to her again to see how she was doing. Her story, exam, and testing did not define the problem. So now I tried different medications.

Checking on her at 4:00 a.m., I found her still in pain. I listened to her heart and lungs again. As I bent over her heart, I noticed the gold cross that hung from her neck. For some reason I asked her how things were going with her church. She grimaced a bit and said, "Horrible." I asked her how that could be. She replied that four days earlier had been the birthday of her dearest granddaughter. She had raised this beautiful, vibrant child on her own. (I regularly see grandparents like her, raising children for a second time. When they arrive in the emergency department, these grandparents are often burned-out.)

This woman had helped her granddaughter through school, college, and even pharmacy school. But then, three years ago, this joy of her life, her investment of love and time, had committed suicide. People in this woman's church told her emphatically that people who take their lives end up in hell. And the confluence of that comment, the precious memories, a birthday, and whatever horror hell meant to her, had seared her mind for four long days.

In careful response I asked her if she could think of a time that her church, or its leaders, had been wrong. She immediately mentioned an issue. I paused and then continued that all people make mistakes, even irreversible mistakes. And God forgives them. Her granddaughter's desperate choice could not be undone, but it could be forgiven.

Did Jesus love her granddaughter? Has Jesus forgiven people who make mistakes? Did Jesus ever say that any one mistake, even suicide, meant hell? I gave her some time to ruminate. When I came back, it was closer to 5:00 a.m. I was adamant and stated plainly, "Your granddaughter is not in hell. She could, in fact, go to heaven." The woman looked up at me, surprised. She smiled, and the smile lasted longer than I expected. She took some deep breaths. Then she took my hand on the railing beside her and cried. Then appeared a hopeful peace in her eyes, "My pain is gone." She didn't need any medications to take home with her. "The truth sets us free."

Victor Wallenkampf, LLUSM class of 1976-A, practices emergency medicine in Roseburg, Oregon. He is involved in getting 85 percent of his rural county residents to complete advanced directives. His wife, Janet (piano teacher), and son Karl (LLUSM class of 2021) approve this message.

December 21

> *"God's purpose is not to destroy us,*
> *but to save us through the Lord Jesus Christ."*
> 1 Thessalonians 5:9, Clear Word

"Man, Alaska is GNARLY!": a quote from Shaun while studying up on geography and flying routes in Alaska. This would be one of several trips to Alaska after many months of preparation. His initial wonder and excitement paled only in comparison to the passion and enthusiasm he experienced with each ensuing trip.

Having grown up with a pilot father, transportation for any distance was delegated to the family's Cessna 172. With time Shaun achieved his own aviation skills obtaining instrument, commercial, and multiengine ratings. But it was flying his Super Cub in Alaska over the mountains and glaciers that he encountered the freedom of an untethered bird as he sighted with awe and reverence the beauty of God's creation on the terrain beneath his wings. With the use of oversized tires, Shaun was afforded the joy of landing atop mountains, in valleys, and on gravel strips in the middle of rivers. Viewing such breathtaking beauty, he later inscribed on a photo taken from his cockpit around midnight with the sun still glowing a multiplicity of pink and golden hues on the horizon, "God has a paintbrush."

To my delight, Shaun invited me to join him on his fourth adventure for a week of elevated living in a pilot's ultimate playground—Alaska! One day while we were flying, Shaun chose to set his plane down on a sandy beach alongside the Bering Sea, where we played the game Hangman. Picking up a stick, he drew the framework with the noose hanging from the top. At the bottom of this sandy artwork he drew five straight lines—one for each letter of the mysterious word he had chosen for me to, hopefully, get hung on. And sure enough, I was unable to spell the word "Kenai" (a region in the Gulf of Alaska).

The game of Hangman is just that—a game. Thankfully, God does not play games with our salvation. Nor do we have to play Hangman with our lives. Many choose to play loosely with life and not accept the reality of God choosing us for salvation. It can become laborious to fill in all the letters so as to "not be hung," and we can become discouraged at trying to find the right word. But when we accept this beautiful gift of salvation, we will find the word that negates Hangman—a word called love. And it is this love that chose us for salvation.

Months after Shaun's plane went down in Alaska in the summer of 2008, we received a forwarded message he had written earlier to a friend. It echoed his exuberance and joy over knowing, assuredly, that we had been created for the gift of salvation. "He's brought us here to win, with His help—to succeed over all the struggles by His grace. Born with a purpose—somehow that feels good!"—Shaun Lunt.

Margie Lunt is a retired RN from LLUMC radiation medicine department, where she served as proton research manager; Shaun Lunt, her son, was an anesthesiologist. This is written in memory of Shaun (December 21, 1973–June 6, 2008 [LLUSM class of 2001]) to honor a life well-lived for God and for others during his 34 years. Shaunlunt.typepad.com is the blog site featuring Shaun's exquisite photography of Alaska.

December 22

The following is based on a story by Maria L. La Ganga that was featured on the front page of the Los Angeles Times, June 17, 2021:

I want to write about Karl because Karl deserves to be noticed.

Karl is an all-but-invisible man. For 16 years, he has worked in our massive medical center's dispatch department, wheeling patients to tests and procedures, moving supplies and medications, and transporting blood and plasma. He does not like attention and describes himself in one sentence: "I'm just a regular guy who loves life and loves people." I want the world to know who Karl is and what he does. I call him "this health care hero." Due to the pandemic, Karl became the person who moved dead bodies from their rooms, then took them to the morgue. And on the surface, this doesn't seem that bad. But in a pandemic, Karl became the body collector.

During the winter surge, the cardiac ICU became the COVID ICU to handle the crush of catastrophically ill patients. The morgue just wasn't big enough so the hospital brought in refrigerated trucks and parked them about a mile away.

I began to help care for Loma Linda's sickest COVID patients on a regular basis. I would see them during morning rounds, and not long after that they would die. It was so many, and it was terrible. That's when my path crossed repeatedly with Karl's—when the hospital was in such dire straits that obstetricians were treating men and body collectors were a regular presence in the ICU. Whenever I saw Karl, he always had a smile and an unassuming approach. He had a way of seamlessly sliding on and off the unit with his morgue transport operation, while everyone else was hustling around.

One day I had come up to the seventh floor to check on two of my struggling patients. As I watched from afar, I realized that no one looked up or said hello to Karl or moved to let him get on with his somber job. Did they really not see him? Or was it that it was too painful to say "hi" to a sign that we didn't save yet another.

I do not remember exactly what kept me from sleeping on that particular February night when I lay in the dark and decided to write about Karl. Maybe I had finally seen so much death and suffering that I could no longer compartmentalize the pain. About a week before that, when I ran into him, I asked him how he was doing now that the pandemic was starting to abate. I wanted to know how he had managed the difficult winter weeks, realizing that he would come to work and spend most of his time transporting the dead. I wanted to thank Karl. When he answered my questions, I almost lost it.

He said he kept going during all of it because he felt like, when all the dust settled, the monitors were turned off, the sheet pulled over the face of a former life, that someone needed to make sure the deceased still got care.

Someone needed to make sure they were put on the metal gurney tenderly, arms positioned comfortably, feet and legs covered. Someone needed to take them down to the morgue with dignity and care. Someone needed to escort them, go with them. Someone needed to be their guardian.

No, not someone.

Karl.

Courtney Martin graduated from Western University of Health Sciences in California and completed her OB/GYN residency at LLUH in 2015. She is an assistant professor in LLUSM's department of gynecology and obstetrics and medical director of maternity services at LLUCH. Mother of three and wife of a wonderful husband, she loves to write and read about the stories of medicine, both as a physician and as a mother.

December 23

"Consider it pure joy, my brothers and sisters, whenever you face trials of many kinds, because you know the testing of your faith produces perseverance. Let perseverance finish its work so that you may be mature and complete, not lacking anything."

James 1:2-4, NIV

Thomas Edison once said that "opportunity is missed by most people because it is dressed in overalls and looks like work." I understood medical school would be a challenge unlike any other I had faced before. What I did not expect was that I would find myself struggling to stay afloat during my first year because of my health. I knew something was wrong fairly quickly, that my current state of "trying hard" was not actually my best work even after accounting for the new level of difficulty. Something was just . . . off. I was falling asleep in odd places and forgetting where I was; memory and concentration were a challenge. I feared seeking help because I thought it might be depression; I've seen my own family struggle with the illness. Was I next?

And so an internalized battle ensued. I doubted God frequently—why did He open the door to medical school when He knew I would develop an illness affecting my mind? Was He really going to close this door? I would soon realize that God knew the best way to teach me a grand lesson in personal growth was through subtlety and a test of patience. It took falling asleep standing up and again in my car at a stoplight to finally seek medical help. During this trying time I learned what it meant to be the frustrated patient, to experience significant failures, and to be humble. Months of evaluation led to the conclusion that I was experiencing persistent symptoms from a meningitis-related brain injury sustained shortly before I graduated college. While I could anticipate a recovery, it would not be a rapid one; adaption was necessary.

Instead of allowing my diagnosis to dissuade me from my medical education, I used it as an opportunity to make positive changes in the way I approach learning, mindfulness, and health care as a whole. With the help of my university, family, learning coach, and physician, I was able to surpass even my own expectations as I recovered. I developed a greater respect and appreciation for patients with complex or vague symptoms, for the struggling student, and for the social support system whose members never failed to stay with me through it all.

Reflecting on this journey reminds me of how God frequently works behind the scenes. Sometimes His answers come much later than we expect or are not immediately clear at the time we pray. Without the trials I was given, I would not have developed a deeper empathy for my patients, a greater appreciation for my friends and family, or a true passion for education. Facing our worst trials can often lead to the greatest blessings God can give us. With this appreciation in mind, my main hope as a physician is that I am able to truly serve my patients with compassion, understanding, and genuine empathy.

Gabrielle Kahler, LLUSM class of 2020, is currently an internal medicine resident at the University of Kentucky Medical Center. In her free time she enjoys scrapbooking and bookbinding.

Christmas Eve
December 24

> *"But then I recall all you have done, O Lord;*
> *I remember your wonderful deeds of long ago."*
> Psalm 77:11, NLT

The beeping of my beeper reminded me that Christmas Eve will not be a quiet call night. Instead of calling the ER, I got up and walked down the hallways of the Jerry L. Pettis Memorial Veterans Medical Center. The nurses' stations had their Christmas decorations in force. Yes, the Christmas spirt was alive.

His name was John, and he was lying on a gurney with a nasal cannula and an IV in his arm. From afar he was not in any acute distress. I went to the ER physician and asked the reason for admission.

Social admission. (In the 1980s we admitted veterans to the hospital for social reasons. Things have changed.) There was not much information in his paper chart, except for the letters ALS. Lou Gehrig's disease.

John was a vet in his early 30s. He had had ALS for some time, and he knew what it was all about as I gathered his medical history. One thing that came across as I was asking questions was the look of peace in his face.

"I know my end is near," he whispered.

"So why come to the hospital this Christmas Eve?" I asked. "Don't you want to be with your family?"

"We already gathered together earlier for Christmas," he shared. "My two daughters already opened their gifts. We had a good time." They were young children.

"I told my wife to take me here once the girls were asleep. A friend took me here."

He shared the reasons he wanted to be admitted to the hospital. His wife also knew.

"If something happens to me tonight or tomorrow, I don't want my girls to see the face of death at home," he reasoned.

"I want them to have a merry Christmas and remember me during the times we were happy," he added.

I wrote admitting orders and wrote DNR.

As I tried to get a few hours of sleep that Christmas Eve, my thoughts turned to John. Beyond the material gifts he gave to his girls, he wanted to give a lasting gift of happy memories to them. I did get a few hours of sleep after midnight, wondering if I would have to endorse John to the incoming team on Christmas Day.

My beeper woke me up 4:00 a.m. on Christmas morning. I called the nurses' station from our call room.

"Could you pronounce our DNR patient?" I heard a nurse's voice over the phone.

I won't have to endorse John to the next team on Christmas Day, but I will endorse his story to them.

Happy memories could be as much a gift for Christmas as gifts we wrapped for each other.

Bevan Geslani completed his internal medicine residency at LLUH in 1987 and is now an assistant professor in LLUSM's department of medicine. He graduated from LLUSPH class of 2009 with an MBA. He is married to Maysie Gerona (SAHP class of 1980) and has two married children: Van Geslani (LLUSM class of 2008) and Alison Geslani Chong (LLUSN class of 2008). His training at LLUMC and the Jerry L. Pettis Memorial Veterans Medical Center in Loma Linda, California, prepared him for the 24 years they spent serving at the Guam SDA Clinic. He believes that the Lord sometimes places us in unexpected situations to be a blessing to others.

December 25

Christmas morning

"Christmas, my child, is love in action. Every time we love, every time we give, it's Christmas."
Dale Evans Rogers (1912–2001): American singer, songwriter, and actress

Sometimes the simplest of ideas morph into wonderful—no, make that WONDERFUL—ideas! A week before Christmas 2016, with no "major" plans, I called up Uncle Frank, one of my dearest friends, and said, "Let's go to Loma Linda University Children's Hospital Christmas morning!"

"Brilliant" was the response, and we quickly went into overdrive.

Our first call was to the volunteer office at the hospital. And once again, the Loma Linda University Children's Hospital, with the biggest heart, staff, administrators, and volunteers, said Yes! On such short notice, we were disorganized, but our heart was in the right place. We canvassed stores for fleece blankets, socks for patients and mom and dad, stuffed animals, books, crayons, cards, preemie knit hats …

Stuffed in a roller duffel, giant bags in tow, dressed in our Santa attire, we descended upon the hospital, met the life-care specialist who would escort us from room to room, and away we went. After visiting a few rooms, we quickly realized what was needed—more Santas! But we forged on. Some children were too sick to sit up or were in isolation; so we gave hugs to their parents. We thanked the staff for their work. We got shy little ones to smile. We watched parents cry, knowing there would not be another Christmas for their child. And we prayed with parents. There were 168 patients on the census that Christmas Day in 2016.

We walked out with our empty bags. We were a little emotionally drained, but we knew we had done something right. Same time next year, we said. And so, on December 26, 2016, we began planning for what would be dubbed the Santa Stroll.

Our official count for Santa Stroll 2017 was 42 Santas and elves visiting 238 patients. We had a first-year medical student making his first rounds as Santa. Senior administration had arrived at 6:00 a.m. to make cider for the gang and serve doughnuts. People came armed with gifts and good cheer.

Any hardships I might have had were put into perspective that day. All my joys were put into perspective as well. We have created a beautiful community that gathers on Christmas morning; many we see only on that one day each year. Every day we teach the children that they are important. Even on holidays when families gather at home, we show the children that complete strangers will take the time to recognize them.

Perhaps the reading of this passage is the inspiration for you to join us or start your very own Santa Stroll wherever you might be in the world on Christmas morning. It's that simple. And it will be the best gift you can give yourself on Christmas Day.

Jill Golden began her master's degree in public health with an emphasis in health education at LLUSPH in January 2019. She currently serves on the Children's Hospital Foundation Board, the Desert Guild Board, and the Indio Advisory Council. This was written in loving memory of Uncle Frank.

Christmas evening *December 25*

> "For unto us a child is born, unto us a son is given: and the government shall be upon his shoulder: and his name shall be called Wonderful, Counsellor, The mighty God, The everlasting Father, The Prince of Peace."
> Isaiah 9:6, KJV

I feel blessed and joyful tonight. It's Christmas Eve 2017. A year ago today I learned I had a cancerous tumor in the head of my pancreas. As the church choir and orchestra took the platform that Sabbath, I was wheeled into a procedural room to place a biliary stent and obtain biopsies to confirm my diagnosis.

I felt shock, anxiety, disbelief, fear, and panic. I kept telling myself, "But my Katie is only 11. My son, Scott, still needs me." I feared not sharing another Christmas with my family.

My journey since has been complex, emotional, educational, challenging, and spiritual. I've changed. I'm more patient and grateful. I firmly believe I'm a walking miracle. I am alive and enjoying everything Christmas.

For over 36 years a Christmas tradition each year has been playing Handel's *Messiah* and sharing a viola stand with my husband. My favorite Christmas carol, "Little Drummer Boy," says, "I am a poor boy too.... I have no gift to bring ... that's fit to give our King.... I played my drum for Him.... Then He smiled at me." I so wanted to play the *Messiah* yesterday for the two church services—to bring my humble gift to Him.

I feel the devil wanted to keep me from doing that. My husband, Larry, had a major health scare earlier this week, my parents' garage caught fire on Wednesday (they're both OK), and my neuropathies this past week were more significant and persistent than usual. My neuropathic therapist, Mark, provided extra therapy, and specific prayers were sent heavenward by me and close friends—as well as a prayer team this past Friday morning.

I was determined to play, regardless how I felt. A quote from General George S. Patton kept running through my head: "Make the mind run the body. Never let the body tell the mind what to do. The body will always give up."

Call time for the orchestra was 8:00 a.m. The church sanctuary was very cold. In spite of hand warmers, my thumbs spasmed inward, reacting to one of my chemo drugs. I teared up because I really wanted to play.

I pushed through anyway, adjusting my viola technique and playing the best I could for my God. As I did so, the music and words of the *Messiah* washed over me. Tears welled in my eyes as I played the "Hallelujah Chorus" and "Worthy is the Lamb."

I woke up this morning with barely any neuropathies—as if the devil had said, "Oh, well, that didn't work." Thank you, my prayer warriors around the world from a variety of faiths; thank you for being God's angels on my path. Above all, I praise and give thanks to my God. *Soli Deo gloria.*

Handel's *Messiah* reminds me: "For unto us a Child is born ... Hallelujah ... I know that my Redeemer liveth [because] worthy is the Lamb that was slain ... Amen." Christ's birth is what gives me hope, and this Christmas I am at peace. Merry Christmas!

Melissa Kidder, LLUSM class of 1994, is an assistant professor in LLUSM's department of gynecology and obstetrics. As the daughter of missionaries, she spent ages 3 to 12 in South America. She joined the New England Youth Ensemble in high school and married her viola stand partner, Larry. Their two children are her life. She was chair and residency program director of OB/GYN at LLUSM when pancreatic cancer changed everything.

December 26

> *"Are they [angels] not all ministering spirits, sent out to render service for the sake of those who will inherit salvation?"*
> Hebrews 1:14, NASB1995

The year was 1995, and we were headed to the island of Cuba on our first project overseas. We were taking thousands of pairs of eyeglasses to support the great ophthalmic needs in that country. We were received by the Cuban authorities and given a place for our temporary clinic, which was attached to the famous Cuban Institute of Ophthalmology Ramón Pando Ferrer in Havana. A police officer controlled the entrance, and only a person with a pass given by the government was granted access. Already hundreds, if not thousands, of persons were standing in lines to have the opportunity to be seen and, hopefully, helped. I knew it would be a difficult task to serve so many people and to do so without growing weary.

On our last day an elderly woman was brought to me accompanied by a companion dressed in white. Neither of them had a pass, but I started the eye exam anyway. I found that the patient previously had a cataract removed without the placement of an intraocular lens (it needed a +12-diopter correction), and she also had advanced optic nerve damage. To correct these conditions, she needed a pair of high-power glasses that sadly we did not have. As I told her I was sorry that we could not help her, she grasped my arm and exclaimed, "But I need to read my Bible!" In talking with her further, I discovered that she conducted Bible studies. "I still can read," she said as she took out an old scratched loupe held with wires and started reading her Bible with much difficulty.

I told my wife, Gloria, to please go find the highest power eyeglasses we had. She found a +4 bifocals, and I said to the patient, "This is all we have," and placed them on her. As I did so, I saw her face immediately start to glow, and a huge smile came across her face. With tears of joy she wept, "I can see! I can see again!" Her companion cried with the patient as she started reading her Bible, but this time without halting and hesitating. As my ecstatic patient stood to leave, I gave her a big hug and prayed with her in glorifying God.

The next day one of our team recognized the patient when she returned and asked how she had entered the building the day before without a pass. She relayed that she was outside in the crowd when the passes had all been handed out. She continued, "A woman grabbed my arm and quickly took me past the officer and control point without any questions being asked."

"And who was the woman who brought you in?" asked my teammate.

"I don't know," she replied, "but I know she brought me here to you."

I am convinced that I had witnessed an angel at work.

Pedro Gomez-Bastar is currently chair of Instituto de la Vision Universidad de Montemorelos, Mexico, and is married to Gloria. Together they have three children and one grandchild.

December 27

"I expect to pass through life but once. If therefore, there be any kindness I can show, or any good thing I can do to any fellow being, let me do it now, and not defer or neglect it, as I shall not pass this way again."
William Penn (1644–1718): *founder of Pennsylvania and English author*

"Loma Linda saved my life." I can't tell you how many stories I've heard over the years that began with those very words. They may start the same, but then the stories vary somewhat, with a surgery in the operating room, or a quick-minded emergency medical physician, or maybe a prolonged proton treatment. In fact, I heard another such story just yesterday from a man sitting in my office. His story also began with "Loma Linda saved my life." With early detection followed by surgery two days later, the survivor was telling me his story after living 20 years cancer-free. There are countless others. Indeed, our health care professionals save lives in our hospital every day.

One day quite some time ago I heard it again, and it started the same as the others: "Loma Linda saved my life." But after that infamous opening line, this story was very different. Different because the lifesaving measure did not take place in the operating room. It did not take place in the emergency department or even in one of our clinics. It took place in an office. It took place on the sidewalk. It took place in the conference room and in the hallway. This story was different because it did not involve a medical treatment, procedure, or a medication. It happened over the course of many years as an employee of the university.

The subject of this story, like many others, came to Loma Linda looking for a job. After other candidates were eliminated, she was selected for the position. Her co-workers were happy with the decision. She was friendly and reliable, and performed her assigned tasks well. She was easy to get along with and fit in well with her group of co-workers. Honestly, from that day forward everything seemed pretty routine. We got caught up in the daily grind and lost track of time as the years passed us by.

Unbeknown to those around her, her life had been heading in the wrong direction. Fate would bring her to Loma Linda, a place where people would care about her, a place where people live an example of God's love for us. Simply put, a place where we care about others. Yes, we take care of and care about our patients, but we also care about our fellow co-workers. A single life-altering event could not be identified; there were no radical discussions from colleagues where advice was given—a recipe to turn her life around. Rather, it was long-term daily examples of humanity and kindness. So simplistic in its delivery. "This place is different," she would often say. Indeed, it is different, and it made a difference in her life—the specific details need not be shared.

We often go through our day not realizing the real impact we have on those around us, both positive and negative. This story reminds me that one does not need to be a skilled surgeon or a knowledgeable nurse; one does not even need a medical background to save a life. Each one of us is capable of impacting another in a positive way, a way that can reflect the image of Christ for life-saving measures. I would like to thank all of the employees of this institution I have come to love for making a daily difference in the lives of others. Yes, I would say this place is different and very special, and I am very proud to call this place home.

Darrell Petersen, DrPH, MBA, is an assistant professor in LLUSM's department of pathology and human anatomy, division of anatomy. He is also director of anatomical services and the Bodies for Science program at LLUSM. Both he and his wife are graduates of Loma Linda University. They have two daughters, and in 2020 they celebrated their twentieth wedding anniversary.

December 28

> *"Rejoice always, pray continually, give thanks in all circumstances; for this is God's will for you in Christ Jesus."*
> 1 Thessalonians 5:16-18, NIV

On December 28, 2018, a beautiful sunny day at Mammoth mountain in California, I went down a ski run with my two daughters (Charlene and Cheryl), and then the next thing I knew, I woke up in an ambulance with a paramedic talking to me. What had happened? Per my daughters' account, I had stopped halfway down the run to rest and wait for them, and in an instant a snowboarder had lost control and collided into my back. When Charlene got to me, I was facedown, unconscious and limp. Thus began my transition from being a physician of 23 years to being an ICU patient for the first time.

In the emergency department the diagnosis came back: cerebral contusion with mild subarachnoid hemorrhage and lumbar spine 1-4 transverse processes fractures. I immediately saw the concerns on the faces of my family. Then came the next major decision: Should I be airlifted to the closest trauma center in Reno (3½-hour drive) or be observed overnight at Mammoth Hospital (17-bed facility with two ICU beds)? I was cognitive enough at this point to call my neurosurgery colleague by phone for advice. After reviewing the texted copies of the CT scan, he assured me that the head injury was relatively minor and that the likelihood of neurosurgical intervention was low. So I was admitted to the ICU at Mammoth Hospital. The ICU stay was a new experience: every-hour neurological checks, BP cuff inflating every hour, sequential compression devices inflating/deflating regularly, beeping monitor sound because of transient low oxygen saturation requiring oxygen, and medications for back pain. No Foley catheter was needed (a great relief, even though I am a urologist). The morning could not have come any sooner. Repeat head CT showed improvement of the hemorrhage, and with no worsening neurological changes, I was given the good news of hospital discharge.

In reflecting upon my experience as a patient, I am grateful to:

1. God for His protection and mercy, as the outcome could have been much worse.
2. My family for taking charge and care of me when I was down (Cheryl insisted on staying in the room with me overnight, while Mom and Charlene packed up the car to be ready to leave for Reno at a moment's notice).
3. My neurosurgeon friend who was on call for me remotely for any questions.
4. The entire medical staff (physicians, nurses, CT technicians, phlebotomist) at Mammoth Hospital for their professionalism and compassionate care.

As I transition back to be a physician, I have a new perspective from the "other side" of the bed. Being a health care provider can be demanding, time-consuming, draining, and even routine. As a result, we may lose sight of our calling, thus leading to burnout. However, having a priceless peep from the patient's perspective, I am grateful and privileged to be part of a profession that truly makes a difference in someone's life daily. You don't need to be involved in a skiing accident to be reminded of the noble cause: to be the hands and feet in the healing ministry of Jesus Christ.

Yu Wang, LLUSM class of 1987, practices urologic oncology and is chief of urologic surgery at Kaiser Permanente, San Bernardino County. His two daughters, Charlene (LLUSM class of 2022) and Cheryl (LLUSM class of 2024) are current medical students. He believes that being a physician is a noble calling to service and healing in his patients.

December 29

"Yet in all these things we are more than conquerors through Him who loved us."
Romans 8:37, NKJV

Gazing into starry skies makes me feel directly connected to God, not caught up in what's around me: busy city or unknown, dark jungle. In the Bible God instructed Noah's family to build one window in the roof of the ark so that in the midst of mass destruction and storms around them, they could only look up to God, their sole source of strength and hope. God knows how lost we can get in the worries of this world and provides hope. I've always heard about the "storms" a life in medicine brings, and I was wrestling with my decision one particular moonlit night on a mission trip.

Mosquitoes buzzing in my ear, I'm on the Amazon River trying to tune out the boat's engine so I can get some rest before another clinic. No one knows their future, but everyone worries about it. Familiar fears grabbed hold of me: possible wasted time, failure, the feeling of lacking faith in God to pursue medicine. Hours creeped by; out of desperation I left my hammock searching for an answer to my anxiety. While the rest of my mission crew slept soundly, I stood at the front of the boat where there was no roof covering the sky. I looked up and literally started talking to God as to a close friend. No one knew I was awake. Without any reception, no one at home even knew where I was in this foreign country. It was so dark I felt as if no one in the world could see me, but God could.

Fast-forward one year, I'm sleep-deprived and spending the majority of 24 hours on campus buried in my first-year studies. I'm falling behind in lectures, failing classes, lashing out at loved ones, and plagued by the guilt of not studying enough. In this cycle I often find myself right outside of Centennial Complex looking up for His reassurance. Exhausted, I sigh out a prayer and choose to trust God to empower me. When I go back to study, I see my best friend persevering beside me, remember my family who believes in me, and realize the sacred opportunity to make eternal differences in someone's life each day. God listens to the deep groanings of my heart and answers them in His perfect way.

My favorite promise is Romans 8:37 because it tells us that we are conquerors. He has extraordinary plans for every one of us even if you're like me and feel … well, extremely average. We are a part of a cosmic battle, the great controversy, between God and Satan, and each of our unique lives is an important testament to prove God's character true. All of us have tough journeys, but never forget that we can overcome, because He's on our side. With God holding our future, despite inevitable troubles, look up! No matter what battles you face each day, rejoice in the wins, learn from the losses, and know that you are a conqueror.

Laura Tobing, LLUSM class of 2022, was born and raised in Loma Linda with her parents, sister, brother, and their Maltipoo pup. She attended Southern Adventist University in Tennessee, where she took hold of her personal relationship with Jesus and now hopes to encourage others daily.

December 30

> *"Seek opportunities to show you care. The smallest gestures often make the biggest difference."*
> **John Wooden (1910–2010): American legendary college basketball coach**

It is interesting to note that there are two stories of Creation given in the book of Genesis. The first one that comes to our minds describes an all-powerful God (Adonai) that merely has to speak, and things are created. But soon after, there is a second story of Creation:

"Then the LORD God formed the man from the dust of the ground. He breathed the breath of life into the man's nostrils, and the man became a living person" (Genesis 2:7, NLT).

In this story we have the relational picture of God (Yahweh), who, with a touch and a breath, creates humanity. Each year LLUH trains, prepares, and graduates hundreds of health professionals who are provided with the power of science, the best technology and insights to treat disease and chronic needs. But sometimes those are not enough to bring about healing.

I was a young man of 20 years. I was in an intensive care unit fighting for my life from a gunshot wound that had pierced my stomach, liver, spleen, and intestines, and totally severed my vena cava. I was afraid that whoever had shot me would find out that they hadn't accomplished my death and would come to finish the job. I was terrified, but I played tough and hardened. No one saw past my mask of false bravado to see frightened "me." No one, that is, except my nurse. After my doctor and others had left the room, she remained. She stood by my bed and asked if I was all right and if I needed anything. "No, I don't need anything. I'm fine," I lied. She asked if I'd mind if she just stayed awhile. I replied, "Do what you want. I can't do anything about it."

She stood quietly. Then she did for me what no medicine could have done. She reached down and held my hand. She looked me in the eyes and said, "I'm here, and I will stay with you until you go to sleep. Then I'll check back with you throughout the night." Her presence, her touch, her love, shone as a heavenly light into the darkness of my heart and life. She helped heal me. She helped my broken, dark, distrusting life to find the first step on the pathway back to wholeness and God. That experience helped me to write a little phrase that I include at the end of my emails and phone texts: "The darkest room is powerless against the light of a single candle flame."

This world is a dark place with broken, lonely, frightened, hurting people. All of the technology, all of the glitz of entertainment, all the material things, all the wisdom of the world, cannot show them the way out of darkness.

They need someone.
They need a loving touch.
They need transforming love.
They need just a single candle flame.
They need . . . you to show them God and His love still lives.

Terry Swenson, DMin, serves as director of university spiritual care and is an associate professor in LLUHSR. Working with young adults and building connections between cultures and races through a deeper relationship with Jesus have been a constant focus throughout his 37 years of pastoral and chaplain ministry. The opportunity to focus his ministry on students at a university level attracted him to his current position 23 years ago.

New Year's Eve — **December 31**

> *"And if I go and prepare a place for you, I will come again, and receive you unto myself; that where I am, there ye may be also."*
> John 14:3, KJV

If you knew this man as I did, you'd be struggling now to capture the warmth, the joy, the challenging conversations, the stories, and the memories that his life encompassed. You might have learned to sail or to paddle a canoe with him at Lake Nojiri in Japan. You might have trudged across your snowy Michigan backyard, leaving tracks as you went to join him for an early-morning jog. You might have shot a BB gun at a wooden match across the basement family room, until, to your amazement, he shot one and lit the match at 30 feet. Bull's-eye!

You might have learned to ride a bike, to drive a stickshift, to weed a garden, or to sing in harmony. You might have joined him in the Princeton chapel to experience a rollicking celebration of God's love, complete with Old Testament-style cymbals and tambourines. You might have tried with him to play harmonica, or clarinet, or slide trombone. You'd have shared goose bump moments with him and Marjorie as she played and they harmonized together at the piano, singing everything from "Jacob's Ladder" to "Brazen Little Raisin." You may have learned some words of Japanese, which he spoke fluently; you might have read in Greek. You could have borrowed books from his vast library. You would have passionately discussed them, and most likely lent him one of yours. You might have sung beside him in a choir or led song service with him in the youth tent at a Soquel, California, camp meeting.

If you were one of his three girls, you would have learned to pray. First with toddler hands clasped reverently, later peeking through your fingers during church, and finally as you grew into adulthood, when you'd have your own private dialogues with the One whom you had come to love yourself.

Because this man loved Jesus. He was a preacher, professor, parishioner, and lifelong student. His entire life was lived in the context of the single fact that guided all his longings, thoughts, and actions—Jesus was his friend. You couldn't sit with him or jog with him or walk with him or talk with him without having a sense that he had heard you, and that you mattered deeply to him. Sooner or later, depending on your readiness, not his, you also learned you mattered deeply to his best friend, Jesus.

And if you knew him as so many people did, you'd miss him now with aching heart, and want to be with him again. Losing him has made me imagine those friends of Jesus who had gathered with their broken hearts after His brutal death, and to whom He then appeared. He promised them He'd come again, and Dad knew He would. Dad liked to remind us of "the prayer at the back of the book," Revelation 22:20: "Even so, come, Lord Jesus" (KJV).

It's true; we love and miss you, Dad, but in your own words this is only, "Bye for now. We'll see you in the morning."

Elizabeth Venden Sutherland is a writer and project facilitator who consulted on various LLUH projects for nearly 30 years. More germaine, she's the eldest daughter of Louis Venden, who was senior pastor of the Loma Linda University Church; professor in the LLUSR; eagerly compliant patient of several talented, caring LLUSM physicians; and active, involved member of the Calimesa Seventh-day Adventist Church. He fell asleep in Jesus on December 8, 2020.

Epilogue

This book you hold in your hands started as an idea in 2007. It was seen as one way to involve as many students, alumni, faculty, and friends of Loma Linda University School of Medicine as possible in anticipation of the 2009 centennial of the founding of the school. Now, three books, 14 years, 1,096 stories, and over 800 authors later, that idea has culminated in tangible inspiration beyond what any of us could have dreamed.

To those who shared their stories of joy, sorrow, success, failure, transparency, and vulnerability, you have made us better people because of the lessons you have taught us. You have shared your humanity, and you have expanded ours. May all of us who read these stories be reminded to choose love above all else, *always*.

— Donna R. Hadley
Editor

Index of Daily Scripture and Quote References

Scripture

Genesis
2:7, NASB .... December 15
3:15, NIV .... April 3
16:13, KJV .... July 29
21:16, NIV .... September 9
50:20, NKJV .... March 17

Numbers
6:26, NIV .... January 12

Deuteronomy
10:21, NIV .... July 27
31:6, NIV .... January 30
31:8, NIV .... June 25

Joshua
1:9, NIV .... March 21

1 Samuel
16:7, ESV .... August 30

1 Kings
4:29, NIV .... August 2

1 Chronicles
21:2, NLT .... August 20

2 Chronicles
7:14-15, ESV .... June 18
15:7, NIV .... October 21
16:9, ESV .... September 12

Esther
4:14, ESV .... July 23

Job
5:8-9, NIV .... December 6

Psalms
3:4, Remedy .... September 24
5:11, NIV .... November 25
17:6-7, 15, ESV .... September 25
19:14, KJV .... January 24
23:1-4, NIV .... March 15
23:4, MSG .... March 30
27:1, NKJV .... November 22
30:5, NKJV .... August 23

32:8, KJV .... December 22
33:22, NIV .... April 20
34:7, GNT .... February 4
34:7, KJV .... June 29
34:18, GNT .... July 19
37:23, NLT .... July 12
37:23-24, KJV .... February 8
39:7, NLT .... January 23
47:3, ESV .... April 6
51:10, NIV .... May 23
54:4, ESV .... June 13
75:1, ESV .... July 15
77:11, NLT .... December 24
77:12, ESV .... August 25
89:46, NIV .... March 13
90:12, NIV .... July 31
90:17, ESV .... May 4
91:4, NLT .... July 4
91:4, GNT .... October 18
102:17, NLT .... May 21
103:1-5, KJV .... August 13
103:2-4, ESV .... September 10
104:24, AMP .... August 27
112:7, NIV .... November 30
121:3, ESV .... July 25
121:7-8, ESV .... August 7
127:1, ESV .... May 11
127:3, NLT .... May 6
139:10, ESV .... June 30
139:13-14 ESV .... March 25
139:16, NIV .... October 31
145:18, ESV .... October 23
147:3, NIV .... May 10
147:4, ESV .... November 9

Proverbs
3:5-6, KJV .... October 26
3:5-6, NKJV .... April 24
3:13-14, NIV .... January 13
4:5-6, NIV .... April 11
6:6, KJV .... August 1
11:14, KJV .... August 31
17:22, ESV .... February 10
18:22, NLT .... May 14
19:17, ESV .... July 13
22:6, NKJV .... November 14
23:15-16, NASB .... May 18

386

27:17, NASB .... October 17

Ecclesiastes
1:2, NIV .... February 15
3:1, 7, MSG .... October 28
3:11, NIV .... September 27
11:1, NKJV .... June 12
11:5-6, KJV .... June 15
12:3-5, CEV .... May 1

Isaiah
1:17, NIV .... January 16
9:6, KJV .... December 25
26:3, GNT .... June 14
26:3, NIV .... August 26
30:21, KJV .... July 5
40:31, NASB .... February 23
41:10, NKJV .... August 17
41:13, ESV .... January 5
43:1, KJV .... March 14
43:2, NIV .... November 29
43:19, NASB1995 .... October 15
46:4, NLT .... September 19
49:6, NKJV .... October 13
49:15, NIV .... May 8
49:16, ESV .... March 28
53:5, KJV .... May 26
55:6-7, KJV .... October 6
58:9, WEB .... July 6
58:13-14, NKJV .... December 17
61:1, NASB .... December 4
65:24, GNT .... January 20
65:24, NIV .... May 27

Jeremiah
1:5, ESV .... May 16
9:23-24, NKJV .... August 18
24:7, ESV .... March 7
29:11, GNT .... August 8
32:27, KJV .... June 10
33:3, ESV .... February 7

Lamentations
3:25-26, NKJV .... April 28

Ezekiel
36:26, NKJV .... August 6

Micah
6:8, NIV .... February 22

Nahum
1:7, ESV .... February 6

Habakkuk
2:4, ESV .... December 11

Zephaniah
3:17, ESV .... November 7

Zechariah
2:8, NIV .... March 23
4:6, NKJV .... March 18

Matthew
6:9-13, ESV .... April 23
6:10, KJV .... April 25
7:7, NIV .... October 12
7:12, NASB .... April 5
9:12-13, KJV .... October 24
9:35, NIV .... June 22
11:28, NIV .... October 27
11:29, NIV .... January 26
18:33, NASB .... June 17
19:26, ESV .... November 23
19:26, GNT .... June 4
19:26, NLT .... July 7
20:26-27, ESV .... June 8
22:37-39, MSG .... January 2
25:37-40, GNT .... November 10
27:45-46, 50, NRSV .... July 1
28:20, NKJV .... March 24

Mark
1:35, NKJV .... January 10
3:1-5, ESV .... February 13
4:35, NASB .... February 5
6:31, NKJV .... October 10
8:36, NKJV .... May 5
10:45, ESV .... July 18
12:31, NIV .... December 12
16:15, ESV .... April 22

Luke
2:7, NRSV .... December 16
3:10-11, NIV .... January 28

Reference	Date
6:38, ESV	August 29
9:2, KJV	August 16
10:27, NKJV	February 28
12:15, ESV	April 14
13:13, NIV	August 19
14:11, NASB	June 11
15:20-24, ESV	June 19
17:15-18, NLT	November 16

John

Reference	Date
3:16, KJV	June 21
4:10, NIV	February 19
5:24, KJV	February 2
6:37, KJV	January 3
6:68, NKJV	May 31
8:6-9, NIV	March 1
8:12, KJV	June 1
8:32, NKJV	December 20
8:36, KJV	June 6
11:4, NASB1995	November 20
11:25-26, NIV	July 24
11:33, 40, NIV	May 13
11:35, NIV	July 28
12:26, ESV	July 17
13:12-15, ESV	June 3
13:34-35, NKJV	May 15
14:3, KJV	December 31
14:9, NET	October 22
14:27, KJV	August 24
15:5, NKJV	May 19
15:12, NIV	August 15
15:13, NIV	December 9
15:17, NLT	September 1
16:21, NKJV	September 21
16:33, NIV	September 5
17:23, NASB1995	September 6
20:25, NIV	February 27

Acts

Reference	Date
2:3, NASB	November 19
20:35, ESV	April 9
27:31, KJV	April 19

Romans

Reference	Date
1:16, KJV	September 28
2:1, NIV	January 25
5:3-5, NIV	March 12
5:8, NASB	March 31
6:9, NASB	April 17
8:26-27, ESV	November 13
8:28, KJV	April 10
8:37, NKJV	December 29
10:14, NLT	January 11
12:2, ESV	August 14
12:10, KJV	April 7
13:10, NIV	June 20
14:9, ESV	September 20
14:19, NIV	April 26
15:5, NIV	July 16

1 Corinthians

Reference	Date
4:9, NIV	January 31
12:5-6, NIV	March 20
12:15-19, NLT	July 8
13:11, NASB	April 2
13:13, NIV	September 4
15:58, NKJV	March 19

2 Corinthians

Reference	Date
1:3-4, ESV	September 29
1:6, ESV	January 21
3:2-3, NIV	February 3
4:8-9, NLT	January 14
4:16, ESV	December 13
4:17, BSB	April 27
4:18, NIV	October 25
5:17, NIV	December 10
6:2, KJV	January 29
9:12, NIV	November 17
12:9, ESV	February 16

Galatians

Reference	Date
5:13, CEV	November 4
5:22-23, NASB	November 3
6:10, ESV	April 8

Ephesians

Reference	Date
2:8-9, ESV	July 22
3:14-15, ESV	August 10
3:20, NASB	April 1
4:1, NIV	February 18
5:1, ESV	March 9
5:2, GNT	September 23
6:12, ASV	July 11

5:15, ESV .... October 7
6:18, NIV .... January 18

Philippians
1:6, NASB1995 .... February 14
1:21, ESV .... April 15
4:6-7, NKJV .... March 6
4:13, ESV .... March 10
4:13, NKJV .... April 18

Colossians
3:17, ESV ....June 9
3:23, NIV ....February 21
3:23, NLV .... March 4

1 Thessalonians
4:13, NIV .... March 2
4:13-14, ESV ....June 7
4:16-17, KJV ....December 14
5:9, Clear Word....................December 21
5:16-18, ESV ....May 20
5:16-18, NIV ....December 28
5:23-24, NKJV .... March 29

1 Timothy
4:12, NIV ....June 26

2 Timothy
1:7, NKJV ....September 18

Hebrews
1:14, NASB1995 ....December 26
2:17, NIV ....February 20
4:12, NIV ....February 24
4:14-16, ESV .... April 13
6:10, NIV ....June 23
11:1, ESV .... November 26
11:1, NIV ....February 17
12:1-3, NIV .... December 5
13:2, NLT .... December 8
13:7, NIV ....May 12
13:14, NLT......................................July 26

James
1:2-4, NIV ....December 23
1:19, NIV ....June 27
5:13-15, NASB ....May 25
5:16, KJV .... March 22

1 Peter
3:8, NIV ....September 11
3:18, NASB1995 ....November 21
5:6-7, NKJV ....October 16

1 John
1:5, NKJV ....July 30
3:1, ESV..May 3
3:1, NIV ....July 21
4:7, ESV................................December 1
4:11, ESV .... October 8
4:12, NIV ....September 22
4:16, NIV ....June 5
5:14, GNT..................................March 16
5:14, NIV .... November 11

3 John
2, NIV.. March 3

Revelation
2:10, GNT...............................June 16
3:18, ESV .... October 20
7:9, NIV ....September 14
21:4, ESV .... November 27
21:5, ESV ....January 9

Quotes

African proverb ....March 11
Angelou, Maya .... September 30
Anonymous ....January 15, January 27,
April 4, May 9, July 3, August 3,
November 8, December cover
Ashton, Marvin J. .... February 12
Beecher, Henry Ward .... December 18
Boese, Paul.. May 30
Bonhoeffer, Dietrich .... September 26,
October 5
Brock, Jared..................................October 29
Buck, Pearl S. ....May cover
Buscaglia, Leo ....January 17
Carter, Kim ....January 19
Chambers, Oswald .... May 2
Chapman, Steven Curtis .... June 28
Childress, Alice .... September 16
Cohen, Alan H. .... November 1
Curie, Marie............................ February 26
Einstein, Albert ....October 3
Elliot, Walter .... August 12
Fosdick, Harry Emerson .... July 10
Fulghum, Robert............................June 2
Fuller, Janet ....January 7
Gardner, John W. .... January cover
George, Elizabeth........................ August 11
Grosz, Bill .... May 22
Hay, Louise ....October 4
Hays, Richard B. .... May 7
Heschel, Abraham .... March 26
Hippocrates ....January 1
Keller, Helen...........................August cover
King, Jr., Martin Luther .... October 8
Kingma, Daphne Rose ....October 11
Kübler-Ross, Elisabeth..................April 12
Kushner, Harold S. ....September cover
Lawson, Douglas M. ....November 15
Lewis, C. S. .... February 25
Lincoln, Abraham .... June cover
Luther, Martin................................ April 16
McCartney, Colin .... July 14
Milton, John .... November cover
Moore, Thomas........................ February 11
Musser, Mark J. ....April 30
Niebuhr, Reinhold .... December 7

Nouwen, Henri ....October 19
Olsen, V. Norskov...............................July 9
Osler, William .... January 4, April 21
Palmer, Parker J. ....October cover
Parks, Rosa .... April cover
Peabody, Francis W. .... Sep 13
Penn, William........................ December 27
Phipps, Wintley ....August 5
Prieto, Adolfo .... November 6
Roberts, Stewart R. .... January 8
Rodríguez, Carlos A. .... April 29
Rogers, Dale Evans .... December 25
Rogers, Fred.............................November 24
Roosevelt, Theodore .... September 8
Salley, Jerry....................................... June 28
Sartre, Jean-Paul............................August 9
Scholtes, Peter Raymond ..... December 19
Schweitzer, Albert.........July 20, August 21
Seneca the Younger.................... August 28
Sheldon, Arthur F. .... November 2
Spurgeon, Charles..........................March 5
Stewart, Potter .... February cover
Stoddart, John ....August 5
Stott, John.................................... June 24
Ten Boom, Corrie .... January 22
Teresa, Mother .... July cover
Thoreau, Henry David .... September 17
Tico, Rose .... May 17
Tomlin, Chris ....March 8
Tutu, Desmond .... March cover
Van Gogh, Vincent ....February 1
Vineyard, Sue ....October 14
Ward, William Arthur .... November 5
Wesley, John.................................January 6
White, Ellen G .... March 27, April 23,
May 28, August 22,
September 3, December 2
Wooden, John........................ December 30

Index of Authors

Afolayan, Oluwatobi 358
Aitken, April Angelique 144
Akamine, Christine 200
Albano, Bobbi 332
Alexander, Kelcie 36
Anderson, Bruce N. 364
Angkadjaja, Julia 82
Angkadjaja, William 217
Anonymous SM Student 58
Ask, Mickey 288
Aveling, Leigh 224
Babienco, Ryan 88
Bacchus, Austin 303
Bacon, Barry 158
Bailey, Josianne 192
Barnes, Gladys Snyder 85
Batin, H. Roger 341
Belensky, Sarah 261
Bhattacharjee, Arlin "Larry" 284
Blanchard, Jason 208
Bland, David 118
Blue, Cheri 336
Boloix-Chapman, Ester 42
Bond, Robert 194
Borovic, Josif 218
Boskovic, Danilo 277
Boudreaux, Patience 334
Boyd, Caroline 3
Briggs, Burton 128
Brisbane, Wayne 222
Brockie, Darren 282
Brockmann, Doug 166
Broeckel, Philip 221
Brooks, Dilys 145
Broomes, Lloyd Rudy 80
Browne, Genise 18
Bunnell, William P. 57
Burghart, Victoria "Tori" 291
Cacho, Bradley 212
Calaguas, Daniel 133
Calaguas, Shannon Fujimoto 35
Campbell, Andrene 263
Cao, Jeff 64
Carlson, Donna 52
Carter, Kim 20
Charles-Marcel, Zeno L. 352

Chastain, Cody 90
Chen, John E. 247
Chen, Sam M. 271
ChenFeng, Jessica 55
Cherepuschak, Kelsey 81
Chi-Lum, Bonnie 313
Chong, Esther G. 201
Choo, Daniel 162
Chow, Eric C. 321
Chujutalli, Ricardo 345
Chung, Paul Y. 132
Church, Christopher 214
Cipta, Andre 110
Clark, Jane 174
Clem, Kathleen 154
Cotton, Adrian 161
Crandell, Kristy 245
Dalley, Matt 71
Damazo, Benjamin 149
Daniel-Underwood, Lynda 152
Daniyan, Adegbemisola 54
Diehl, Shani Judd 49
Dixon, Linda Harsh 324
Dorotta, Ihab 170
Duerksen-Hughes, Penelope 59
Durbin, Eva Ryckman 240
Dysinger, P. William "Bill" 92
Ejike, Janeth 6
Elkins, David 209
Elloway, Richard 273
Endeno-Galima, Elizabeth 316
Eng, David 311
Engdahl, Anders 150
Estes, Molly 106
Evans, Dwight C. 66
Ezeribe, Hazel 169
Fedusenko, Ashley Evans 72
Ferry, Linda Hyder 368
Fitch, Klaireece 184
Flynn, Thomas 177
Folkerts, Andrew 168
Folsom, Lisal Stevens 268
Forde, Esther 298
Foster, Kristoff 28
Frederick, Dexter 267
Freed, Spencer 12

Geslani, Bevan 375	Hodgkin, John E. 195
Giang, Daniel 98	Hodgkin, Steven E. 153
Gibson, Quince-Xhosa 86	Holloway, Christopher 370
Gobble, Tim 23	Hong, Denny 228
Gold, Philip M. 101	Hoxie, Russell E. 329
Golden, Jill 376	Hrdina, Robin 280
Gomez, Jesse 325	Hughes, Jill 189
Gomez-Bastar, Pedro 378	Hussey, Maddison Ulrich 47
Goodge, Brent 108	Isaeff, Dale 9
Goorhuis, Jonathan 272	Ito, Shiho 317
Gow-Lee, Guillermo 31	Johnson, Denise Roberts 361
Green, Morgan 142	Johnston, Chris 173
Green, Tedean 241	Kahler, Gabrielle 374
Greene, Briana 344	Kam, Nathan 53
Gulley, James 250	Kellar, Jesse 353
Guthrie, Laurel 146	Kelly, Ted Martin 97
Haase, Shari 252	Ketting-Weller, Ginger 104
Hadley, Beverly 266	Kettner, Sid 183
Hadley, Craig 328	Khuc, Thi 346
Hadley, Roger 155	Kidder, Melissa 377
Hamel, Loren 61	Kim, James S. 178
Hamel, Lowell 111	Kim, Lindsey N. 238
Hamilton, Ted 322	Kim, Paul P. 116
Hankins, E. A. "Billy" 289	Kim, Young-Min 60
Hansen, Kent 123	Kime, Wesley 160
Harris, Wayne B. 285	Kimmel-McNeilus, Mary Ann 196
Hart, Elaine 205	Ko, Edmund 138
Hart, Richard 91	Kozik, Paul 157
Hartman, Matthew 310	Krause, Marianne 79
Hayton, Amy 112	Krause, Raymond 78
Hayton, Ryan 270	Laack, Torrey 29
Hayton, Sharlene 204	LaBore, Bill 239
Hegstad, Doug 193	Lalas, Angela Manalo 198
Heinrich, Kerry 231	Lam, Carrie 147
Heldt, Jonathan 315	Lamberton, Henry 320
Hellsten, Bjørg Irene Harvey 70	Lamberton, Tessa 256
Henry, Gina 15	Landless, Peter 32
Herber, Steve 244	Langley, Shawna McCarty 172
Hernandez, Barbara Couden 83	Lau, Benjamin H. 171
Herrmann, Paul 283	Lau, Kathleen 14
Hewes, Judi Lacy 363	Lee, Cameron M. 75
Hewes, Robert 229	Lee, Michael Z. 34
Hilliard, Anthony 131	Lohr, Jason 117
Hilliard, Jolene Lang 40	Lopez, Merrick 210
Hilliard, Tammy 10	Luh, George 30
Ho, Matthew 73	Lunt, Margie 372

Magloire, Victoria 67	Palmer, Sharon Michael 4
Mannoia, Kristyn 51	Pandit, Dipika 137
Manns, Ryan 197	Pang, Nilmini 243
Marais, Ryan 102	Park, Dennis 357
Markel, Kory 294	Park, Eunice 367
Marpaung, Eunice 5, 156	Parker, Bonnie R. 230
Martin, Courtney 373	Patee, Allen 253
Martin, Jerome 248	Pauldurai, Jennifer 305
Matus, Michael 93	Paulien, Jon 258
McGrosky, Dale 301	Payne, Kimberly 203
McHan, Steve 77	Peckham, Miriam 13
McMillan, Jim 265	Pelton, Cyndee 43
McMillan, Kathy 24	Peoples, Christopher 296
McRae, Joyce 207	Perez, Rubicelia 281
McSherry, Carissa 16	Petersen, Darrell 379
Meelhuysen, Delbe 249	Petersen, Floyd 354
Miles, Ethan 48	Peterson, Myra 37
Miller, Cheyanne 251	Peverini, Ricardo 264
Miller, David K. 314	Piñango, Kyra Brusett Eddy 215
Miller, Paul 226	Price, Sharmila 38
Milosavljevic, Filip 27	Quave, Brett 139
Mindoro, Ken 340	Raines, R. Marina 180
Miot, Christelle 50	Ranzolin, Susan 134
Mitchell, Gayle 2	Rauser, Michael 96
Moody, Richard 275	Reeves, Mark 175
Moores, Don 100	Reichert, Zachary 306
Moores, Michael 45	Reimche-Vu, David 246
Moran, Matthew 356	Rich, Jennifer Renaud 140
Moreno, Cheri 105	Richards, Jon 124
Moretta, Dafne 165	Richards, Winston 114
Murrell, Suzonne Weeks Meek 347	Rigsby, Ryan 103
Nadarajan, Sarah 107	Ritland, Sandra 355
Namm, Jukes 339	Rittenhouse, Robert 129
Ndlela, Emily 74	Rivera, Aimee Hechanova 299
Nelson, Donovan C. 342	Rivera, Benjamin 333
Nelson, Scott 242	Rogers, John R. 279
Netteburg, Danae 202	Rogstad, Daniel 186
Newman, Naeem 41	Roquiz, D. Andrew 318
Ngan, David A. 182	Rose, Kenneth 148
Ngo, Khiet 185	Rosenquist, Robert 121
Nguyen, Van 308	Ruff, Lloyd 188
Nishikawa, Christal 365	Rusch, Joyce Johnston 225
Nishino, Toshihiro 181	Sagadraca, Remy 94
Nist, Laura 130	Sakala, Elmar 135
Olson, Linda 235	Sanchez, Randy 312
Orr, Barbara 26	Sandoval, Mark 360

Santana, Monique Freire	76
Saunders, David	236
Sayler, Landon	89
Schmidt, Wally	327
Schrader, Jeanne	22
Scofield, Merrilee	349
Seheult, Craig	254
Seton, Gillian	211
Shadle, Sr., Eric	167
Shannon, Kevin	206
Sharley, Jonathan	297
Shawler, William R.	68
Shen, Christine	151
Small, Mary	39
Smart, Danae	125
Sobrinho, Giovanna	232
Spady, Heidi	44
Speyer, Garrett	99
Stecker, Rheeta	234
Stevens, W. Tait	343
Stoll, Shaunrick	292
Stottlemyer, Debra	331
Studer, Karen	304
Sutherland, Elizabeth Venden	383
Swensen, Waylene Wang	227
Swenson, Terry	382
Tan, Laren	87
Tatosyan-Jones, Kristine	348
Thomas, Tamara	323
Thomas, Wilson	163
Thompson, Connie Eller	274
Thorp, Kandus	21
Thorp, Stephen	176
Tjandra, Christine	113
Tobing, Laura	381
Torrey, Melissa	330
Tran, Mai-Linh	143
Tsao, Bryan	136
Turay, David	220
Tyler, Lance	362
Ubah, Chibueze	213
Udonta, E. Dan	278
Underwood, Matthew	7
VanderWel, Rachel	260
Vassantachart, Basil	119
Veltman, Jennifer	164
Villegas, Cristian	11
Von Walter, Astrid	25
Wagner, Marian	141
Wai, Andrew	326
Walker, Jasmine Turner	187
Wallenkampf, Karl	233
Wallenkampf, Victor	371
Walters, Nick	338
Wang, Betty Hwang	293
Wang, Marilene	65
Wang, Yu	380
Ward, David	84
Warren, Mark	109
Warren, Nichelle	199
Waterbrook, Stephen	300
Watkins, Dixie Marcotte	216
Watkins, Hubert C.	257
Watson, WayAnne	366
Weber, Shelby Tanguay	237
Wendt, Joshua	307
Whittaker-Allen, Janette	69
Wiafe, Adwoa	8
Will, Ruth	302
Williams, Jennifer	17
Williams, Shammah	122
Williams, Va Shon	179
Wilson, Don	269
Wilson, Thaddeus	262
Winslow, Dwight	335
Winslow, Gerald	115
Wise, Gregory	219
Wolcott, Deane	259
Wonoprabowo, Jeffrey	295
Wood, Chanel	369
Wood, Virchel	46
Woodruff, Brianna	19
Woodruff, Krista	56
Woodruff, Roger D.	309
Woolcock, Ruth B.	290
Yi, Zane	120
Yorozuya, Lauren Ivey	359
Yu, Jack	276
Zinke, Nancy Carter	337

COVID-19 Stories

January 22 .... Tim Gobble
March 13 .... Monique Freire Santana
March 24 .... Laren Tan
March 30 .... Michael Matus
April 4 .... Garrett Speyer
April 16 .... Lowell Hamel
April 24 .... Basil Vassantachar
May 17 .... April Aitken
July 1 .... Josianne Bailey
July 2 .... Doug Hegstad
July 9 .... Christine Akamine
December 16 .... Eunice Park
December 22 .... Courtney Martin

Awareness Dates and Related Stories

January

Cervical Cancer Awareness Month
September 17 ....Jonathan Goorhuis

Glaucoma Awareness Month
July 8................................ Nichelle Warren

February

American Heart Month
February 4............................ Myra Peterson
March 12...........................Cameron M. Lee
June 5....................................Eric Shadle, Sr.
November 22...................... H. Roger Batin

Congenital Heart Defect Awareness Week
(every February 7–14)
June 24 ....Sid Kettner

National Organ Donor Day (February 14)
February 20............................Nathan Kam
August 28 ....Cheyanne Miller
November 11....................... Melissa Torrey
December 13 .... Bruce N. Anderson

Rare Disease Day (last day in February:
February 28, 2022)
June 24 ....Sid Kettner

March

Blood Clot Awareness Month
January 6 .... Matthew Underwood
January 12.......................Miriam Peckham

Child Life Month
August 1................................ Leigh Aveling

National Colon/Colorectal Cancer
Awareness Month
June 22 ....Toshihiro Nishino
July 12............................... Kimberly Payne
December 17 .... Linda Hyder Ferry

April

Alcohol Awareness Month
March 8....................................Matt Dalley
June 19 ....James S. Kim

Child Abuse Prevention Month
February 27...................... Young-Min Kim

Donate Life Month
January 13 .... Kathleen Lau

National Cancer Control Month
September 1.........................Tess Lamberton

National Infertility Awareness Week
(April 24–30, 2022)
May 11 .... Edmund Ko

National Occupational Therapy Month
January 18 ....Brianna Woodruff

Parkinson's Awareness Month
February 4............................ Myra Peterson

National Retina Awareness Month
April 1 ....Michael Rauser

World Malaria Day (every April 25)
July 11.............................Danae Netteburg

May

Amyotrophic Lateral Sclerosis (ALS)
Awareness Month
July 26..........................William Angkadjaja
December 24 .... Bevan Geslani

Bladder Cancer Awareness Month
June 7..............................Doug Brockmann
July 18................................. David Elkins

Bone Marrow Donation Awareness Month
November 21........................ Ken Mindoro
January 21 ....Jeanne Schrader

Brain Tumor Awareness Month
February 16 .... Shani Judd Diehl
August 31 .... Craig Seheult

Drowning Awareness Month
November 5 .... Linda Harsh Dixon

Guillian-Barré Syndrome Awareness Month
October 29 ...... Elizabeth Endeno-Galima

Mental Health Awareness Month
February 9 .... Ester Boloix-Chapman
August 9 .... Giovanna Sobrinho
September 8 .... Andrene Campbell
October 25 .... Randy Sanchez
December 4 .... Sandra Ritland

National Day of Prayer (every May 6)
January 7 .... Adwoa Wiafe
January 18 .... Brianna Woodruff
January 22 .... Kristoff Foster
January 31 .... Peter Landless
February 25 .... Anonymous LLUSM student
March 8 .... Matt Dalley
March 10 .... Matthew Ho
March 15 .... Raymond Krause
March 16 .... Marianne Krause
March 22 .... Gladys Snyder Barnes
April 1 .... Michael Rauser
April 8 .... Ryan Rigsby
April 10 .... Cheri Moreno
May 5 .... Paul Y. Chung
May 19 .... Laurel Guthrie
June 15 .... Jane Clark
June 28 .... Jasmine Turner Walker
July 29 .... David Turay
August 11 .... Rheeta Stecker
August 30 .... Allen Patee
September 5 .... Rachel VanderWel
October 13 .... Stephen Waterbrook
October 23 .... Matthew Hartman
November 7 .... Andrew Wai
November 22 .... H. Roger Batin
December 2 .... Jesse Kellar
December 12 .... Judi Lacy Hewes

National Nurses Month
March 22 .... Gladys Snyder Barnes
April 4 .... Garrett Speyer
August 2 .... Joyce Johnston Rusch
November 6 .... Jesse Gomez
November 18 .... Nancy Carter Zinke

National Stroke Awareness Month
January 29 .... George Luh

Postpartum Depression Awareness Month
October 15 .... Ruth Will

Pre-eclampsia Awareness Month
December 26 .... Wilson Thomas

Skin Cancer Awareness Month
March 19 .... Julia Angkadjaja

June

Acute Myeloid Leukemia Awareness Month
January 23 .... Kathy McMillan
September 4 .... Deane Wolcott

Alzheimer's and Brain Awareness Month
February 13 .... Gerald Winslow

National Scleroderma Awareness Month
April 23 .... David Bland

July

Bereaved Parents Awareness Month
January 21 .... Jeanne Schrader

Glioblastoma Awareness Day (every Wednesday in 3rd full week of July: July 20, 2022)
July 25 .... Dixie Marcotte Watkins

August

Grief Awareness Day (every August 30)
March 2 .... Marilene Wang
July 14 .... Elaine Hart
August 23 .... David Reimche-Vu
October 26 .... Bonnie Chi-Lum

Psoriasis Awareness Month
June 15..Jane Clark

September

Childhood Cancer Awareness Month
March 28.............................. Richard Hart
May 13 ....Jennifer Renaud Rich

Children's Cardiomyopathy Awareness Month
January 13............................. Kathleen Lau

Leukemia and Lymphoma Awareness Month
May 13 ....Jennifer Renaud Rich
September 16 ....Sam M. Chen
October 19.....................Zachary Reichert

Muscular Dystrophy Awareness Month (September 7—World Duchenne Awareness Day)
January 2 ....Caroline Boyd

Pain Awareness Month
July 21...................................Bradley Cacho

National Addiction Professionals Day (every September 20)
October 1................................ Mickey Ask

National Prostate Cancer Awareness Month
August 27 .... James Gulley
September 10 ....Jim McMillan

National Recovery Month
October 24................................ David Eng

Rheumatic Disease Awareness Month
July 3.. Robert Bond

October

National Breast Cancer Awareness Month
June 6................................. Dafne Moretta
June 30 ....Jill Hughes
October 21.............................. Van Nguyen

National Depression Awareness Month
October 18.....................Jennifer Pauldurai

Domestic Violence Awareness Month
January 9 ....Tammy Hilliard
September 25 .... Robin Hrdina

Eye Injury Prevention Month
October 23...................Matthew Hartman

Liver Awareness Month
February 20...........................Nathan Kam
December 13 .... Bruce N. Anderson

Liver Cancer Awareness Month
March 28............................... Richard Hart
May 21 .... Kenneth Rose

National Pregnancy and Infant Loss Awareness Month
February 6................................ Mary Small
March 15........................Raymond Krause
May 8 ....Elmar Sakala
July 6..Ryan Manns

Respiratory Syncytial Virus (RSV) Awareness Month
December 10 ..... Denise Roberts Johnson

National Substance Abuse Prevention Awareness Month
August 30 .... Allen Patee

Sudden Cardiac Arrest Awareness Month
March 6..............Janette Whittaker-Allen

November

Adoption Day (every Saturday before Thanksgiving: November 19, 2022)
November 7...........................Andrew Wai
November 14................... Benjamin Rivera
December 6............................ Dennis Park

Bone Marrow Donation Awareness Month
November 21.......................Ken Mindoro

Crohn's and Colitis Awareness Month
April 13 .... Brent Goodge
July 12 .... Kimberly Payne

Diabetes Awareness Month
February 24 .... William P. Bunnell
April 26 .... Robert Rosenquist

National Chronic Obstructive Pulmonary Disease (COPD) Awareness Month
March 31 .... Remy Sagadraca

National Family Caregivers Month
October 4 .... Victoria "Tori" Burghart

National Hospice and Palliative Care Month
January 15 .... Carissa McSherry
April 15 .... Andre Cipta
December 18 .... Chanel Wood

Lung Cancer Awareness Month
October 26 .... Bonnie Chi-Lum

Pancreatic Cancer Awareness Month
September 29 .... Arlin "Larry" Bhattacharjee
December 14 .... Christal Nishikawa
December 25 .... Melissa Kidder

Prematurity Awareness Month
March 15 .... Raymond Krause
March 16 .... Marianne Krause
March 28 .... Richard Hart
June 28 .... Jasmine Turner Walker
December 10 ..... Denise Roberts Johnson

Stress Awareness Day (1st Wednesday of November: November 2, 2022)
January 11 .... Spencer Freed
January 27 .... Kristoff Foster
October 4 .... Victoria "Tori" Burghart
October 27 .... David K. Miller

Pneumonia Awareness Month
September 12 .... Dexter Frederick

December

National Drunk and Drugged Driving Prevention Month
January 14 .... Gina Henry

National HIV/AIDS Awareness Month
January 25 .... Barbara Orr
June 27 .... Daniel Rogstad

Influenza Vaccination Week (1st full week in December: December 4 –10, 2022)
October 29 ...... Elizabeth Endeno-Galima

Twin to Twin Transfusion Awareness Month
March 15 .... Raymond Krause